D0146086

Introduction to BIOMEDICAL ENGINEERING TECHNOLOGY

Laurence J. Street

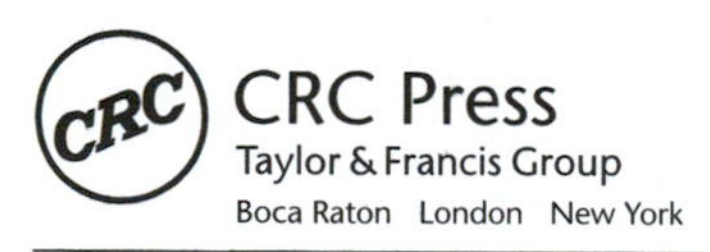

CRC Press is an imprint of the
Taylor & Francis Group, an informa business

CRC Press
Taylor & Francis Group
6000 Broken Sound Parkway NW, Suite 300
Boca Raton, FL 33487-2742

Printed in the United States of America on acid-free paper
10 9 8 7 6 5 4 3 2 1

International Standard Book Number-13: 978-0-8493-8533-9 (Hardcover)

Library of Congress Cataloging-in-Publication Data

Street, Laurence J.
Introduction to biomedical engineering technology / Laurence J. Street.
p. ; cm.
"CRC title."
Includes bibliographical references and index.
ISBN-13: 978-0-8493-8533-9 (hardcover : alk. paper)
1. Medical instruments and apparatus. I. Title.
[DNLM: 1. Equipment and Supplies. 2. Biomedical Technology. WB 26 S915i 2008]

R856.S77 2007
610.28--dc22 2007015248

Visit the Taylor & Francis Web site at
http://www.taylorandfrancis.com

and the CRC Press Web site at
http://www.crcpress.com

Dedication

To my family, who make it all worthwhile. I love you!

Table of Contents

Preface

PURPOSE

SCOPE OF THIS BOOK

Medical devices are often very complex, and while there are differences in design from one manufacturer to another, the principles of operation, and more importantly the physiological and anatomical characteristics on which they operate, are universal. In this book, more attention will be paid to the commonalities of equipment than to differences. With the many details specific to a given manufacturer, it would be impossible to cover all such material in a text of this nature; it is meant to serve as an overview.

As such, the book is not intended as a substitute for service or operator manuals; the specifics of operation of any device are too complex and idiosyncratic for this to be practical. Factory and self-guided training courses, and the study of manuals, are required for individual devices.

Details of electronic circuits are not covered, since these vary greatly not only from one manufacturer to another but also from one generation of equipment to another. Moving from vacuum tubes to transistors to integrated circuits to microprocessor-based systems, the details of electronic design and function have become less and less relevant to technical support staff, while the overall function and integration of equipment into the medical system have become more and more important.

With the goal of giving students a clear idea of the function and application of the various medical devices, extensive descriptions of theory have been avoided, since these can obscure the overview. Where theory is directly relevant to function and application, an appropriate description has been provided.

The main focus of the book is on clinical equipment, devices that are used directly with patients in the course of their care, for diagnostic or treatment purposes.

Seven chapters are used to describe medical devices, three covering clinical diagnostic equipment, one for diagnostic imaging systems, and three for treatment devices. There is some overlap between diagnostic and treatment devices; for example, a bronchoscope can be used to diagnose respiratory diseases, and in conjunction with an electrosurgery machine, it can be used to remove lesions from the bronchial passages. In such cases, both functions are described together.

Imaging technology is given only an overview, because of its high degree of complexity; these devices are covered in much more detail in other texts, as referenced in the bibliography.

Many laboratory devices are also very complex and very manufacturer-specific; because of this, and because of their distance from direct patient care, they are not covered in this text. Again, please refer to the bibliography for other sources of information.

Regarding photographs in the text, some of them are from a stock photo company, some were very graciously supplied by equipment manufacturers, and the rest were taken by me in the hospital where I work. The latter are not studio-quality images. I trust they are clear enough, but they are "in the field," and so there may be the odd cable or box of paper or telephone in the background. This was not a negative, in my opinion, because biomeds working in a hospital are much more likely to find equipment beside a coffee cup or under a stack of papers than on a pedestal in a perfectly lit, perfectly tidy studio.

Acknowledgments

I would first like to thank Tony Galvin of EMCParadigm Publishing, for his initial interest and encouragement with this whole project. I might not have followed though on my ideas if not for Tony's positive attitude.

Then Michael Slaughter of Taylor and Francis picked up the ball and ran with it — thank you, Michael, for seeing the potential, and for your patience.

Thank you also to Laurie Wakefield of Philips Medical Systems, Peter Seo of Inmagine, Heidi Stuelpnagel of Fluke Biomedical, and Terry Follett of Valleylab/Tyco for all their help in arranging access to images for me to use in the text. I truly appreciate all who helped out in this regard.

Thanks, Frank, for you-know-what and for believing.

And finally, thank you to my family for putting up and filling in while I have been "away" working on this project. Sheri, Jordan, and Shannon — I couldn't have done it without you.

Author

Laurence Street earned a diploma in biomedical engineering technology at the British Columbia Institute of Technology in Vancouver, BC, Canada, in 1979, and has since worked continuously in a variety of hospitals, from the very large Shaughnessey/BC Children's/Vancouver Women's complex, to a regional hospital in the British Columbia interior, to (1991 to present) the Chilliwack General Hospital, a mid-sized community hospital outside Vancouver, and part of the Fraser Health Authority. In the latter two cases, he was solely responsible for setting up and implementing the biomedical engineering departments.

He received a B.Sc. degree in zoology from the University of British Columbia (1974), as well as a British Columbia teaching certificate, also from UBC (1975). He taught junior high school science at Trafalgar Junior Secondary in Nelson, BC (1975–1976), and a number of electronics and math courses to electronics and computer technology students at East Kootenay Community College in Cranbrook, BC, including several courses that he developed himself (1983–1991).

Mr. Street's hospital work involves the repair and maintenance of all patient care electronic devices in the hospital, as well as close involvement in planning for future technological directions and the evaluation and acquisition of equipment. He also provides in-service education to medical staff regarding the safe and effective use of patient care devices. As Chilliwack General is a well-equipped acute care and teaching hospital and is also part of a regional medical community, he works with an extremely wide variety of both older and very modern equipment. He has taken a large number of factory training courses on the various devices that he services.

1 Introduction

I. HISTORY OF MEDICAL DEVICES

The history of medicine is a story of humans trying to better understand and treat the various diseases and injuries that befell themselves and their companions. From simply providing comfort and empathy, medical care evolved with ever more effective means of diagnosing and treating illnesses. Pharmacology was likely the first tool to be developed, thousands of years ago, as shamans or medicine women or simply mothers caring for infants found that certain plants had beneficial properties (Figure 1.1). In *The Clan of the Cave Bear,* Jean Auel describes how a Neanderthal medicine woman treated the wounds of a small Cro-Magnon child:

> "This destroys the evil spirits that make infection," Iza motioned, pointing to the antiseptic iris-root solution. "A poultice of the root draws out poisons and helps the wound heal." She picked up a bone bowl and dipped in a finger to check the temperature. "Clover makes the heart grow strong to fight evil spirits — stimulates it." ... "Alder bark cleans the blood, purifies it, drives out the spirits that poison it."
>
> **(From *The Clan of The Cave Bear* by Jean M. Auel, p. 21)**

Even though Iza did not understand the true nature of infections, she recognized that there were tools she could use to ward them off. Though many later developments in medicine were fraudulent, generally medical practitioners looked for better and better ways to diagnose and treat their patients. They recognized that there were different, specific maladies, and that these maladies caused specific symptoms. The location, type, and degree of pain or tenderness; localized or systemic heating; swellings; skin color; eye appearance; the color, texture, and odor of bodily discharges; heart, lung, and digestive system sounds — all served to help diagnose ailments and guide treatment. Adept physicians knew that the better they could identify symptoms, the better their chances of curing their patients, and so they searched for better methods of determining symptoms.

Just as pharmacology developed from observing the effects of various foods, to trial and error of natural substances, through outright quackery, to the scientific research, testing and analysis used by modern drug companies, so too has medical hardware evolved (Figure 1.2).

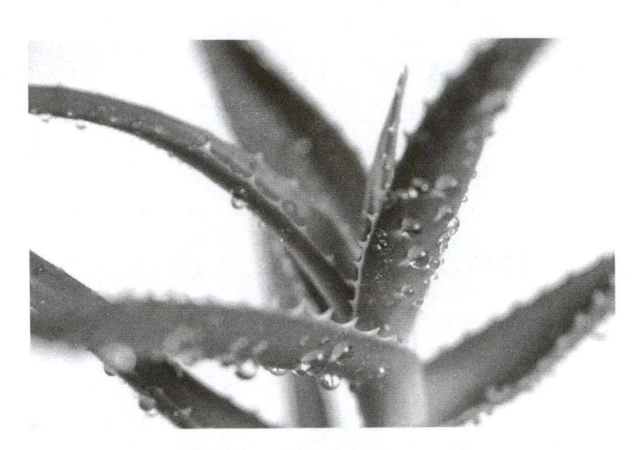

FIGURE 1.1 Aloe vera, an ancient medicinal plant. (Modified from Inmagine Corp, www.123rf.com, with permission.)

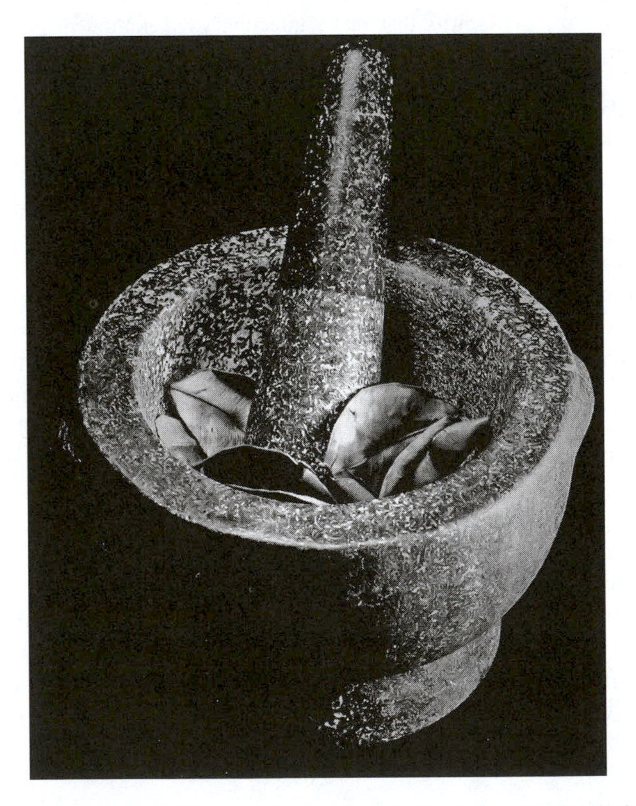

FIGURE 1.2 A mortar and pestle used to prepare medications. (Modified from Inmagine Corp, www.123rf.com, with permission.)

A Patient from the Past

Robert Smith entered Dr. James Llewelyn's surgery in London and collapsed into a chair, moaning and clutching his abdomen. Dr. Llewelyn's nurse, Mrs. Peabody, bustled out to him and managed to get him up from the chair and into the Doctor's examination room, where he lay upon the table, still moaning.

Dr. Llewelyn entered and immediately looked the patient over, noting that he was pale, breathing shallowly, and perspiring profusely.

"Well, sir, what have we here?" he enquired.

"It's me belly, Doctor, it hurts so!" replied Smith, grimacing.

"All right, let's have a look shall we? Come on, I'll unbutton your vest and loosen your belt. There. Now I'm going to press on different parts of your belly and you tell me where it hurts most, will you?"

Gentle probing revealed extreme tenderness in Mr. Smith's lower right side, and the Doctor noted a recently healed wound in the area.

"Mrs. Smith, laudanum, please," ordered the Doctor, and his nurse produced a bottle of syrup from which she poured a spoonful and fed it to their patient.

Dr. Llewelyn took his stethoscope from a side table and listened intently to Smith's heart, lungs, and abdomen. He then asked Mrs. Peabody to help get Mr. Smith into the next room, where they assisted the poor man, now quite groggy from the laudanum but at least not moaning so much, onto another table.

A strange and marvelous device, called a Crookes tube, was mounted above the table, and it was connected to more machinery that the good doctor referred to as "My lovely Rhumkoff coil," though Mr. Smith was, by this time, less than impressed. Mrs. Peabody brought out a glass photographic plate, which she slid into a space under the tabletop. Dr. Llewelyn implored his long-suffering patient to remain as still as possible, and then he energized his contraption. There was a loud humming sound, which went on for many minutes, and after a while a hot electrical smell filled the room. Finally the machine was shut off, and Mrs. Peabody retrieved the plate from beneath the nearly comatose Smith.

Dr. Llewelyn took the plate into a side room and proceeded to develop the image of Smith's abdomen. Though blurry, the plate confirmed the good Doctor's suspicions — Smith had a lead ball lodged in his belly, the result, no doubt, of a bar-room brawl gone too far.

"Right then, Mrs. P., let's get him to the surgery," the Doctor said cheerily, and they struggled to get Smith onto yet another table in a third room.

It hardly seemed necessary, but Llewelyn used ether to render Smith completely unconscious. Then, after bathing the area in carbolic acid and donning thick rubber gloves and a cloth mask, he used a scalpel (Figure 1.3) (which had also been soaked in carbolic acid) to deftly slice through the layers of tissue near the wound. Mrs. Peabody, masked and gowned, valiantly mopped up blood, and finally Dr. Llewelyn reached into the surgical opening and extracted the lead ball with a cry of victory. More carbolic acid washed out the area, and Llewelyn stitched up his patient layer by layer.

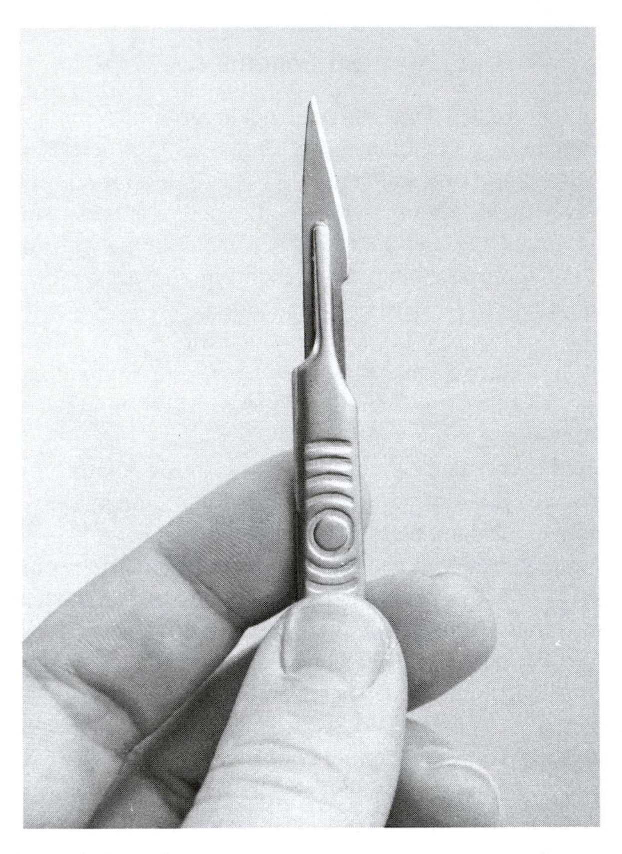

FIGURE 1.3 Surgical scalpel. (Modified from Inmagine Corp, www.123rf.com, with permission.)

The Roentgen Rays, the Roentgen Rays,
What is this craze?
The town's ablaze
With the new phase
Of x-ray's ways.
"I'm full of daze,
Shock and amaze;
For nowadays
I hear they'll gaze
Thro' cloak and gown — and even stays,
These naughty, naughty Roentgen Rays."

A. Stethoscopes

Perhaps the first medical diagnostic device was the stethoscope. Medicine men knew that the sounds made by a patient's heart, the noises of breathing, and the gurgling of the intestinal tract all could provide clues as to the patient's condition. Rapid

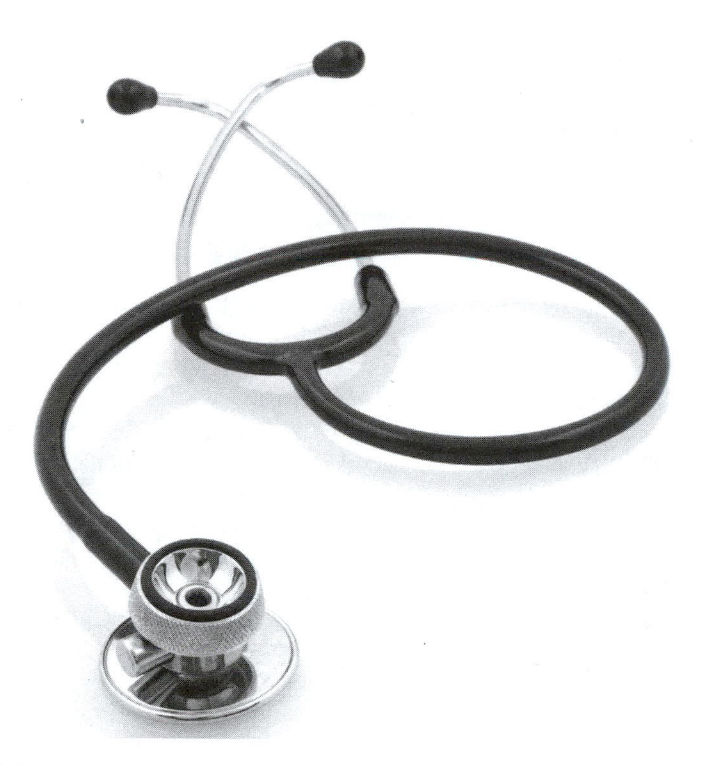

FIGURE 1.4 A modern stethoscope. (Modified from Inmagine Corp, www.123rf.com, with permission.)

heartbeats could signal infections, unusual beat sounds could mean a heart structure defect, and wet-sounding inhalations might point to pneumonia or tuberculosis. Laying an ear on the patient provided the first means of detecting such sounds, but this was often inconvenient, inefficient, or messy, and so mechanical means of listening were devised. The first stethoscopes might have been cones of bark, but someone discovered that sounds were carried quite well by wooden sticks, and even better by hollow tubes. A cup on the end of the tube helped to gather more sound, providing more information, and when the tubes were split into a "Y" and brought to both ears at once, external sounds were shut out, and the important internal ones amplified, allowing ever more refined discernment and interpretation of bodily sounds.

The shape and size of the cup, or bell, has been improved, a diaphragm added, and better materials used to make the modern stethoscopes a vital tool for physicians and nurses (Figure 1.4). It is used to listen to not only heart, lung, and intestinal sounds, but also to pick up the Korotkoff sounds made by blood vessels in determining blood pressure (in conjunction with a manometer), and the sounds of a fetal heartbeat within the mother's abdomen.

With the advent of electronics, stethoscope evolution took another large step. Sensitive microphones, acoustically coupled to the skin with special gel, provided signals that could be amplified and filtered and then reproduced with either headphones or larger speakers.

Of course, such devices are more expensive than traditional mechanical stethoscopes. They are more fragile, and they need batteries, so the old style continues in common use except where the additional capabilities of electronic versions are required.

Doppler Fetal Heart Detectors

A device related to the stethoscope became available with electronic technology, and it used a principle discovered in 1842 by Christian Andreas Doppler. The "Doppler effect" is that waves produced by a moving object will be compressed or expanded relative to a stationary observer depending on whether the source is moving toward or away from the observer (the classic change in pitch of a train whistle as it passes by is a good example of the Doppler effect.) The phenomenon was first used practically with radar systems, in which radio waves were bounced off objects such as airplanes. If the returning wave was of a higher frequency than the emitted wave (i.e., it was compressed), the reflective object was moving toward the radar installation; if it was of a lower frequency, the object was moving away. Comparing the values quantitatively allowed a calculation of the speed of the object.

In medicine, it was found that this principle could be applied using ultrasonic waves. When sound waves are sent into a patient's body, they are reflected by the various structures within. If the surface that reflects the waves is moving, such as the components of the heart during each beat, or the walls of blood vessels as they expand and contract when blood pulses through them, or blood cells themselves as they flow through vessels, the reflected sound waves will show the Doppler effect. The motions of the internal structures can therefore be determined and represented, as a sound or an image or both (Figure 1.5).

B. Microscopes

Technology was adopted in many other ways as the practice of medicine evolved.

Lenses were discovered thousands of years ago, but their magnifying ability was not likely put to use by medical practitioners until perhaps the time of Roger Bacon in the thirteenth century. Hans Jansen, Robert Hooke, and Antonie van Leeuwenhoek contributed to the development and use of microscopes (Figure 1.6).

Microscopes evolved, with better glass and optical coatings, improved mechanical features, binocular eyepieces, and more effective and varied lighting methods, including polarization and ultraviolet light. Adapters have been created to allow a second person to observe the image (Figure 1.7), or a video camera can be attached so that images can be displayed on video monitors or computer systems.

Electronics really entered into the realm of microscopy with the advent of the electron microscope in the 1930s. Using an electron beam instead of visible light waves, these devices enabled greater magnification of images.

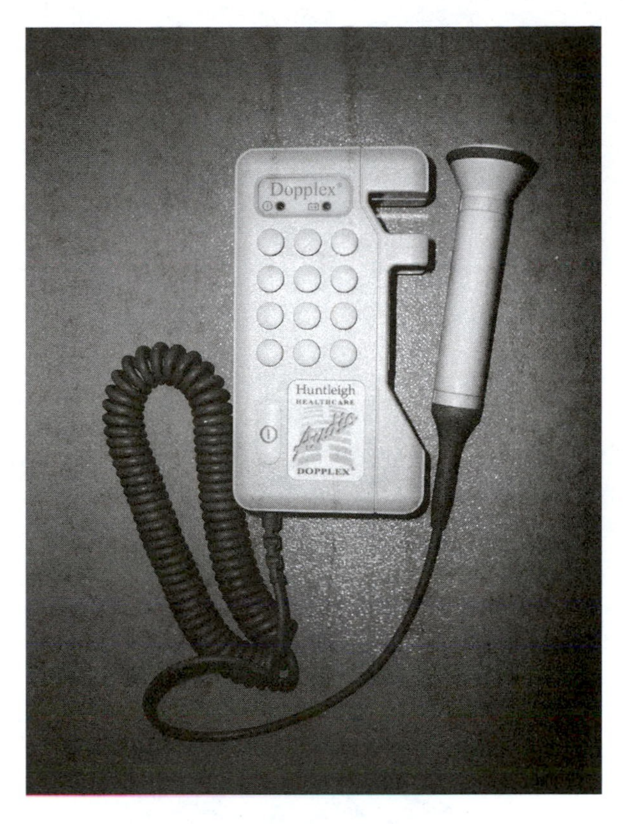

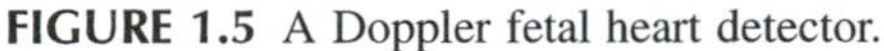

FIGURE 1.5 A Doppler fetal heart detector.

C. Surgery

Surgical devices were in use many thousands of years ago, as evidenced by the discovery of human skulls that had been cut open and later healed over.

Stone or obsidian scalpels were used to peel back the scalp and then to carve a hole in the patient's skull. A section of bone was removed, and evil demons (or perhaps pressure from a subdural hematoma) could then escape.

The age of metals saw the development of scalpels that were easier to form and manufacture than those of stone, and that could also be sharpened when necessary. Steel became the ultimate physical scalpel material, but again electronics entered into the picture. It was found that high frequency electrical signals could not only cut tissue, but cauterize it as well, helping to reduce both bleeding and the chance of infection. These electrosurgery units (ESUs) were at first simply a power supply and connectors. Cushing and Bovie refined the equipment, creating a "spark-gap" device that became widely used; even today, ESUs are often referred to as "Bovies" (Figure 1.8).

ESUs, since they employed electrical currents to produce cutting and cauterization, required a return path for the current to carry the electricity from the cutting site, through the patient's body (which is filled with conductive fluids) and back to

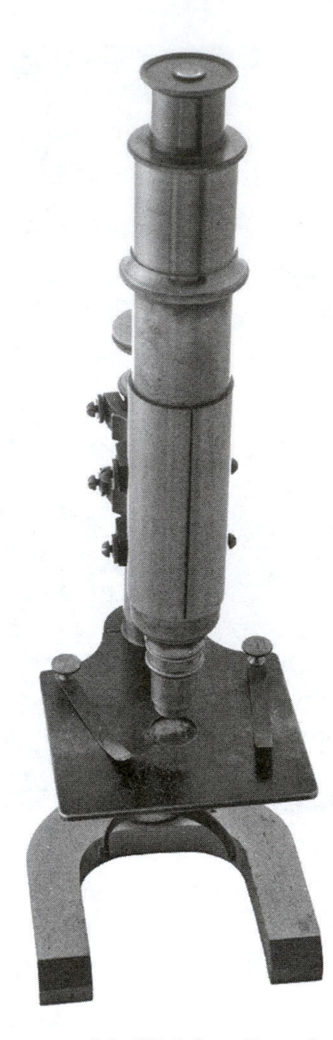

FIGURE 1.6 An early microscope. (Modified from Inmagine Corp, www.123rf.com, with permission.)

the ESU or a common ground point. This return path had to be arranged so that the current leaving the patient's body was spread over a large enough area that burning or overheating didn't cause damage. The requirement of a return path also meant that safeguards were needed to prevent alternate paths, either through other parts of the patient's body or through staff members. ESU evolution produced devices with output waveforms optimally shaped to provide the best combinations of cutting and coagulation with minimal collateral tissue damage and minimal risks to both patients and staff.

Further developments of this technology included the use of beams of ionized gas to provide the contact for cutting and coagulation, rather than a metal blade as in previous units. ESUs are often used in conjunction with laparoscopic procedures,

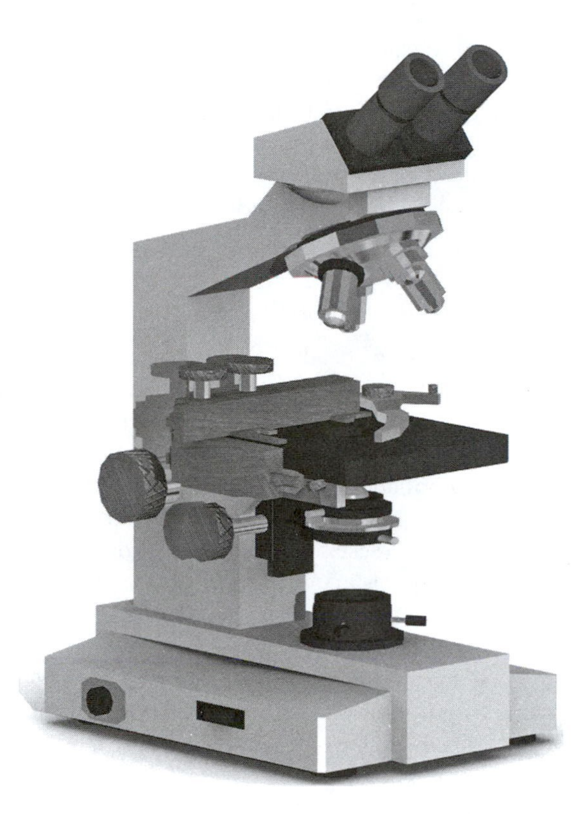

FIGURE 1.7 A modern binocular microscope. (Modified from Inmagine Corp, www.123rf.com, with permission.)

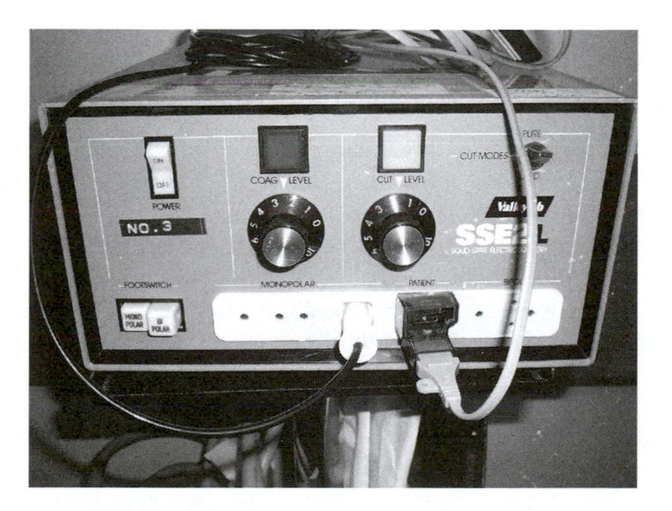

FIGURE 1.8 Electrosurgery unit.

since appropriate accessories can carry the surgical current through small tubes and into the patient's body without the need for large incisions.

A further development in surgical technology involves the use of laser beams instead of electrical current. By controlling the power, wavelength, and width of laser beams, various surgical effects can be achieved, from cutting and/or coagulation, to tissue ablation, to "welding" detached retinal tissue to the inner surface of the eye.

D. Defibrillators

Cardiac arrest is a major cause of death, and as soon as scientists discovered the electrical nature of heart contractions, and especially the characteristics of fibrillation, they began to devise means of restarting or recoordinating the cardiac rhythm. Electrical shocks seemed to be the logical means of accomplishing this, especially since they could induce fibrillation in some circumstances. Electrically induced fibrillation was discovered in 1849, and 50 years later it was found that another applied shock could sometimes reestablish a normal cardiac rhythm. Dr. Claude S. Beck from the University Hospitals in Cleveland used a defibrillator to save a human life for the first time in 1947.

Since that time, defibrillators have become more sophisticated and effective, using precisely designed waveforms to provide optimal efficacy with minimal electrical current (Figure 1.9). They have integrated ECG circuitry, which allows observation of patient waveforms as well as synchronization to abnormal rhythms. Some include pacemakers or pulse oximeters; some have been miniaturized enough to be implanted within a patient's body, so they can provide shocks directly to the heart whenever needed; and some have been automated and simplified in operation sufficiently that they can be placed in public places or private homes to be used by untrained personnel (Figure 1.10).

II. THE ROLE OF BIOMEDICAL ENGINEERING TECHNOLOGISTS IN HEALTHCARE

As medical technology evolved, a need arose for people to take care of the equipment involved. Devices had to be designed and built, their use had to be demonstrated and explained to the end users, functionality had to be checked and maintained, and these devices had to be repaired when they failed. At first, much of this was done by whoever invented the equipment, but eventually specialization was required, and specific individuals were assigned responsibility for the maintenance of medical technological devices. Depending on the equipment, these people might have been electricians, or technicians who would normally operate the devices, or simply someone in the medical facility who had an interest and aptitude for hardware.

Further development of equipment made it more complex and varied, and this meant that the people taking care of it had to be more highly trained and experienced. Electronic circuits became critical and powerful components of many medical devices, so an in-depth knowledge of electronics became a necessity (Figure 1.11).

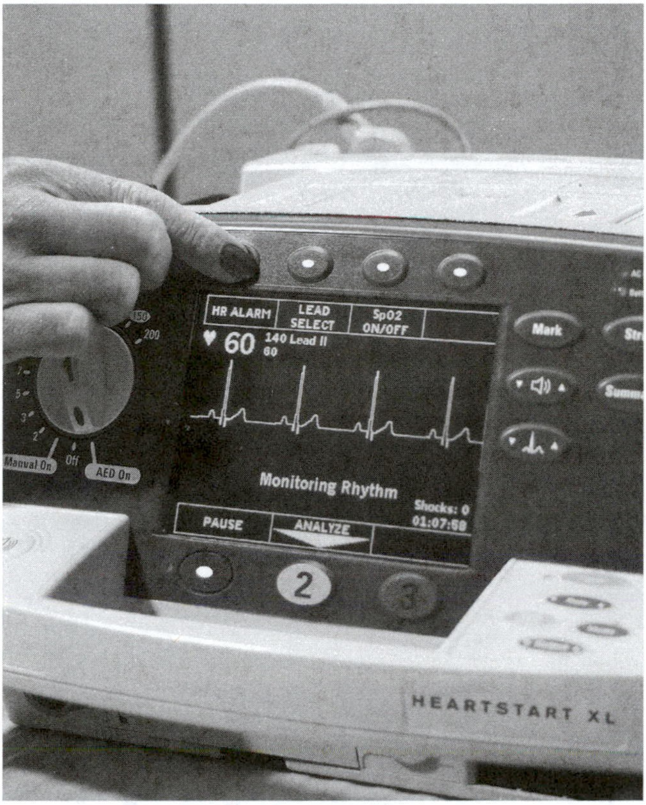

FIGURE 1.9 Philips HeartStart XL defibrillator. (Modified from Philips Medical, CD provided directly, with permission. © 2006 Koninidijke Philips Electronics N.V. All rights reserved. Reproduction in whole or in part is prohibited without prior written permission of the copyright owner.)

Sometime after World War II, the field of medical equipment support became sufficiently specialized that a title was given to those who practiced it: BMET, or BioMedical Equipment Technician. Gradually the "E" changed to mean first "Electronics" and then "Engineering," while the "T" moved from Technician to Technologist, all of these changes reflecting the changing roles and responsibilities of BMETs in the medical community.

Today, most BMETs receive their initial training in a two- or three-year program at a community college, technical school, or university, or through an Armed Forces training school (Table 1.1). A listing of most of these programs in the United States and Canada is provided in Appendix C.

The evolution of medical technology continues, and this means that BMETs continue to learn throughout their careers, with on-the-job experience and mentoring, continuing education classes, and factory training courses on specific devices.

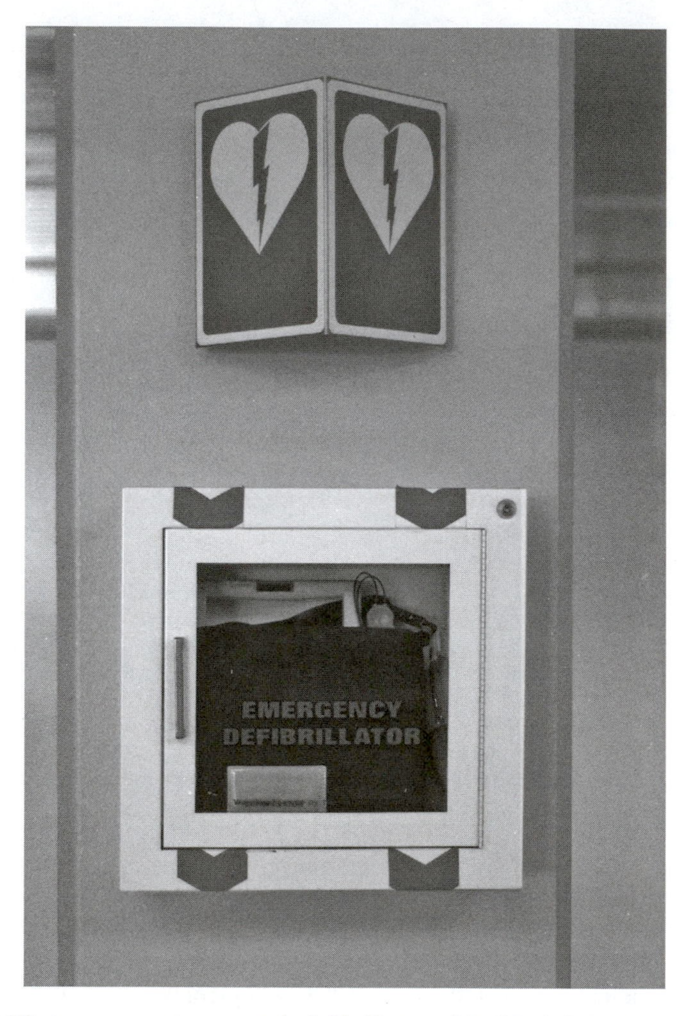

FIGURE 1.10 An automatic external defibrillator. (Modified from Inmagine Corp, www.123rf.com, with permission.)

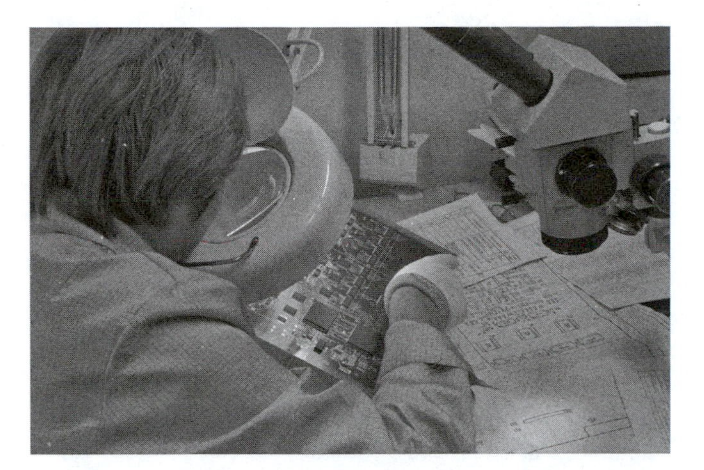

FIGURE 1.11 BMET at work. (Modified from Inmagine Corp, www.123rf.com, with permission.)

A Day in the Life of Joe Biomed

7:30 a.m. — Joe Biomed arrives at work, the Biomedical Engineering Lab at Hippocrates General Hospital, a mid-sized community hospital in a mid-sized semirural town. He greets Angela Jones, one of the two other BMETs on staff, who had arrived earlier that morning. Joe checks for phone messages and then signs onto the hospital computer intranet to check for e-mail and to see if any work orders have been assigned to him for the day. He notes that he is scheduled to do a preventive maintenance (PM) test on a defibrillator from the Cardiac Intensive Care Unit, or CICU. Then he discusses events of the previous day with Angela, and they go over plans for the day (Figure 1.12).

7:45 a.m. — An IV pump arrived at the lab overnight. It has a note taped to it that says "Not working." Joe looks up the pump in their database and finds that it came from the third floor nursing unit. He marks that on the pump and retrieves the service manual for that model from their departmental library. Being familiar with the pumps (there are over sixty of them in the hospital), Joe sets it up on the IV pump analyzer and starts it running at 125 ml per hour. After a few minutes, the pump stops, and an alarm sounds, accompanied by an alarm code on the LCD screen. Joe looks up the code in the service manual. The manual suggests testing the voltage at a particular test point, which Joe does. The voltage is lower than it should be, and the manual indicates that, in that case, the CPU board of the pump needs to be replaced. Joe asks Angela if there are any CPU boards left in stock, and she informs him that the last one got used two weeks ago. Joe orders several CPU boards, since they have been a common source of problems with these pumps, and then puts all the parts for the pump in a container and sets it aside, with a note on it explaining that parts

TABLE 1.1
Typical Course Outline for a Two-Year BMET Program

	Credits
Level 1 (15 weeks)	
BHSC 1101 Anatomy and Physiology 1 (BMET)	4.0
BMET 1100 Electronics Principles and Practice 1	9.0
COMM 1178 Technical Writing 1 for Biomed Eng Tech	3.0
COMP 1120 Intro to Computer Architecture & Config	4.0
MATH 1781 Technical Math for Biomed Engineering	7.0
PHYS 1178 Physics: Biomedical Engineering	4.0
Level 2 (20 weeks)	
BHSC 2201 Anatomy and Physiology 2 (BMET)	4.0
BMET 2200 Electronics Principles & Practice	29.5
BMET 2215 Digital Electronics	6.5
CHEM 1205 General and Organic Chem for Biomed Eng	6.5
COMM 2278 Technical Writing 2 for Biomed Eng Tech	2.5
ELEX 2860 Electronic Prototype Manufacturing	5.5
MATH 2782 Calculus for Biomedical Engineering	6.5
Level 3 (15 weeks)	
BMET 3300 Electronics Principles and Practice 3	7.0
BMET 3301 Biomedical Devices Technology 1	6.0
BMET 3302 Quality Assurance and Systems	5.0
CHEM 2305 Biochemistry/Instrumental Analysis	6.0
COMP 3151 Software Engineering	5.0
Level 4 (15 weeks plus practicum)	
BMET 4401 Biomedical Devices Technology 2	6.0
BMET 4402 Biomed Engineering Technology Project	3.0
BMET 4403 Medical Imaging Systems	5.0
BMET 4415 Digital Systems and Microprocessors	5.0
BMET 4420 Practical Experience in Biomed Eng Tech	7.0
COMM 3478 Technical Writing 3 for Biomed Eng Tech	1.0
ELEX 4855 Electronic Image Displays	4.0
MATH 3782 Statistics for Biomedical Engineering	3.0
NURS 1182 Patient Care	2.0
Total Credits:	137.0

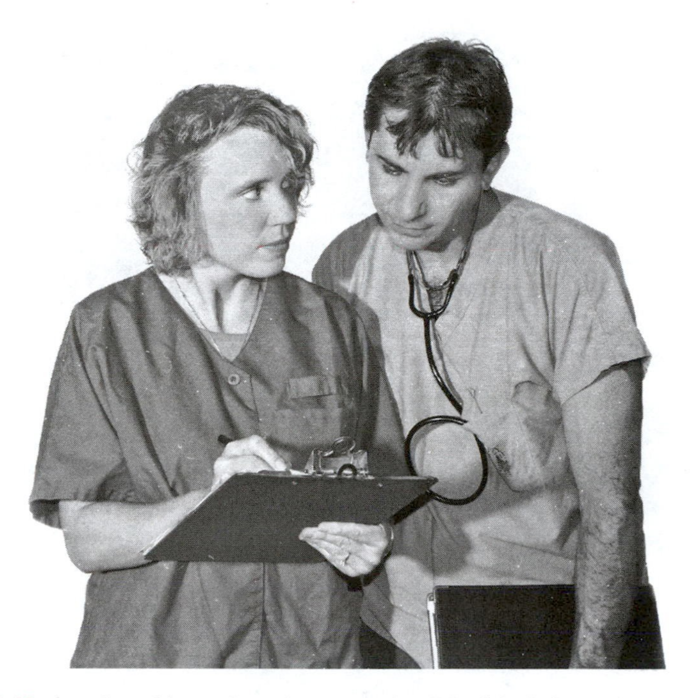

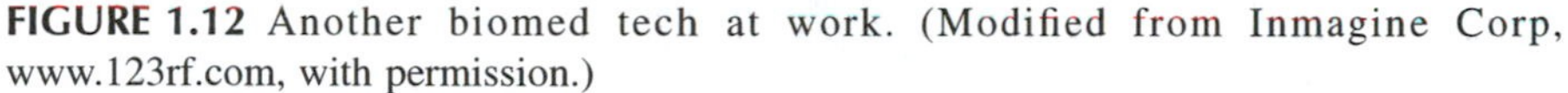

FIGURE 1.12 Another biomed tech at work. (Modified from Inmagine Corp, www.123rf.com, with permission.)

were on order and giving the order number. He returns the service manual to the library.

8:15 a.m. — Joe greets Mike Cho, the third member of the team, as he arrives at work. Then he reads over the work order for the defibrillator, noting the equipment number. He takes a small cart and makes his way through various corridors and up an elevator to the CICU, where, after observing the proper infection control protocols, he chats with the nurses at the central monitoring station. Joe tells them he needs the defibrillator for testing, and after going over the current patients and expected admissions, they tell Joe he can take the unit away, but he has to have it back by the afternoon.

Joe unplugs the defibrillator, removes any charts as well as accessories that he will not need, then transfers the unit from the CICU crash cart to his own cart and places a note on the crash cart indicating where the unit has been taken and when it should be back. Returning to the Biomed lab, Joe does a thorough visual inspection of the unit and accessories, then connects it to their defibrillator analyzer (Figure 1.13) and runs through a series of preprogrammed performance tests.

These test results are transferred to the equipment control database on the department computer (Figure 1.14). Joe then uses an automated electrical safety analyzer to check that the unit meets grounding and electrical leakage standards; these tests also feed into the equipment control database. Testing complete, Joe types a few notes into the work order then closes it. The program prints out an

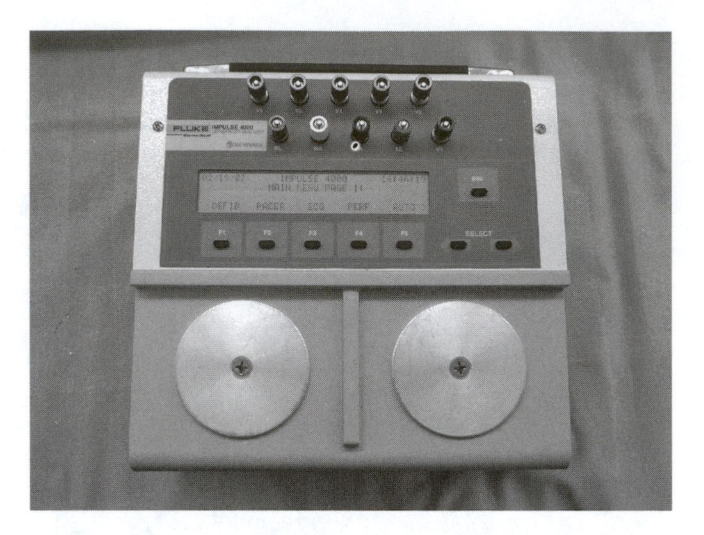

FIGURE 1.13 Defibrillator analyzer.

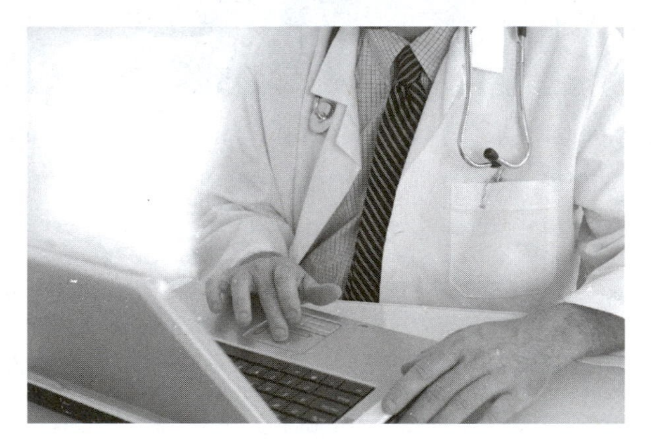

FIGURE 1.14 Yet another Biomed at work. (Modified from Inmagine Corp, www.123rf.com, with permission.)

inspection label, which Joe affixes to the unit. Then he returns it to the CICU, replaces it on the crash cart, reconnects the AC cord, and does a quick operational check, noting especially that the AC indicator is lit. He informs the nursing staff that the unit is back in service and then returns to the lab.

9:30 a.m. — Coffee break.

9:45 a.m. — Joe answers a phone call from a supplier regarding changes in part numbers for feeding pump batteries. He notes these changes in the database.

9:55 a.m. — Another phone call, this time it's an ER nurse asking about changing the order of the waveforms on their bedside monitors. Joe describes the procedure for changing the order temporarily and asks if they want this to be their default configuration. He is transferred to the ER manager, who agrees that it should be changed, so he makes a note in Microsoft Outlook to perform the configuration change when convenient.

10:20 a.m. — A porter brings some boxes, one of which contains parts for a pulse oximeter that Joe was working on last week. He enters the parts in the database, and then completes the repair and does a performance assurance test on the pulse-ox. Test results are entered in the database, and the work order for the unit is signed off and closed; a repair label goes on, and the unit is sent back to its home ward.

10:55 a.m. — "Code Blue, CICU" is called over the hospital PA system, and since the defibrillators there are relatively new to the hospital, Joe decides to attend. He is passed in the hallway by the primary Code Blue team on the run to the CICU, and by the time he gets there, they are just getting the defibrillator in place (Figure 1.15). The resident doctor in charge recognizes him and asks how many charges they can get from the battery. Joe informs him of the number specified by the manufacturer and adds that they have confirmed that in testing.

The patient is resuscitated successfully, so Joe returns to the lab, where he has to fill Angela and Mike in on the excitement.

11:50 a.m. — Lunch break

12:30 p.m. — Joe attends a meeting as member of the hospital's equipment acquisition committee, to discuss the replacement program for their IV pumps. Joe will arrange with purchasing to have several demo units from different manufacturers brought in for evaluation. He explains some of the new features of the pumps to the other committee members.

1:35 p.m. — Joe's pager goes off, indicating the number for the OR. He calls them, and is told that there has been a possible patient burn incident involving an electrosurgery unit (ESU). He asks the OR staff to tag the unit that was involved and to keep all the accessories and cables that had been used during the operation. He gets a list of the doctors and nurses involved in the case and asks that they call him as soon as possible. He begins the incident report process, and then the ESU and accessories arrive at the lab. Joe performs a visual inspection of the items and then does a detailed performance test, especially noting areas that might have been involved in a possible patient burn. He receives a phone call from one of the OR nurses that was working with the patient; she tells him that the burn appeared to be under the return electrode pad. Joe finds no faults with the equipment, so he goes to Post-Op Recovery Room where he talks to nurses and asks them if they could put a section of ESU return electrode pad on the patient's leg. Shortly afterward Joe has a look at the patient's leg and finds that there is definite reddening under the electrode pad. He discusses this with the OR staff, and together they conclude that the "burn" was actually a sensitivity reaction to the electrode adhesive. Joe completes the incident report and sends both paper and e-mail copies to the OR supervisor, the safety committee, and Biomed.

4:00 p.m. — End of the day

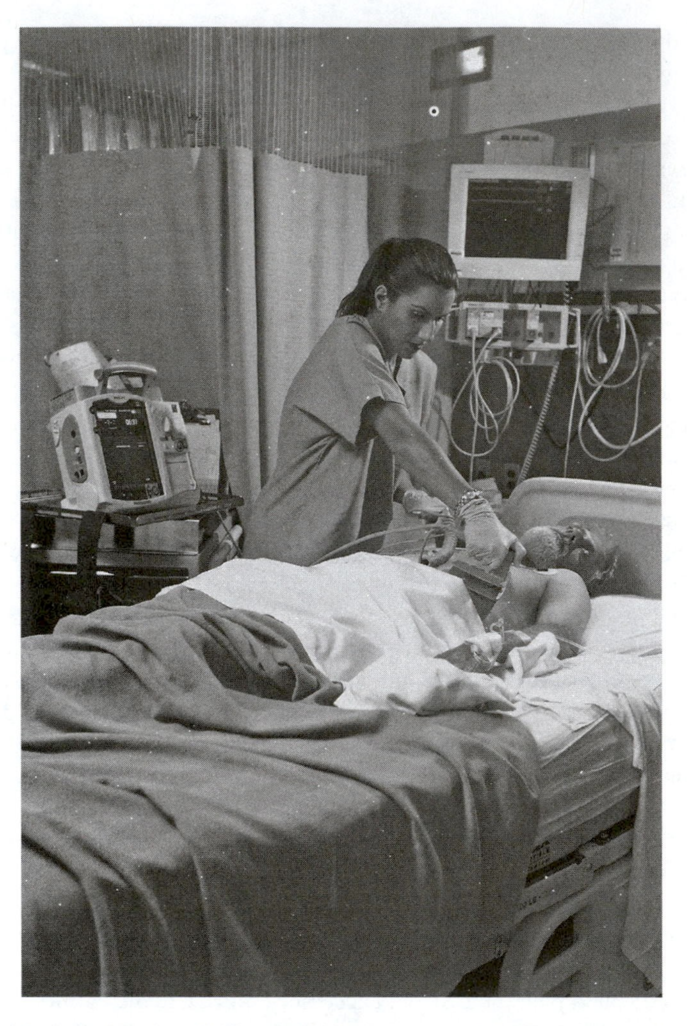

FIGURE 1.15 Code Blue! A Philips defibrillator in use. (Modified from Philips Medical, CD provided directly, with permission. © 2006 Koninidijke Philips Electronics N.V. All rights reserved. Reproduction in whole or in part is prohibited without prior written permission of the copyright owner.)

While the majority of biomedical engineering technologists will likely work in a hospital setting, there are many other career paths. Equipment manufacturers and vendors (which are sometimes one and the same) need experienced professionals to help design and test new devices and to market them. Equipment installation, user training, and hospital BMET staff training is often performed by other BMETs employed by the equipment manufacturer. Vendors/manufacturers also employ field or bench service technologists. Research facilities may need BMETs to design, build, and maintain specialized research devices. And finally, because of the increasing need for BMETs in the medical system as a whole, instructors for training programs are required, and these are often BMETs with work experience who have a desire and ability to teach.

III. CHARACTERISTICS OF HUMAN ANATOMY AND PHYSIOLOGY THAT RELATE TO MEDICAL DEVICES

A. Electrical Signals and Conductivity

Much of the function of the human body depends at least in part on electrical signals. Nerves carry signals throughout the body via chemical reactions and electrical impulses, and these impulses can act on muscle tissue to cause muscle contractions, ranging from skeletal muscle action involved in movement to sphincter muscle control, to the beating of the heart. Within neurons, signals travel by simple conduction within the ionic solution inside the cells. In order for the signal to move from one nerve cell to another, or between nerve cells and muscle cells, a chemical reaction must occur. This has a number of consequences that are relevant to biomedical devices.

The chemicals involved in conveying nerve signals, or action potentials, between cells are called neurotransmitters and include such molecules as acetylcholine, epinephrine (adrenaline), dopamine, and nitric oxide. When an electrical nerve impulse arrives at the junction, or synapse, between the conducting nerve and the next nerve cell in the particular pathway, molecules of neurotransmitters are released into the space between the nerve cells. The neurotransmitter molecules then connect with a receptor structure on the receiving nerve cell, and this causes an electrical signal to be generated in the new cell. Signals thus travel along a chain of nerve cells to their target tissue. With the neurotransmitter steps involved, nerve signal transmission is far slower than electrical conduction speed, in the range of 200 meters per second as compared to 3×10^8 meters per second.

Electrical signals are generated by the flow of calcium, sodium, and potassium ions into and out of cells; this flow is controlled or mediated by the neurotransmitters and their receptors. Due to the nature of the receptor mechanisms, nerve cells can become desensitized; that is, transmission can be reduced or blocked after prolonged stimulation.

Muscle action also has an electrical component, with a wave of polarization proceeding in one direction through the muscle tissue as it contracts, followed by a wave of depolarization in the opposite direction as the muscle relaxes again. This polarization and depolarization involves movement of calcium ions in a complex process, but relevant to biomedical instrumentation, it produces flow of electrical current, which in turn causes a voltage signal to be developed in proportion to the muscle contraction.

Various conditions can affect nerve and muscle activity, such as exercise levels, blood gas levels (especially oxygen and carbon dioxide), electrolyte levels, hormones, temperature, physical trauma, toxins, and disease processes. An accurate measure of the different signals present in the body, followed by effective analysis, can give direct or indirect indications of the factors that are affecting these signals,

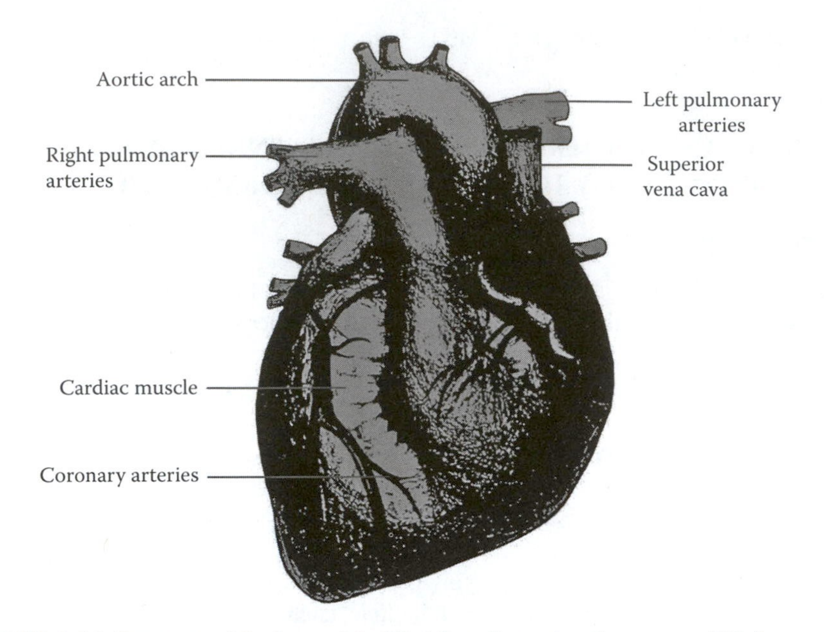

FIGURE 1.16 Structure of the heart. (Modified from Inmagine Corp, www.123rf.com, with permission.)

thus aiding in the diagnosis of disease. These topics will be examined in more detail in the sections that describe specific biomedical devices.

B. Circulation

The function of the heart is to pump blood throughout the body, from the heart to the lungs and back, and then from the heart to the rest of the body and return.

It is made up of four chambers, each of which has muscle tissue, conduction pathways, connecting vessels, and a valve. The four chambers, the right and left atria and right and left ventricles, effectively form two pumps, each with an atrium and a ventricle. The two pumps contract in synchrony (Figure 1.16).

Blood is pumped from the right atrium into the right ventricle, and from there to the lungs, where excess carbon dioxide is removed and fresh oxygen acquired. Returning from the lungs, the blood passes through the left atrium and then the left ventricle to be distributed to the rest of the body, including the heart itself. Returning from the body, blood is now back at the right atrium. The ventricles do the main work of the heart and are therefore larger and have thicker muscle walls than do the atria.

The rate and strength of contractions of the heart are controlled by a number of factors, including the oxygen demands of the body and blood levels of various hormones such as adrenaline (epinephrine).

Coordination of contractions is critical for pumping to be effective, and this coordination is brought about by a system of tissues within the heart that initiate and distribute electrical signals, or action potentials, throughout the heart muscle

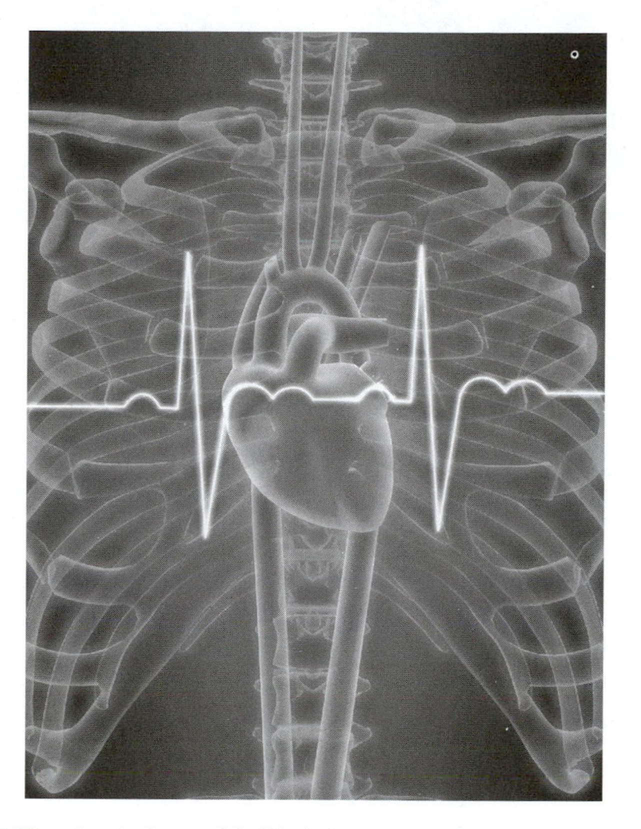

FIGURE 1.17 The electric heart. (Modified from Inmagine Corp, www.123rf.com, with permission.)

(Figure 1.17). Built-in delay mechanisms allow the various parts of the heart to contract at the correct time.

Signals originate in the sinoatrial (SA) node. These signals cause the atria to contract and are also carried to the atrioventricular (AV) node. From the AV node, action potentials travel down a bundle of fibers called the atrioventricular bundle or the bundle of His. This splits into left and right bundle branches, which in turn split into Purkinje fibers, or subendocardial fibers, which ultimately deliver the signals to the ventricular muscles.

The electrical signals within the heart are of relatively small amplitude, in the range of 100 mV. Since the inside of the human body consists of electrically conductive tissue, a part of the cardiac contraction signals is carried to the skin, where it can be detected by an electrocardiogram (ECG). At the skin, the signals are much lower in amplitude than at the heart, approximately 1 mV. However, these signals at the skin surface can be amplified and filtered sufficiently to provide a clear representation of the original signals from the heart. Special electrodes allow for optimal contact between the skin and the measuring wires, or leads. Depending on the placement of the electrodes on the body, the signals coming from the heart can be viewed in a number of different orientations — for example, from left to right

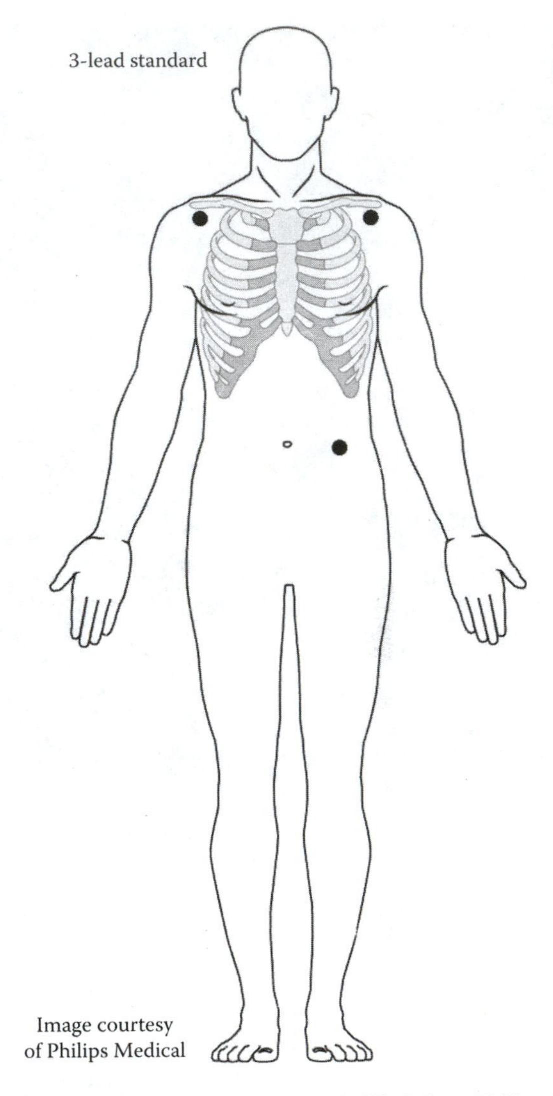

FIGURE 1.18 3-lead ECG electrode placement. (Modified from Philips Medical, CD provided directly, with permission. © 2006 Koninidijke Philips Electronics N.V. All rights reserved. Reproduction in whole or in part is prohibited without prior written permission of the copyright owner.)

horizontally, from lower left to upper right, etc. Originally using just the left arm and right leg, to take advantage of the long axis of the heart to maximize signal size, the placement of electrodes has now become standardized in order to allow useful comparisons (Figure 1.18).

The basic ECG electrode placement has electrodes on the left and right shoulders (left arm or LA and right arm or RA), and the left and right lower abdomen (called the left leg or LL and right leg or RL, from earlier times when the electrodes were actually on the legs, or even consisted of a bucket of saline solution into which the

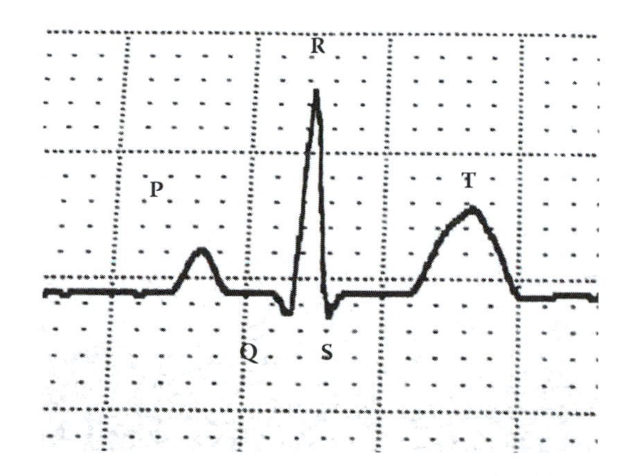

FIGURE 1.19 Normal ECG waveform.

feet were placed.) The wires for these electrodes have been color coded (LA = black, RA = white, LL = red, RL = green.) Depending on which two contact points are used for measurement, various orientations of the ECG signal can be observed. These selections are called "leads," and the first ones in common use were labeled with Roman numerals. Lead I takes the left arm as positive and the right arm as negative. Since this orientation is across a smaller section of the heart, the Lead I signal is usually relatively small. Lead II has right leg positive, right arm negative, and Lead III is left leg positive, left arm negative.

The ECG Waveform

The P wave is generated by contraction of the atria (Figure 1.19).

After this, there is a delay caused by the AV node, which gives blood time to flow from the atria into the ventricles.

When the signal reaches the ventricles, they contract powerfully, producing the QRS complex.

Finally, the ventricles repolarize, producing the T wave, and the cycle can begin again.

Positive and negative were chosen as such because, with the wave of polarization of cardiac muscle proceeding generally from the top of the heart to the bottom, this will give a waveform that is mostly positive-going.

Other ECG leads have been developed, with a chest electrode location (brown) added to make a five-lead system (Figure 1.20). Six-lead and twelve-lead arrangements are also used, with the 12-lead being the standard for complete diagnostic ECG measurements (Figure 1.21). Some manufacturers have developed electrode placement and signal analysis systems whereby near-diagnostic-quality 12-lead ECG waveforms can be derived with only five electrodes.

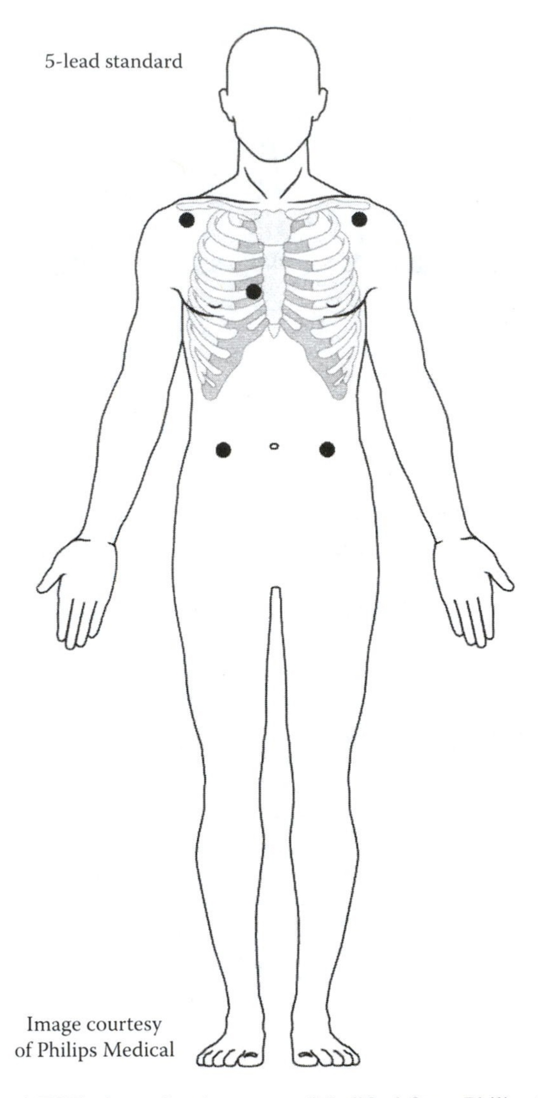

FIGURE 1.20 5-lead ECG electrode placement. (Modified from Philips Medical, CD provided directly, with permission. © 2006 Koninidijke Philips Electronics N.V. All rights reserved. Reproduction in whole or in part is prohibited without prior written permission of the copyright owner.)

ECG lead systems are discussed in more detail in Chapter 2.

Since the focus of ECG measurement and analysis is to aid in the diagnosis of cardiac disease, the changes that disease processes cause to ECG signals are of critical importance. Many of these changes reflect either a reduced blood supply to some areas of the heart muscle or damage to the muscle or conduction pathways caused by a partial or complete blockage of blood flow to an area of cardiac tissue.

Normally one's heart rate is controlled by signals from the autonomic nervous system, which are in turn influenced by exercise, hormone levels, drugs, noncardiac

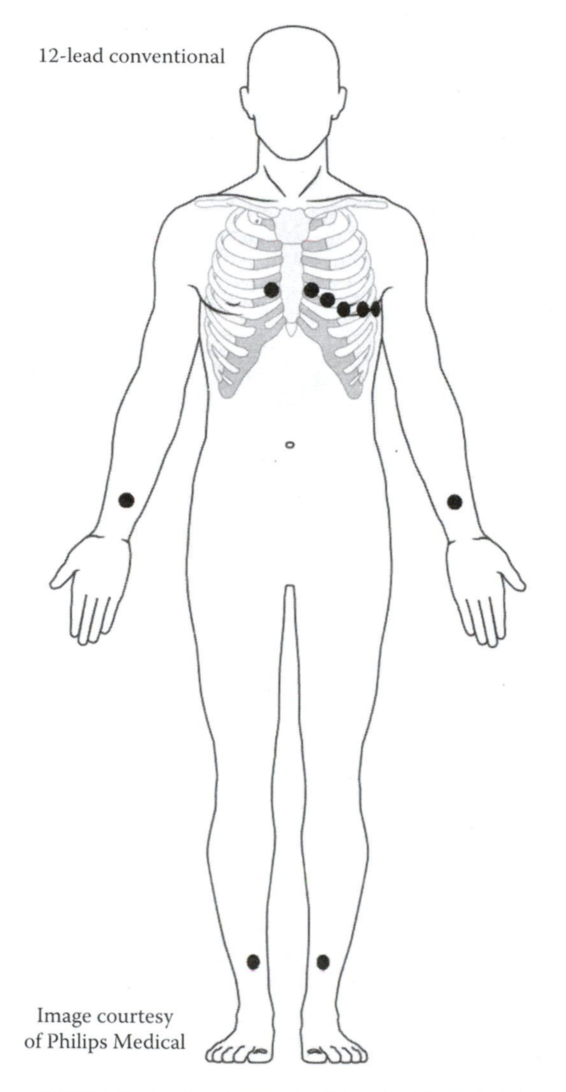

FIGURE 1.21 12-lead ECG electrode placement. (Modified from Philips Medical, CD provided directly, with permission. © 2006 Koninidijke Philips Electronics N.V. All rights reserved. Reproduction in whole or in part is prohibited without prior written permission of the copyright owner.)

disease processes, and other factors. Cardiac muscle cells, however, are unique in the body in that they will contract rhythmically all by themselves. These automatic contractions can be coordinated by an overriding signal, which under normal circumstances results in the proper, effective beating of all areas of heart muscle tissue. If conduction pathways are blocked, either temporarily or permanently (usually by inadequate or no blood flow to part of the heart containing the conductive pathway), then individual areas of the heart can begin beating independently of each other. If these areas consist of small sections of heart muscle, the action is called fibrillation,

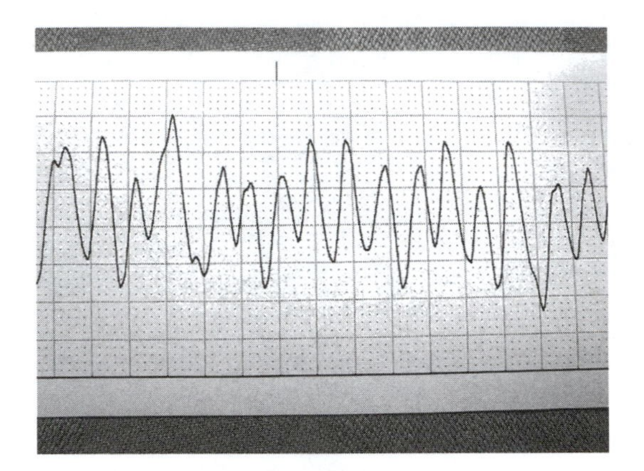

FIGURE 1.22 Ventricular fibrillation waveform.

which can occur either in the atria (atrial fibrillation or a-fib) or ventricles (ventricular fibrillation or v-fib; Figure 1.22). These areas can be resynchronized by an electric shock, a process called defibrillation. In atrial fibrillation, the ventricles are usually beating more or less normally and still pumping blood, though less efficiently than normal. A shock at the wrong time could disrupt the ventricular rhythm, therefore the defibrillation pulse has to be timed to the ventricular contraction signal and delivered at the correct part of the cycle, a procedure commonly called synchronized cardioversion. With ventricular fibrillation, the atria are likely fibrillating as well, and so the defibrillating shock can be delivered at any time.

There are many other types of abnormal cardiac rhythms, or arrhythmias, each of which reflects blockage to some part of the conduction pathways of the heart. By examining high-quality ECG waveforms, experts can learn a great deal about the condition of the heart, and computerized analysis allows classification of arrhythmias by ECG machines and physiological monitors. Arrhythmias will be discussed in more detail in the sections on these devices.

When the heart is beating normally, the rate is controlled by the sino-atrial (S-A) node, which has a natural rhythm of about 70 to 80 beats per minute (bpm). If the atrio-ventricular (A-V) node is controlling contractions, there will be a slower rate of 40 to 60 bpm, while the contractions led by conduction bundles are slower yet at only 15 to 40 bpm.

Some arrhythmias are brought on by chemical, thermal, or electrical disturbances to the heart and will often disappear when the causative factors are resolved. If this process is prolonged or if the problem is caused by permanent damage to part of the heart, it may be necessary to provide continued synchronization of the heart muscle contractions artificially, using a pacemaker. There are three modes of delivering pacemaker pulses to the heart: with a relatively large signal applied through electrodes placed on the patient's chest; through wires connected from an external device directly to the heart muscle; or via wires from an implanted pacemaker device to the heart muscle. These devices will be covered in Chapter 6.

Besides ECG signal measurement devices, a number of other technologies can be used to help diagnose heart problems. Injecting a radiopaque dye into the patient's blood stream and taking x-ray images as the dye passes through the cardiac arteries can show reduced blood flow to parts of the cardiac system. Ultrasound, computed tomography (CT), or magnetic resonance imaging (MRI) scans can provide detailed images of cardiac structures in two or three dimensions. Pressure transducers, introduced to different chambers of the heart by catheters via an artery in the neck, arm, or groin, and sometimes isolated from other areas by a balloon further down on the catheter, can give precise measurements of pressure at different points, which can be clues regarding heart function. Cardiac output can be measured by introducing either dye or cold saline to the heart and measuring dilution at a later point.

Technological means of improving cardiac function include the previously mentioned defibrillators and pacemakers as well as angioplasty devices, which enlarge blocked arteries either by expanding them with a balloon, or cutting out blockages with a mechanical auger or a laser. Faulty valves can be replaced with biological or mechanical implants, and the whole heart can be replaced with either a donor heart or an artificial pump.

C. Blood

Blood performs a number of functions in the body, including gas and nutrient transport, wound healing, disease resistance, and homeothermy. Some of these functions are more important than others from an engineering perspective, and these will be discussed in this section.

Mechanically, blood is a fluid somewhat more viscous than water, made up mostly of water plus various compounds such as sodium chloride, nutrient and waste molecules, a variety of proteins, and several types of cells. The most numerous of these cells are erythrocytes, or red blood cells (Figure 1.23), whose main function is transporting oxygen and carbon dioxide between the lungs and body tissues. Other cells are involved in immune response and tissue cleanup and repair. Being an ionic solution, blood is a relatively good conductor of electricity.

Red blood cells carry various proteins and carbohydrates on their cell membranes, and the type and arrangement of these substances varies between individuals. If the membrane surfaces of two individuals are similar, they are said to have the same blood type. The broadest and most commonly referenced blood types are A, B, AB, and O, each of which can have a particular characteristic (the Rh factor) either present (positive) or absent (negative). If these main blood types are compatible, one individual can accept a blood donation from another. Blood types have a great deal more complexity than this, but the basic descriptions are sufficient for this text.

The movement of blood cells within veins and arteries allows the detection of blood flow by means of Doppler ultrasound, which is described in Chapter 3.

Blood is also involved in clotting, which is the means by which the body tries to prevent excessive blood loss following a breach of blood vessels by trauma or disease. A soluble glycoprotein, fibrinogen, is activated in the presence of an opening in a vessel, and it is converted into fibrin, an insoluble protein that polymerizes to form a mesh. Platelet cells in the blood bind to the fibrin to produce a clot, which reduces and hopefully blocks the escape of blood. Blood clotting is of course critical

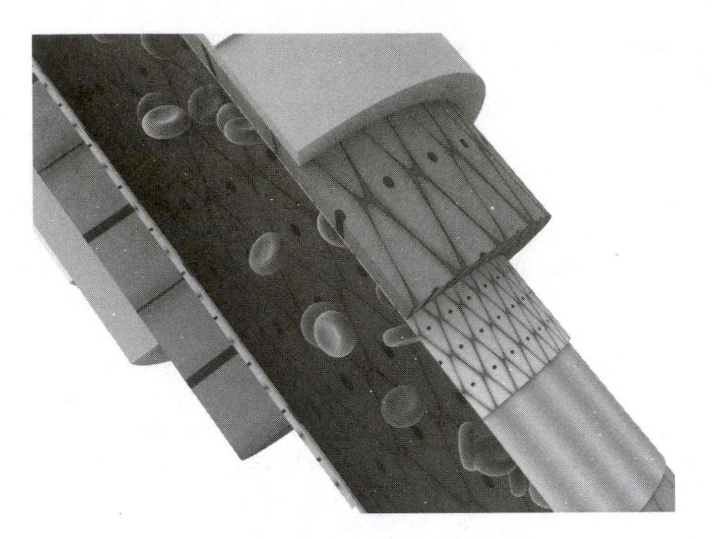

FIGURE 1.23 Red blood cells. (Modified from Inmagine Corp, www.123rf.com, with permission.)

to survival, but can also be a problem when it occurs at the wrong time or place (which can result in an embolism), or when it takes place too slowly, as in a major trauma such as an accident or surgery.

D. Respiration

Respiration is the process by which atmospheric oxygen is taken into an organism so that is can be transported to tissues where it is exchanged for carbon dioxide. The carbon dioxide is then transported so that it can be released from the organism, completing the respiration cycle. Some other gaseous metabolic wastes may also be removed from the body during the cycle. Ventilation is a subset of the respiration process, involving only the movement of gases in and out of the lungs.

The human respiratory system consists of the airways of the nose and mouth, trachea, bronchi and bronchioles, the lungs, the muscles that power the flow of air into and out of the lungs, and associated nervous system control components (Figure 1.24). Passive gas exchange occurs in the alveoli of the lungs, which are the interface between air and blood.

Airways provide additional functions of filtering, warming, and humidifying inspired air.

Both a shortage of oxygen and an excess of carbon dioxide are harmful and potentially fatal, thus the vital nature of the respiratory system. The mechanical nature of the system makes it accessible to medical intervention in case of inadequate function or failure.

Air intake (inspiration) is accomplished mainly by the muscles of the diaphragm and the external intercostal muscles of the rib cage. The diaphragm is normally a sheet of muscle domed up at the bottom of the chest cavity. When it contracts, it flattens out, pulling air into the lungs. The intercostals muscles act to "square up"

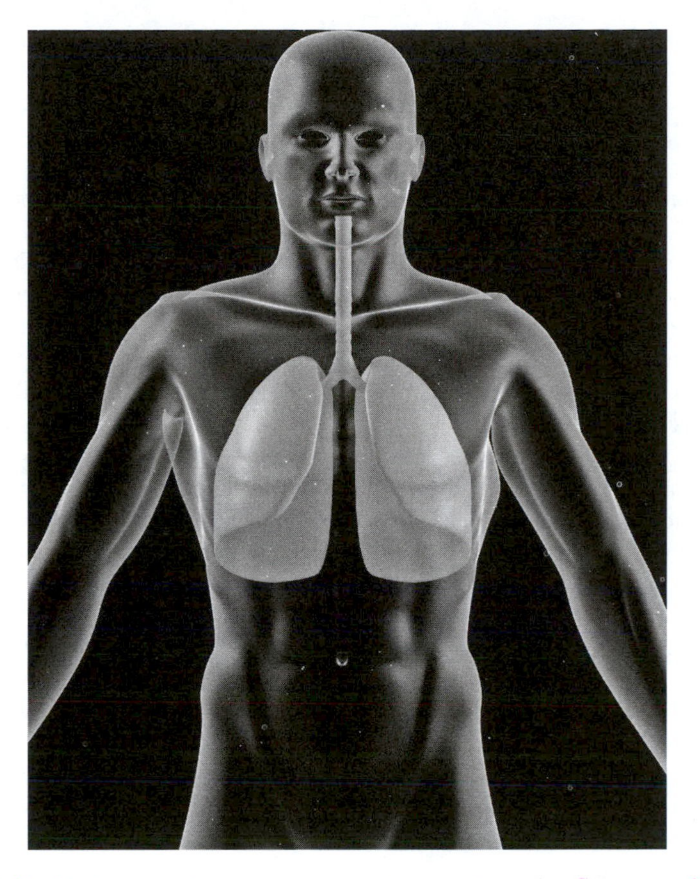

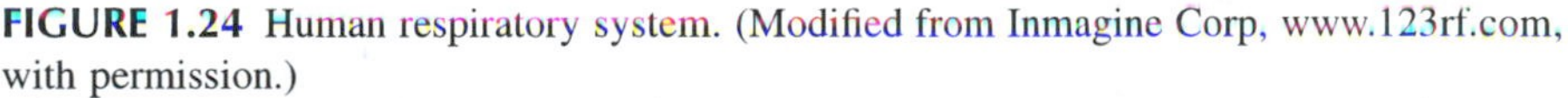

FIGURE 1.24 Human respiratory system. (Modified from Inmagine Corp, www.123rf.com, with permission.)

the chest cavity, thus increasing its volume, again drawing air into the lungs. During maximal inspiratory efforts, some other muscles around the chest cavity may also assist the diaphragm and intercostals.

Expiration is normally mostly passive due to the elasticity of the lungs, though abdominal muscles and external intercostals can provide forced expiration.

Typically, about 500 ml of air is taken in with each resting breath, and about 10–20 breaths are taken per minute, resulting in 250 ml of oxygen uptake and 200 ml of carbon dioxide output per minute. These values can, of course, have a wide range depending on the individual, age, gender, exertion level, and state of health.

Given the important roles of oxygen and carbon dioxide in the body, means have been developed to measure levels of both, in inspired and expired air as well as in the blood. Instruments to perform these measurements are described in Chapter 3.

E. Chemical Balances

All physiological functions involve chemicals as part of their processes, and normal health depends on these chemicals remaining in overall balance. Chemicals in the body range from ions of elements such as sodium, chlorine, potassium, and calcium, to simple molecules like carbon dioxide, water, and oxygen, to more complex sugars and carbohydrates, to convoluted proteins, and to the genetic materials of RNA and DNA.

Gas balances are described in more detail in Chapter 3.

Most protein and genetic material chemistries are outside the scope of this book, but the balance of ions and relatively simple molecules will be examined more closely.

One of the most important organ systems in maintaining chemical balance is the renal system, consisting of the blood supplies to the kidneys, the kidneys themselves, the ureters, bladder, and urethra, and associated control components. This makes the kidneys vital but also vulnerable to damage by disease or harmful chemicals, and thus a large amount of medical equipment is designed to help determine kidney function and to take over some or all of kidney function should they fail. These devices are described in Chapter 7.

Membranes within the kidneys selectively pass different molecules and ions, thus maintaining balance. As an example, sodium intake can vary from one-tenth normal to ten times normal, and the kidneys maintain blood plasma sodium concentrations within a few percent. Just 10% kidney function can maintain health.

Buffer chemicals in the blood help maintain proper pH balance, which is important since a drop from the normal pH of 7.4 to just 6.8, or a rise to 7.8, can be fatal. These buffers are controlled by both the kidneys and the lungs. Equipment to measure pH and other blood chemicals are described in Chapter 3.

The simple sugar, glucose (Figure 1.25), is the means by which energy is supplied to cells in the body. Glucose is produced by the digestion of most foods or by the utilization of body fat, and its levels are controlled mainly by the pancreas and the insulin it produces; insulin operates by controlling the movement of glucose in and out of cells. Chronic inadequate production and/or control of insulin is known as diabetes.

Glucose is normally maintained at concentrations between 4 and 8 millimoles per liter (mmol/l), or 72 to 144 milligrams per deciliter of blood.

The brain is the first organ to show signs of low blood glucose (hypoglycemia). At levels below 3.6 mmol/l, reductions in mental capacity start to become apparent, while levels below 2.2 mmol/l cause significant impairment of judgment and performance. Seizures can result if levels drop further, and a level under 0.55 mmol/l produces a coma state and, if not corrected, death.

High levels of blood glucose (hyperglycemia) in diabetes can also have severe consequences. Intraocular pressure changes result in blurred vision. Patients may also experience extreme hunger and thirst, fatigue, weight loss, impaired wound healing, dry skin and mouth, and impaired infection handling. Eventually, blindness and tissue death in the extremities can occur.

Blood glucose levels can be measured by a variety of devices, as described in Chapter 3, while pumps to help maintain proper insulin levels are discussed in Chapter 6.

F. Densities

The densities of various body tissues and fluids are factors in the function of many biomedical devices. Table 1.2 lists some tissue and fluid densities.

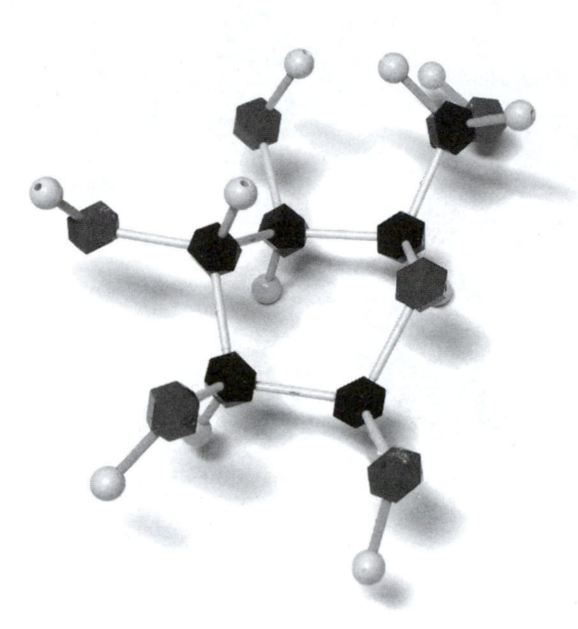

FIGURE 1.25 A model of a glucose molecule. (Modified from Inmagine Corp, www.123rf.com, with permission.)

TABLE 1.2
Tissue Densities

Tissue Type	Density (kg/m^3)
Bone marrow	1810
Fat	920
Bone	1810
White matter	1040
Gray matter	1040
Skin	1010
Eye	1170
Muscle	1040
Blood	1060
CSF	1010
Nerve tissue	1040
Cartilage	1100

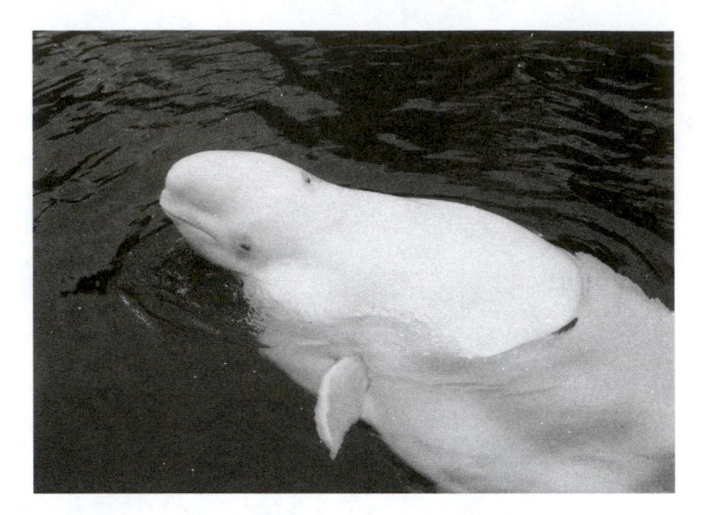

FIGURE 1.26 A beluga whale stays warm. (Modified from Inmagine Corp, www.123rf.com, with permission.)

G. Temperature

Humans are endothermic, or warm-blooded, organisms, which means that internally produced heat helps maintain internal body temperature at a constant level of about 37°C. This means that we can continue to be active when external temperatures are significantly below body temperature, allowing a wider range of habitats. This maintenance of core temperature is called homeothermy; the body has a "set point" temperature, and if core temperature changes significantly from the set point, mechanisms are activated to bring it back in line.

There is some small variation of "normal" body temperatures, both between different individuals and within individuals at different times. Other species can have significantly higher or lower normal body temperatures than humans (Figure 1.26).

Maintaining homeothermy requires a number of adaptations, including a system to monitor temperature and signal variations, circulatory modifications to reduce or increase blood flow to the skin and extremities, structures to increase or decrease heat loss to the environment (such as sweat glands that excrete water to the skin surface, which evaporates and cools the skin, or layers of body fat and/or hair to provide insulation), and behaviors to assist in the process (such as increasing physical activity and/or shivering to produce extra heat, seeking shelter from temperature extremes, or utilizing clothing).

If core body temperature cannot be maintained, severe symptoms will result.

Various means of measuring and monitoring body temperature are described in Chapter 4.

1. Hypothermia

Hypothermia results when core temperature drops significantly, and physiological responses are fairly consistent (Figure 1.27).

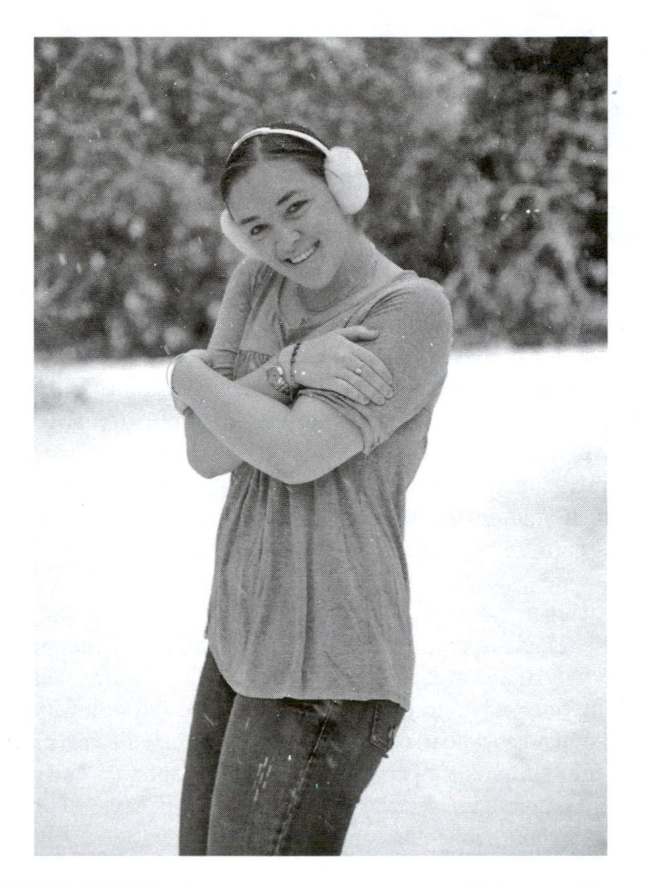

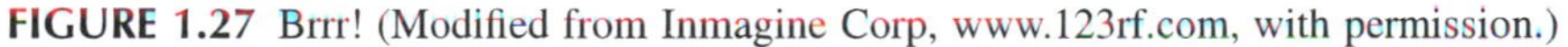

FIGURE 1.27 Brrr! (Modified from Inmagine Corp, www.123rf.com, with permission.)

Below about 35°C, shivering occurs, heart and respiration rates increase, and blood pressure rises. Below this temperature, all of these parameters begin to decline again, and some brain functions may become impaired, resulting in decreased coordination, disorientation, and communication difficulties.

Below 32°C, shivering usually ceases, and decreased metabolism results in reduced oxygen consumption. Cardiac output drops, arrhythmias may appear, and the patient may be in a stupor.

Further drops to below 28°C produce a complete loss of nervous reflexes and greatly reduced brain function, as well as greatly reduced cardiac output and severe arrhythmias. The patient may appear to be dead, and death will certainly result if conditions worsen and/or continue for any length of time, though some extreme cases of survival have been recorded. Some victims of accidental hypothermia have been successfully revived from core temperatures as low as 14°C, while under controlled conditions of induced hypothermia, core temperatures have been as low as 9°C. Cardiorespiratory function has been seen to stop for as long as an hour under these conditions, with no lasting damage, because metabolic rates have been so low. The key to survival in these circumstances seems to be that brain temperature must drop relatively quickly, which is why small children have survived for long periods of extreme hypothermia.

Rewarming extreme hypothermic patients is difficult, as all vital body structures must be warmed quickly and almost simultaneously, but high temperatures of warming materials must be avoided.

2. Hyperthermia

Increases in core body temperature can result from a response to disease processes (fever) or from excessive production or absorption of heat (hyperthermia.)

Fever increases the body's temperature set point by a few degrees, thus initiating responses to bring core temperature up to the new set point. This is why people with fevers may feel chills (their actual core temperature is initially below the new set point) and experience shivering as their body attempts to raise its core temperature. Higher temperatures seem to enhance immune system response and also seem to negatively affect some pathogens such as viruses. Excessively high fever temperatures can be harmful or even fatal and must be reduced by medication and/or external means.

When body temperature rises due to increased internal heat production and/or increased ambient temperature or incident infrared radiation, a number of responses can occur. Behaviorally, any organism might seek shade or water, while humans can alter their clothing or simply turn up the air conditioner. Physiologically, blood flow may increase to skin areas where excess heat can be radiated away, and (in humans) sweat glands in the skin produce perspiration, which evaporates and cools the body.

If human core temperature rises above 39 or 40°C, behavioral changes such as irritability and confusion ("mad dogs and Englishmen") start to appear. As well, the skin reddens, blood pressure drops, and heart and respiration rates increase. Further temperature increases produce still lower blood pressure, which may result in a blotchy appearance of the skin. Convulsions may occur, as well as chills and shivering. At 41°C, brain death begins, and at 45°C, death almost always occurs.

Recovery from extreme hyperthermia is less likely than from extreme hypothermia, but it is important to cool the victim's body as soon as possible to prevent excessive core temperatures. Methods of doing this range from simple moistening of the skin, to cold- or ice-water baths, to the use of special cooling devices.

IV. CHAPTER SUMMARY

Chapter 1 provides a brief look at the history of some medical devices and an outline of some important anatomical and physiological features of the human body, including electrical signals, circulation and blood, respiration, chemical balances, tissue densities, and thermoregulation.

2 Diagnostic Devices – Part One

I. PHYSIOLOGICAL MONITORING SYSTEMS

A. Overview

Various means of examining and measuring the "vital signs" of patients have been developed in the past. Heart rate, ECG waveform, blood pressure, temperature, respiratory rate, blood oxygen content, and other parameters could be determined accurately.

As technology advanced, it became apparent that some of the equipment for these monitored parameters could be integrated into a single unit. This made monitoring more convenient and also allowed direct comparison of values and integrated recording of numeric and graphical data (Figure 2.1).

Electronic data storage allowed systems to store parameter values and waveforms for significant time periods, with times extending as technology advanced. Patient charting became easier and more comprehensive.

Data communications gave the capability of displaying information from one patient on the monitor of another patient, or at a central location, or even off-site.

Changing capabilities led to evolving labels for equipment. What was once called simply an ECG monitor became a bedside monitor, a vital signs monitor, and then a physiological monitoring system or multiparameter monitoring system (Figure 2.2).

B. Integration and Connectivity

The integration of various vital signs monitoring devices into one brought a number of benefits:

1. The monitoring location became much less cluttered, with a single box and power cord and one set of mounting hardware. The number of connections to the patient was not reduced, but at least they all originated in the same area (Figure 2.3).
2. Some functions such as determining heart rate could be adapted to use the best source available. For example, if an ECG signal was noisy, pulse information might be gathered from an invasive blood pressure line or an SpO_2 waveform.

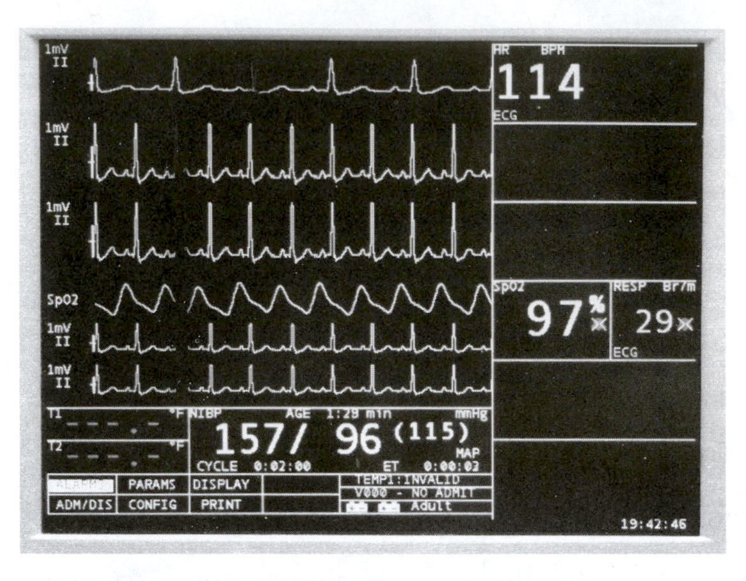

FIGURE 2.1 A physiological monitor screen. (Modified from Inmagine Corp, www.123rf.com, with permission.)

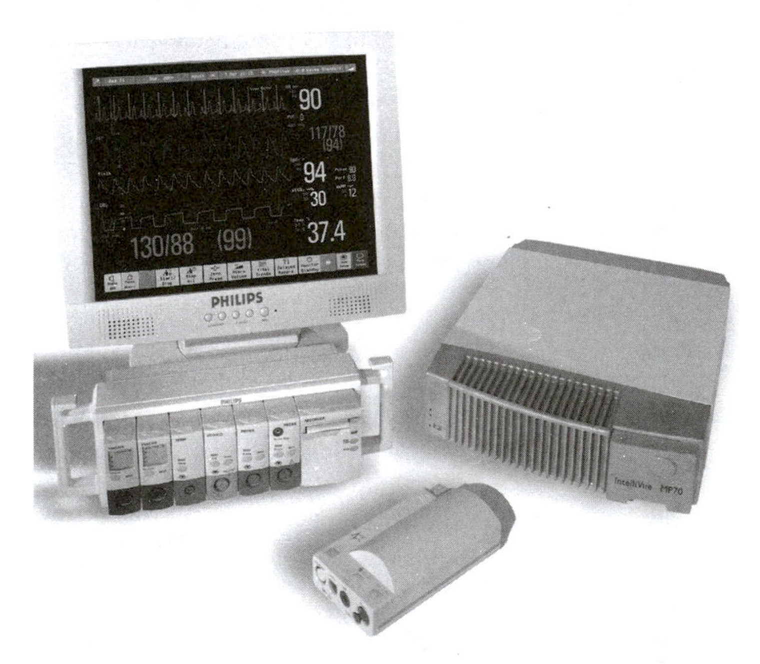

FIGURE 2.2 A modern multiparameter monitor. (Modified from Philips Medical, CD provided directly, with permission. © 2006 Koninidijke Philips Electronics N.V. All rights reserved. Reproduction in whole or in part is prohibited without prior written permission of the copyright owner.)

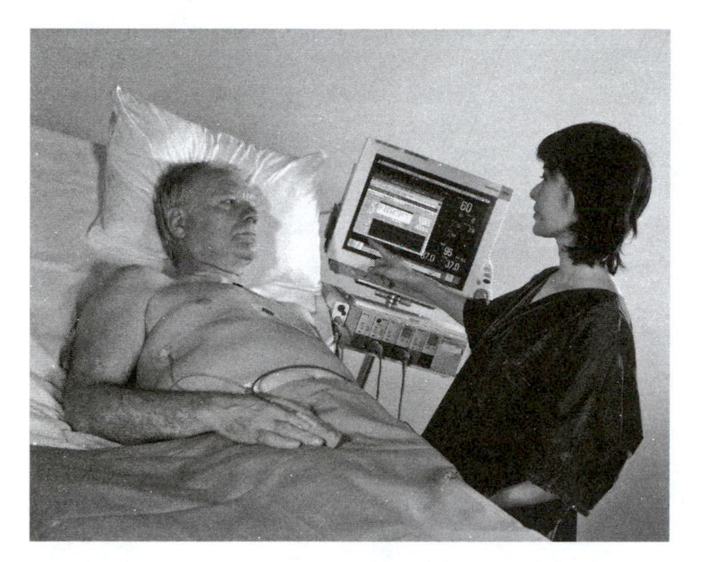

FIGURE 2.3 A monitor at a patient's bedside. (Modified from Philips Medical, CD provided directly, with permission. © 2006 Koninidijke Philips Electronics N.V. All rights reserved. Reproduction in whole or in part is prohibited without prior written permission of the copyright owner.)

3. Comparison of waveforms was much easier. Looking at ECG signals on the same time scale as pressure waveforms can provide useful information.
4. Connecting the monitoring system to other devices, such as central stations or networks, is much easier when all components are in one box and designed with common interface and communication standards.

The earliest interconnected monitoring systems used proprietary interfaces, different for each manufacturer, and utilizing heavy, multiconductor cables. Newer systems use industry-standard serial communications with CAT-5 or optical cables. This allows the use of standard data switches, amplifiers, connectors, and other components. The systems are actually just computer LANs, making that part of system design much more standard and "off the shelf." This also allows easier connections to other networks, such as in-hospital LANs/WANs and the Internet. (See section on networking in Chapter 11.)

C. Central Stations

When more patients were being monitored electronically, special hospital units were developed to have all such patients in the same area, since their medical needs were similar. These areas were called Intensive Care Units, Cardiac Care Units, Special Care Units, and a variety of other descriptive names.

With such a concentration of patients, it became increasingly difficult for nursing staff to watch all the monitors, and indeed most patients went for relatively long periods of time without any critical events occurring. Systems were then developed

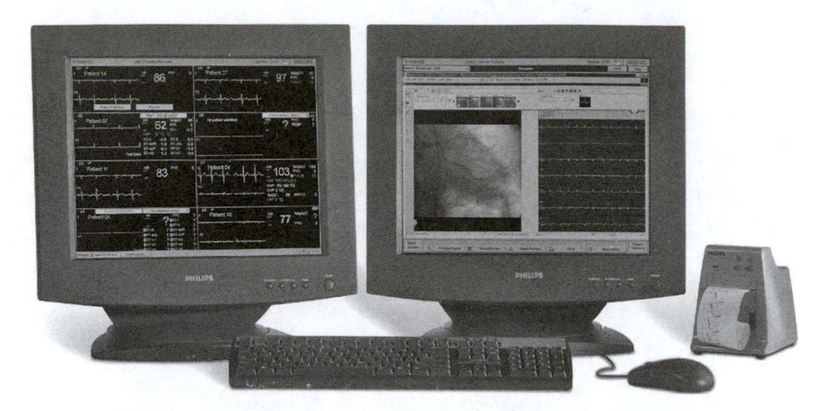

FIGURE 2.4 Intensive care central station displays. (Modified from Philips Medical, CD provided directly, with permission. © 2006 Koninidijke Philips Electronics N.V. All rights reserved. Reproduction in whole or in part is prohibited without prior written permission of the copyright owner.)

to gather data from each bedside monitor and transmit it to a central location such as a nursing station, where it could be displayed on a monitor — a central station (Figure 2.4).

Since there is generally more data from all of the care-unit bedsides than can be simultaneously displayed on one monitor at the central station, only certain data are selected for display. Generally other data can be selected for individual circumstances, taking up a disproportionate amount of screen space for a short time.

Because of its location, it is convenient to be able to enter patient data into the system at the central station when a new patient is admitted, so a keyboard (and perhaps a computer mouse) was added for this function.

Hard-copy recordings are often needed for analysis and to use as part of a patient's record, and the central station arrangement makes this much more convenient. Instead of individual strip chart recorders at each bedside, from which paper strips would have to be collected, the recorders can be located in the central station, printing strips out from whichever bedside originated the request (Figure 2.5). Depending on the amount of recording being requested, two or more recorder modules might be present in the central station.

Larger-format recordings are useful as well, and the bulky recorders (such as laser printers) required for this are located at or near the central station. Multilead ECGs, longer-term waveform recordings, tables of measured values, patient data, and even configuration and troubleshooting information, can all be conveniently printed on the central printer (Figure 2.6).

Multiple screens allow more patients and/or more detailed information to be displayed, though there is a practical limit to the number of patients that can be handled from each central station, so large care units may be divided into groups.

Some other features that may be present with a central station include touch screens for ease of response and information selection, an interface to a nurse-call or paging system so that staff can be alerted when critical alarms occur, the capability of transferring certain data from one bedside to another so that staff can analyze

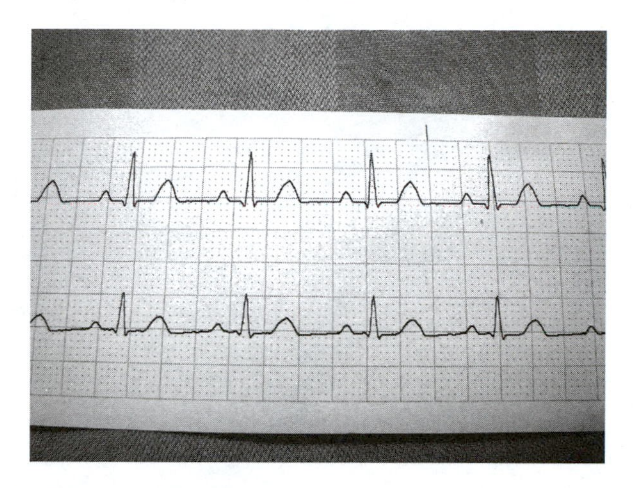

FIGURE 2.5 An ECG recording strip.

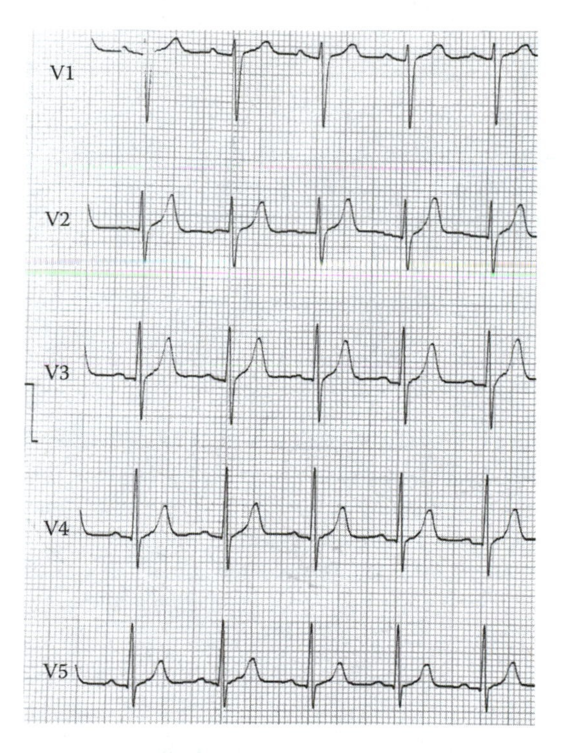

FIGURE 2.6 Printout from a central station printer. (Modified from Inmagine Corp, www.123rf.com, with permission.)

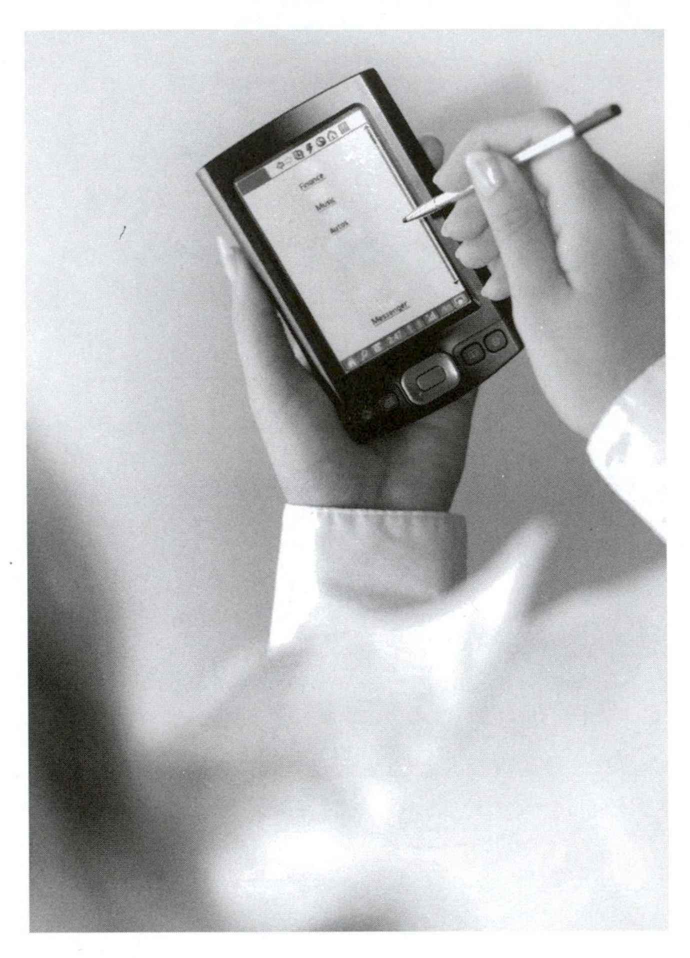

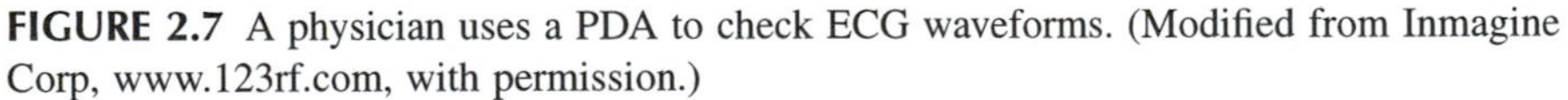

FIGURE 2.7 A physician uses a PDA to check ECG waveforms. (Modified from Inmagine Corp, www.123rf.com, with permission.)

information without necessarily leaving the bedside of the patient they are with, communication with other special care monitoring systems or other areas in the hospital to allow staff to examine patient data from these other areas, integration with hospital admission, discharge, and transfer systems to coordinate the movement and collection of patient information, and the ability to transmit information to remote locations such as another hospital, a physician's office, or a handheld device such as a palmtop computer or PDA (Figure 2.7).

D. Telemetry

As patients, particularly cardiac patients, improve, they often come to a point where it would be beneficial to be able to get out of bed and exercise some, but they still require monitoring in case there are problems. Radio technology came into play, combined with ever-smaller electronic circuits, to allow the development of telemetry units, which combine ECG leads, filters, and amplifiers with a radio transmitter in order to pick up the patient's ECG signal and broadcast it to a central receiver and monitor.

These units have to be small enough to be readily portable, have enough battery capacity to transmit for many hours without battery replacement, have sufficient range to allow adequate freedom of movement to the patient and to supply a clinically useful signal (accurate and free from significant noise or drift) at the monitoring end of the system.

As telemetry systems have evolved, they have grown in capability and quality while shrinking in size. Current systems may include SpO2 monitoring and even noninvasive blood pressure, though the pumps and other mechanisms needed for the latter make the transmitter heavier.

The transmitter portion of a modern "tele" pack includes a set of three or more lead wires (usually not more than five), ECG input and amplification circuitry, sometimes ECG analysis components, components for additional functions such as SpO2 and NIBP if present, a battery compartment and power circuitry including what is needed to generate low-battery signals, a nurse call and/or "event" button for patient use, an RF transmitter including antenna, and interface circuitry to go between the ECG and RF portions (Figure 2.8). Most new telemetry is digital, which means that analog to digital conversion is also included. Many tele packs have some kind of port to allow direct communication with a computer or other device that allows for programming parameters and troubleshooting.

Digital systems have the capability of changing channel frequencies to make the system more flexible, or perhaps to avoid channels that have excess interference.

Telemetry receivers are usually mounted in a rack, with one module for each transmitter channel. The rack is in a chassis that contains conditioning and interface circuitry to connect to the central monitoring station and/or other network (Figure 2.9).

Some systems have dedicated monitors with a single-channel telemetry receiver built in, and/or with another interface to the transmitter such as an infrared link, allowing direct observation of the telemetry signals.

Digital telemetry allows for changing channel assignments and frequencies, within a predefined range. A few RF bands have been allocated for medical telemetry in North America: 608–614 MHz, 1395–1400 MHz, and 1427–1429.5 MHz. Earlier generations used 450–470 MHz; some older systems may still use this band, but all new installations must use the higher bands.

A properly designed antenna system is critical for the effective functioning of a telemetry system. Since power output is relatively low, and signal integrity is critical, the antennas must be fairly close together and distributed in all areas where telemetry patients will be active (Figure 2.10). Impedance matching at all points in the system is vital, and if some antennas are to be mounted at a considerable distance from the central receiver (for example, a system might have antennas in the diagnostic imaging and physical therapy departments so that patients can continue to be monitored when they are temporarily in these locations) then adequate RF signal amplifiers must be used.

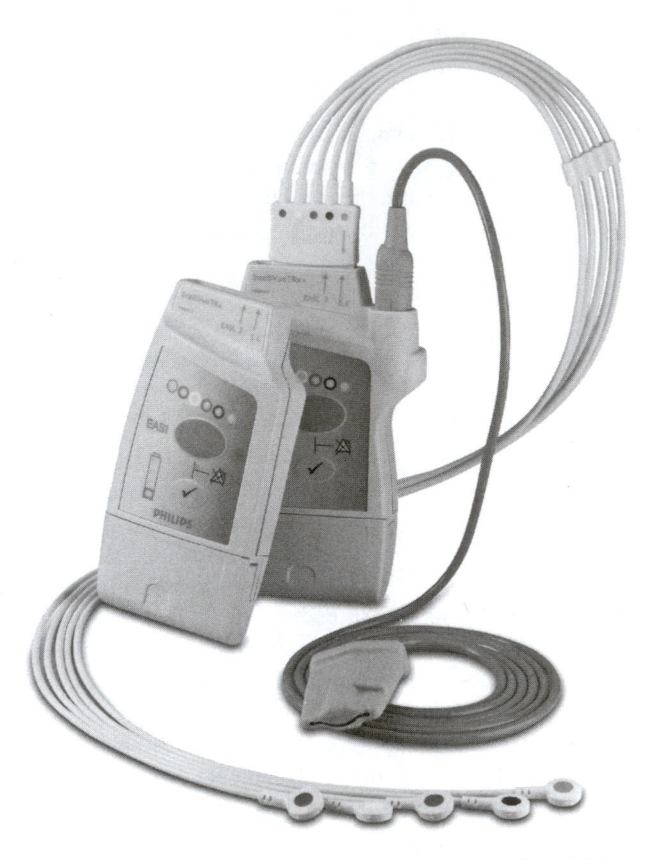

FIGURE 2.8 A modern telemetry transmitter pack. (Modified from Philips Medical, CD provided directly, with permission.

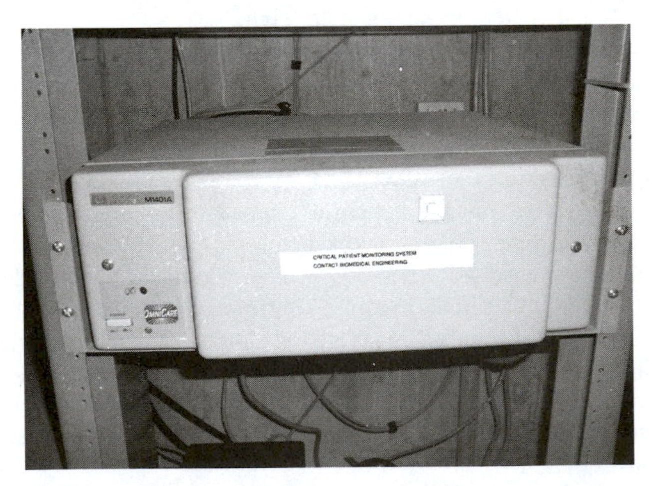

FIGURE 2.9 Telemetry receiver rack.

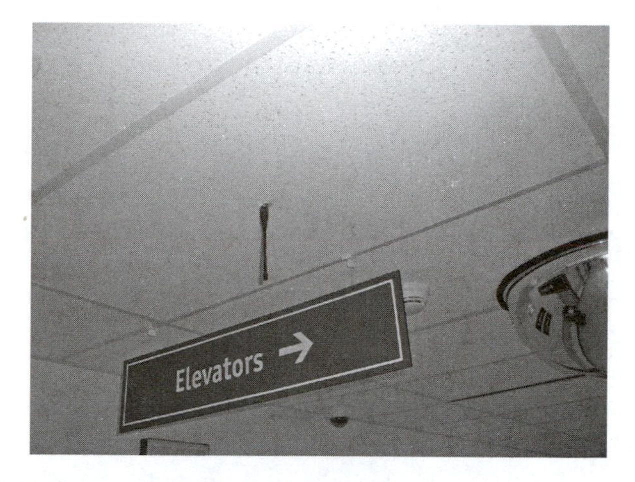

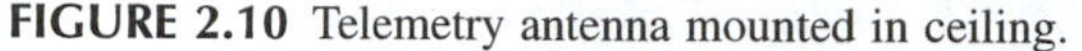
FIGURE 2.10 Telemetry antenna mounted in ceiling.

II. THE HEART

Details of cardiac anatomy and physiology (Figure 2.11) are discussed in Chapter 1.

A. ECG Monitors and Machines

The heart being perhaps the "most vital" of the vital organs, it is important to obtain as much information as possible about its function and condition when assessing a patient. Taking a pulse rate manually and listening for heart sounds have been important tools for medical practitioners for centuries, but as the physiology and anatomy of the cardiac system became better understood, it became apparent that electrical signals could provide very useful information about the heart. Investigators found that the signals within the heart that initiated and coordinated contractions, and were produced by these contractions, could be detected at the surface of the patient. By suitably amplifying and filtering these signals, a waveform could be produced that provided important information about the heart, without any need for surgery. The signals are different at different points on the skin surface, because they originate in different parts of the heart and they travel different pathways to the surface. This means that by placing electrodes at different locations, different types of information about cardiac function can be obtained.

Electrocardiograph (ECG) systems are a common and powerful tool for medical staff and can be found in a variety of configurations and settings. "ECG monitor" generally refers to a device that provides real-time ECG waveforms (Figure 2.12), while an "ECG machine" produces a hard-copy version of these waves. As shall be discussed, the lines dividing these two devices are often increasingly blurred as the capabilities of both bedside physiological monitors and ECG machines grow.

Any ECG system consists of the same basic components: a means of picking up the ECG signals from the skin (or sometimes other tissue) of the patient, an amplifier/filter section to boost the signals to more useful levels and remove electrical interference, some means of displaying the resulting waveforms, and a power supply.

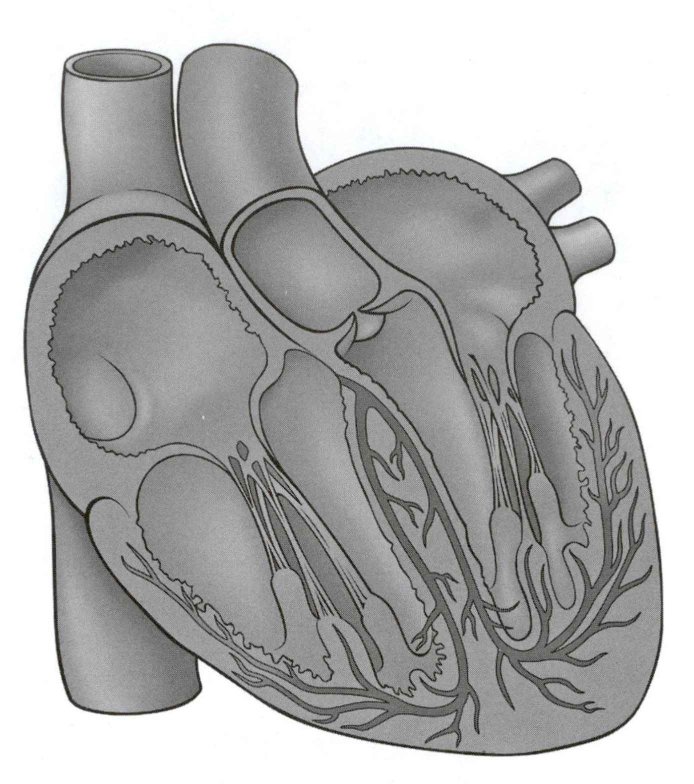

FIGURE 2.11 Cardiac anatomy (Modified from Inmagine Corp, www.123rf.com, with permission.)

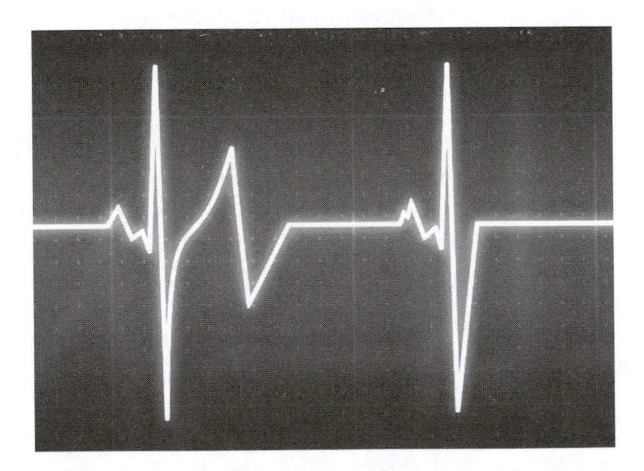

FIGURE 2.12 A stylized ECG waveform. (Modified from Inmagine Corp, www.123rf.com, with permission.)

ECG signals are picked up from the skin through a conductive connection, and so for AC-powered devices an additional feature is necessary for patient safety: a means of preventing potentially harmful electricity (that might be produced by a fault within the circuitry of the device) from flowing back into the patient. A number of techniques were devised for this, and will be discussed in more detail.

ECG History — A Brief Timeline

1838, Italy — Carlo Matteucci demonstrates that an electrical signal is produced each time a frog's heart beats. He uses a section of frog leg muscle as a detector.

1843, Germany — Emil du Bois-Reymond demonstrates that an "action potential" is produced when muscle contracts. His detector is a galvanometer coil with 24,000 windings. He uses the notations P, Q, R, and S to denote the various parts of the observed waveform.

1856, Germany — Rudolph von Koelliker and Heinrich Mueller show that electrical signals are produced with each beat of the heart, and note that the signal is different on diastole and systole.

1869, England — Alexander Muirhead makes the first ECG recording, using an early form of ink-jet printer. (This accomplishment is disputed).

1878, England — John Burden Sanderson and Frederick Page record the first (undisputed) ECG, demonstrating the various phases of QRS and T (Figure 2.13).

1887, England — Augustus D. Waller, first human ECG.

1889, Holland — Willem Einthoven, using jars of saline as electrodes and his dog as a subject, demonstrates ECG signals.

1891, England — William Bayliss and Edward Starling refine ECG technique, identifying the P, QRS, and T components of the signal as well as noting the significance of the PR interval.

1893, Holland — Einthoven first uses the term "electrocardiogram."

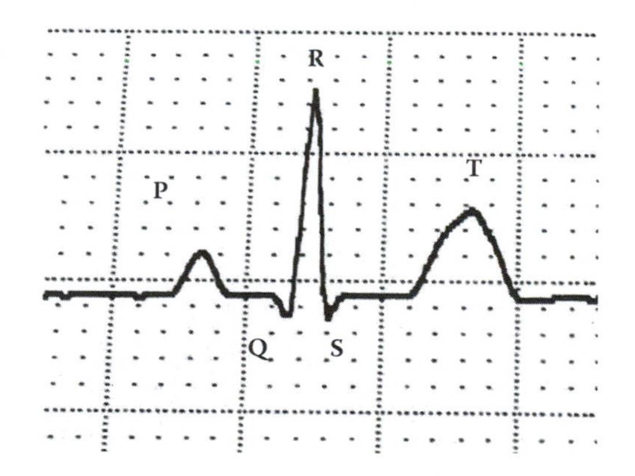

FIGURE 2.13 A normal ECG waveform.

1901, Holland — Einthoven develops a 600-pound "string galvanometer," which is much more sensitive that previous mechanisms.

1905, England — Cambridge Scientific Instruments Company becomes interested in commercial production of ECG machines.

1905–1906, England and Holland — ECG arrhythmias described.

1906, Germany — First fetal ECG.

1912, England — Einthoven introduces his triangle.

1928, USA — First use of vacuum tubes for ECG signal amplification.

1928, USA — Frank Sanborn builds the first portable ECG machine.

1938, USA and England — V1–V6 chest leads defined.

1942 — aVR, aVL, and aVF (augmented) leads developed; when included with Einthoven's three limb leads and the six V leads, this gave the modern 12-lead ECG system.

1949, USA — Norman Jeff Holter builds the first ambulatory ECG recorder, weighing 75 pounds — enough to give someone a heart attack!

1963, USA — The first standard (and still used) protocol for cardiac stress testing is developed by Robert Bruce.

B. ECG Electrodes

The earliest method of making good contact with the patient's skin in order to pick up ECG signals was to immerse hands and feet in buckets of saline. This was obviously a cumbersome technique, and silver plate electrodes were developed, using a conductive paste to help ensure good contact.

A critical part of the conductive pathway for ECG signals is the interface between the skin of the patient and the ECG electrode. High impedance at this point can produce increased interference, wandering baselines, reduced waveform amplitude, or even a complete loss of signal.

The top layer of skin is tough and impervious, which results in higher impedance than is found in underlying tissue. The impedance is significant in all patients, but can be much higher for certain individuals. Dry or oily skin, the use of some skin creams, occupational exposure to insulating oils, and thicker skin layers can all contribute to high impedance.

A coworker once had an uncle who had worked as an auto mechanic for many years. His skin was so impregnated with oil and grease that he could put his finger in a live light socket and feel just a slight tingle. Don't try this at home!

Electrodes are designed to help overcome skin impedance, but for best performance (and sometimes any performance at all), the patient's skin must be properly prepared before electrodes are applied. This includes removing excess hair, cleaning the site, and gently abrading the skin with a gauze pad, a scraping instrument, or sandpaper. Some ECG electrodes come with a section of sandpaper on the cover, and special abrasive tape is available for this purpose. Note that alcohol can dry skin surfaces, resulting in increased rather than decreased impedance, therefore alcohol is not recommended for electrode site skin preparation. One of the biggest sources of medical staff complaints about ECG systems is "poor signal," and often this is a result of inadequate skin prep.

Most ECG electrodes use a silver terminal coated with silver chloride, or a terminal of some other conductive material coated with a silver/silver chloride compound. The electrode may have a conductive paste or gel included, or the paste may be applied separately. Most disposable electrodes come in a package including gel and an adhesive ring, with a metal tab for connecting to the ECG leads.

ECG paste or gel is a material designed to interface between electrodes and skin, usually containing chloride ions. The interaction between the chloride ions in the gel, the silver chloride, and the silver itself creates a stable, low-impedance connection to the leads and then to the ECG input circuitry — as long as the skin is prepared properly.

The adhesive and gel are selected to be nonirritating, though some patients will have sensitivity reactions to one or both. These reactions can sometimes be mistaken for burns.

C. Amplifiers

ECG signals at the surface of the skin usually have an amplitude in the range one millivolt. To be analyzed, manipulate and displayed, the signals need to be about a thousand times larger, so they must be amplified.

An amplifier is basically a feedback electronic circuit, in which the applied signal modifies the conductivity of an element in such as way as to allow a large amount of current to flow through the element in proportion to the input voltage. This current can be applied to further circuitry to develop a voltage that is similar in shape but much greater in amplitude than the input signal.

Early ECG amplifiers used vacuum tubes, but their bulk, high power consumption, and low reliability led to the development of solid-state amplifiers, using transistors. Discrete transistor circuits gave way to integrated circuit (IC) amplifiers, though individual transistors may be used for some stages. Modern ECG systems, even though they use microprocessors for some of their signal modification, still rely on discrete transistor or IC analog amplifiers at the "front end," to amplify the ECG signals to a level that they can be converted to digital.

Amplifiers at any point in the system must be accurate and free from significant internally generated noise.

D. Interference

Ending up with a clinically useful ECG signal from the low-level signal present at the patient's skin requires that all sources of outside interference be reduced to levels much lower than that of the ECG signal itself.

There are many potential sources of interference, or artifact. These can be broadly divided into those generated within the patient, and those generated externally.

1. Internally Generated Artifacts

The two main sources of internal, or physiological, interference signals are muscles and skin.

Skeletal muscles, like cardiac muscles, produce potentials when they contract and relax. These potentials are carried through surrounding tissue to the skin surface, where they are mixed with ECG signals. Fortunately, the characteristics of muscle, or EMG, signals are different from those of ECG signals (EMG signals tend to be mostly higher-frequency spikes), which allows them to be effectively filtered out. Still, it is best to try to avoid placing ECG electrodes over large muscle groups.

Stretching of the epidermis on which electrodes are placed can generate significant low-frequency voltages. This happens when a patient moves or shifts position, and because it is a slowly changing signal, it is harder to filter out. Good skin preparation helps, as can placing electrodes in areas where there is minimal skin stretching during movement.

2. Externally Generated Artifacts

Some early electrode designs formed what was essentially a battery, the electrodes and electrolytes interacting in such a way as to produce a DC voltage. This voltage is known as an offset potential, because it offsets the ECG signal by some amount, possibly even off the screen or chart. It may show up as a rapid shift in the ECG baseline or as a slower drift. Modern silver/silver chloride electrodes are mostly immune to this phenomenon.

Most equipment in hospitals operates on 60-Hz AC (50-Hz in some countries.) This includes patient monitoring and treatment devices as well as lights, motorized lifts, computers, fax machines, floor cleaners, and more. All of these devices, plus the wiring that feeds them, radiate 60-Hz signals. These signals induce a potential in the body that may be up to a few volts in amplitude, far greater then ECG signals. Some of this 60-Hz artifact can be reduced by removing its sources, but the key to the most effective means of reduction lies in the fact that these 60-Hz signals are contacting all parts of the body equally. ECG systems are designed to measure the differences in signals at different points in the skin. If all ECG electrodes in use on a patient have equally good contact with the skin, then the 60-Hz signal should be equal at all of them. Since the amplifiers in use amplify only the difference in potential between sites, the 60-Hz signal will not be amplified, while the ECG signal will be boosted. Good skin preparation and fresh ECG electrodes are necessary for this method to be effective.

Note that ECG electrodes can dry out if they are past their expiry date, if they have been stored improperly (high temperature and/or light levels, torn packages,) or if they have been in place on the patient for too long. Electrode manufacturers will have recommendations as to the time intervals for electrode replacement.

The 60-Hz artifact can be filtered within the ECG system; however some useful ECG information may be in the 60-Hz frequency range and will thus be lost by the action of these filters. A trade-off between artifact and signal accuracy is sometimes required.

Higher-frequency interference can be produced by electrosurgery machines. These devices radiate high-powered signals in the course of their operation, and their power is applied directly to the patient when cutting or coagulating, so the interference is carried throughout the body. Special filters may be used to help reduce such artifacts; also, some ECG lead sets have extra shielding to help block ESU interference.

A final source of artifact is the cable system being used. If signal-carrying wires are compromised, or if contacts at various points in the system are contaminated, or if shield wires are broken and ineffective, then ECG signals may be intermittently interrupted or outside interference may enter the system more easily.

E. Filters

Filters are required within an ECG amplifying system in order to eliminate as much unwanted signal as possible while allowing most of the ECG signal to pass through. How much ECG signal is enough is determined by clinical needs: simple monitoring of rate requires only the basic QRS spike to be available, while such things as arrhythmia detection and analysis and ST segment analysis require the highest possible quality in the ECG signal.

Filters may be simple RC types, or more complex RC or LRC networks. With the advent of digital circuitry, algorithms can be applied to the digitized signals to filter out certain artifacts.

F. Lead Arrangements

ECG systems operate on the principle of differential voltages. The electrical signals generated by the heart travel to the skin. The signals are somewhat different, depending on which part of the heart they are related to, and therefore by measuring signals at various points on the skin, different information about cardiac function can be determined.

The first experimental ECG measurements used buckets of saline solution for electrodes. The subject's limbs were placed in the buckets and measurements taken. The lead arrangements that evolved from this practice were therefore called the "limb leads," with reference points being labeled right arm (RA), left arm (LA), right leg (RL), and left leg (LL). The placement of the electrodes on the extremities was abandoned as better electrodes and equipment became available, and standard locations on the chest were adopted for the four points.

Using LA as a positive reference point and RA as negative is the first standard lead (lead I). Lead II uses LL positive and RA negative, while lead III uses LL positive and LA negative. The three leads together form Einthoven's Triangle (Figure 2.14).

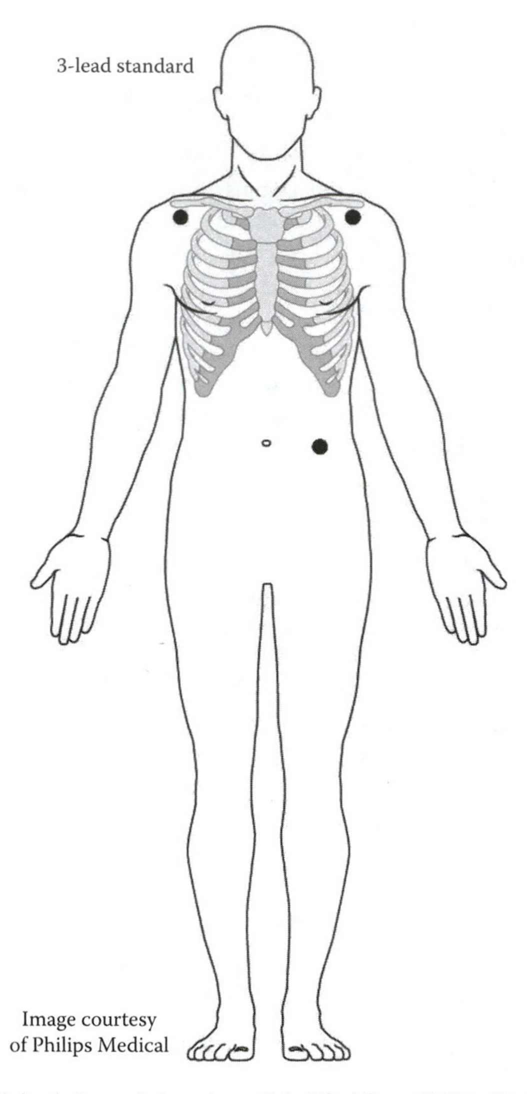

FIGURE 2.14 Limb lead electrode locations. (Modified from Philips Medical, CD provided directly, with permission. © 2006 Koninidijke Philips Electronics N.V. All rights reserved. Reproduction in whole or in part is prohibited without prior written permission of the copyright owner.)

Three additional leads were developed to give more information. These are called the augmented voltage leads, and are similar to leads I, II, and III but moved 30 degrees from each. Instead of a single negative reference point, the augmented leads use pairs of the limb leads as reference. Augmented voltage right arm (aVR) has its positive end toward the right arm and uses lead III as its negative end. aVL is left arm positive, lead II negative, and aVF is left (foot) positive, lead I negative.

These six leads (I, II, III, aVR, aVL, and aVF), use only four electrodes — RA, LA, RL, and LL (Figure 2.15).

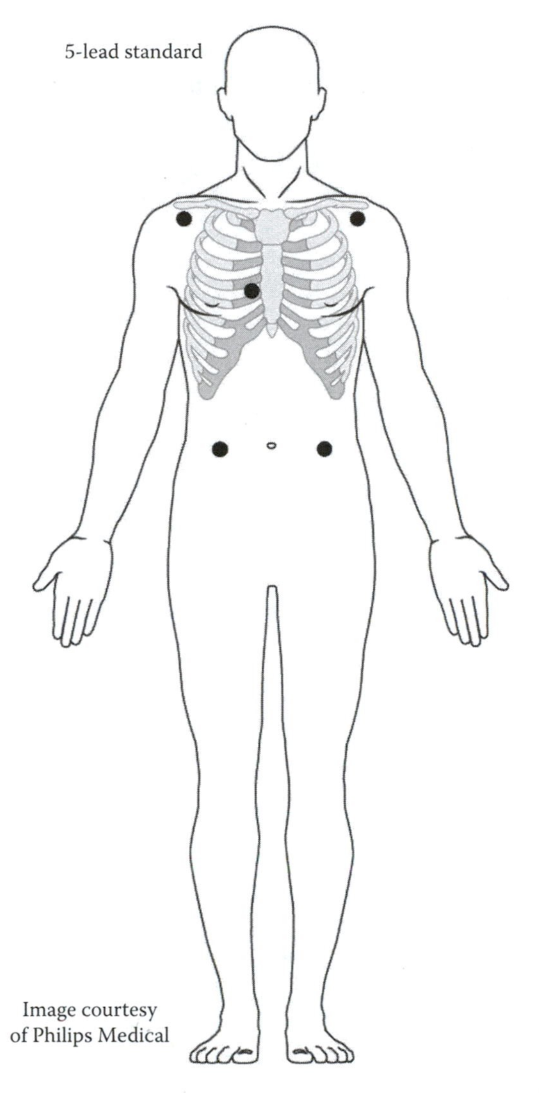

FIGURE 2.15 5-lead electrode locations. (Modified from Philips Medical, CD provided directly, with permission. © 2006 Koninidijke Philips Electronics N.V. All rights reserved. Reproduction in whole or in part is prohibited without prior written permission of the copyright owner.)

Another set of leads provided yet more information, being placed on the chest in front of the heart (precordially). These are the V leads (V1 to V6). These leads use LA, RA, and LL connected together as a reference, and require six additional electrodes.

All together this gives 12 ECG leads (using 10 electrodes), and has long been considered the ultimate in obtaining ECG information, such that a full-featured ECG machine or tracing is still referred to as a 12-lead (Figure 2.16). Typically, a "12-lead" recording measures a few seconds of ECG activity for all 12 leads simultaneously and then prints them out in a grid (see illustration).

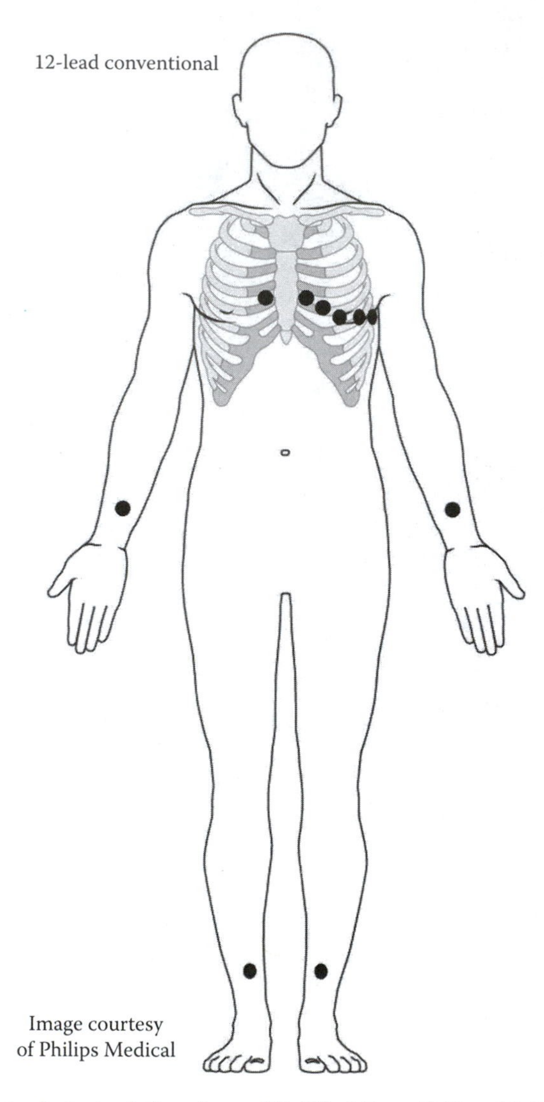

FIGURE 2.16 12-lead electrode locations. (Modified from Philips Medical, CD provided directly, with permission. © 2006 Koninidijke Philips Electronics N.V. All rights reserved. Reproduction in whole or in part is prohibited without prior written permission of the copyright owner.)

Because of their arrangements, the various leads give different characteristic ECG waveforms. For example, in leads II, III and aVF, the main P wave is positive-going, while with aVR the P wave is negative-going.

For many situations, absolute clinical accuracy is not critical, and the 10 electrodes and associated wires are inconvenient. Philips Medical (previously Agilent, previously Hewlett-Packard) developed a means of analyzing the ECG signals from only five electrodes and synthesizing the standard 12-lead information from that. Though this "EASI®" system is generally noted as not being "diagnostic quality," a

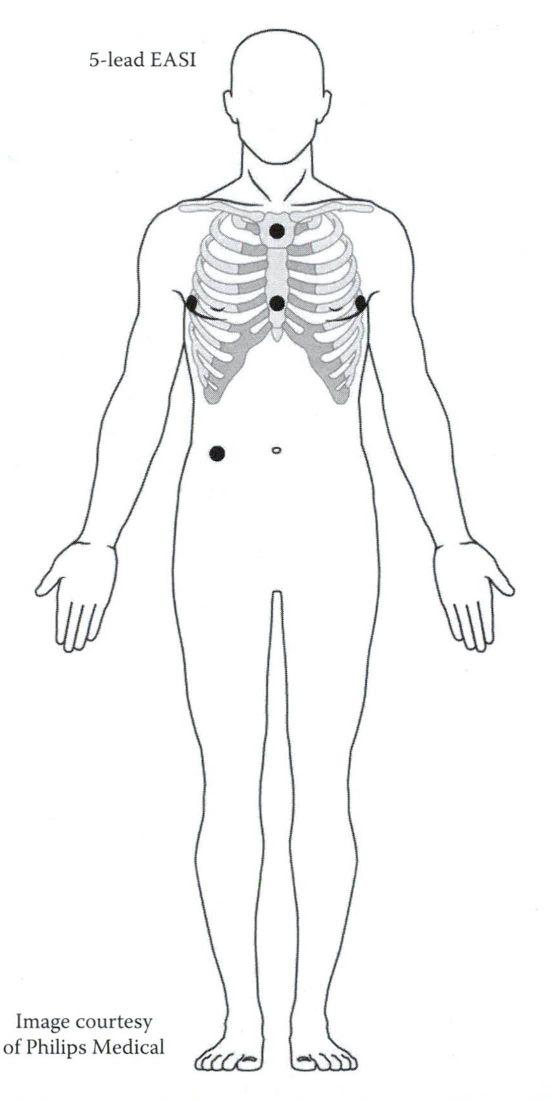

FIGURE 2.17 EASI® lead electrode locations. (Modified from Philips Medical, CD provided directly, with permission. © 2006 Koninidijke Philips Electronics N.V. All rights reserved. Reproduction in whole or in part is prohibited without prior written permission of the copyright owner.)

number of studies have found little difference in the usefulness of waveforms produced with EASI® leads as compared to traditional 12 leads (Figure 2.17).

G. Patient Isolation

ECG monitoring electrodes must make very good electrical contact with the patient in order that adequate ECG waveforms can be obtained. However, this very characteristic poses potential problems in that the electrical contact could provide a pathway for harmful external electrical currents to enter the body and then the heart, causing severe reactions or even death.

These electrical currents might originate from a faulty nonmedical electrical device such as a television, a computer, or an electric shaver, or from a fault in one of the many line-powered medical devices in hospitals, or from the normal function of some medical devices such as electrosurgery machines.

Although such fault currents are rare, especially with equipment of modern design that has been properly maintained, their consequences are so severe that safeguards must be taken.

III. DIGITAL SYSTEMS

Most ECG systems now convert the amplified ECG signal into digital form, using a digital-to-analog converter. The conversion system must have adequate conversion speed and bit depth to preserve all significant components of the ECG signal. Typical systems might use a conversion rate of 250 Hz and 10 bits, much lower than in a music system, since ECG signals have a much narrower bandwidth and smaller dynamic range than do music signals.

Once the signal is converted into digital form, it can be analyzed and stored for future reference.

A. Waveform Analysis and Measurements

Digitizing ECG signals also opens the possibility of automatic analysis by microprocessor systems. This analysis ranges from simple recognition of QRS complexes for beat counting, to the recognition of the major points in the waveform to allow both time and voltage measurements, to the recognition of abnormal waveforms (arrhythmias) and labeling or triggering alarms based on these results.

Arrhythmia analysis is discussed in more detail later in this chapter.

As an example of ECG waveform measurement and analysis, one parameter that is often measured is the time between the S and T parts of the ECG wave, referred to as ST segment analysis (Figure 2.18). This is a relatively straightforward portion of the ECG waveform to detect, and normally it is curved slightly upward and is about 80 milliseconds in duration. ST segment analysis looks at both the shape and duration of this section. If it is flat or sloping downward, or if it is at a lower level than normal, it may mean that blood flow to part of the heart muscles is restricted (cardiac ischemia). If the segment is elevated, it may indicate myocardial infarction (also called cardiac infarction or heart attack, though heart attack can describe other heart problems as well), where part of the heart muscle has necrotized (died) due to loss of blood supply.

1. Alarms

ECG system alarms are generally divided into three levels, corresponding to urgent (life threatening), urgent (non-life-threatening), and nonurgent. Different alarm tones, display colors, and system responses may be assigned to each level, usually with some degree of configurability for different situations.

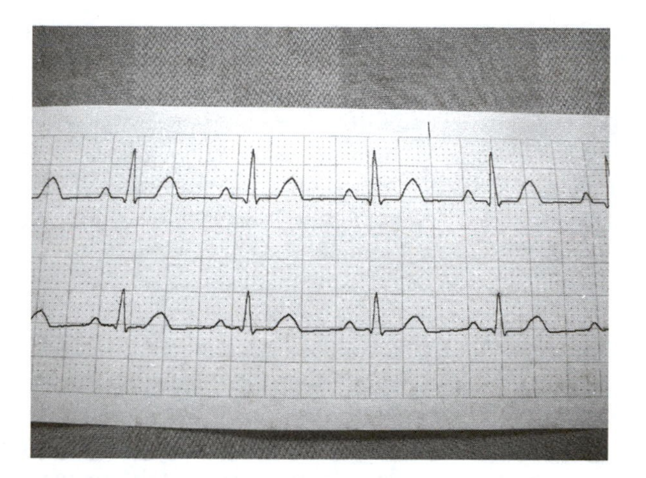

FIGURE 2.18 ECG waveform.

2. Waveform/Event Storage

Digital signals can easily be stored in electronic memory or on disks, the amount being dependent only on the storage capacity. Current ECG systems can store 72 hours or more of full-quality ECG signals. Single-lead or multilead data can be stored, though of course multileads require more storage space.

Stored signals can be retrieved later for statistical analysis, for examination by other medical staff either for diagnostic or teaching purposes, to determine the effects of medication, other treatments, or changes in the patient's condition, or for legal purposes if there is a question about the care given to the patient. Stored data may also be useful for research purposes.

Stored signals can be printed out in hard copy, either in strip form, on a sheet with many lines of tracing, or as individual beats or small sections of signal.

Digitized and stored waveforms can easily be converted into graphical or tabular forms so that trends or responses to medication can be seen more clearly.

3. Arrhythmia Analysis

Any variation from a normal ECG rhythm (or normal sinus rhythm) is called an arrhythmia. Arrhythmias range from occasional odd beats that do not affect the well-being of the patient and can be present for years, to critical patterns that, if not corrected immediately, will result in death.

Arrhythmias may simply be a normally shaped waveform that, in a patient at rest, is too fast (tachycardia) or too slow (bradycardia).

Arrhythmias can arise from a variety of causes: an imbalance in the chemicals that are involved in cardiac function, damage or interruption to the signal pathways in the heart, faults in the systems that control heart activity, or damage to the myocardium, either through inadequate blood flow (ischemia) or complete loss of blood supply to a particular area of the heart, which results in muscle tissue death (necrosis), called a cardiac infarction.

Diagnosis of arrhythmias (or more specifically, their causes) is generally made through a combination of methods. Accurate resting ECG waveforms are examined and analyzed by a cardiologist, perhaps assisted by a computer-based analyzer. Longer-term ECG records are studied (see description in this chapter). Stress-test systems take ECGs at various points in an exercise routine. Catheters may be introduced into the heart, to study cardiac output, or to inject radioopaque dyes for x-ray imaging. Cardiac ultrasound, CT, MRI, and PET scans may all provide information. Finally, analysis of blood samples can provide additional clues.

Two of the more common arrhythmias involve loss of coordinated contractions in areas of the heart, a condition called fibrillation.

In atrial fibrillation (A fib), the atria do not contract in a coordinated manner, with various sections of muscle contracting independently. This makes the heart look as if it is full of wriggling worms, and though it is disturbing to the patient and results in reduced cardiac output, it is generally not life-threatening. A fib can be chronic, presenting continuously until treated successfully, or intermittent, coming and going spontaneously, perhaps in association with sleep or exercise.

Atrial fibrillation can be reversed and the ECG returned to normal by the proper application of a pulse of electrical current, that is, defibrillation.

Ventricular fibrillation results in an almost complete cessation of blood flow from the heart, which means certain death if not immediately corrected, either by the administration of certain drugs or by the use of a defibrillator. A sharp blow to the sternum (precordial thump) can sometimes produce defibrillation as well. This technique is used to great dramatic effect on TV and in the movies.

Fibrillation and defibrillation are discussed in more detail in the section on defibrillators in Chapter 7.

There are a large number of other cardiac arrhythmias, with classifications for general types, though there are often gradations within and between types. Nomenclature is somewhat variable, though, and acronyms abound.

A full study of arrhythmias, their origin and treatment, is beyond the scope of this book; however some knowledge of the basic types is important when working with the diagnostic equipment used.

a. Types of Arrhythmias

There are a large number of different types of arrhythmias, as well as a variety of ways of describing and naming them. Some of the more common types are shown in Figure 2.19. These and some others are described here:

- Asystole: Complete cessation of any contractions; "flatline." No blood flow. Obviously critical, asystole must be treated immediately to prevent death, usually by "defibrillation," even though the heart is not fibrillating.
- Atrial fibrillation (A fib): Discussed above. Blood clots can form in the heart during atrial fibrillation, leading to an increased incidence of strokes.
- Atrial flutter: Atrial contractions are very rapid and are coordinated within the atria, but do not transfer to the ventricles, which continue to contract normally.

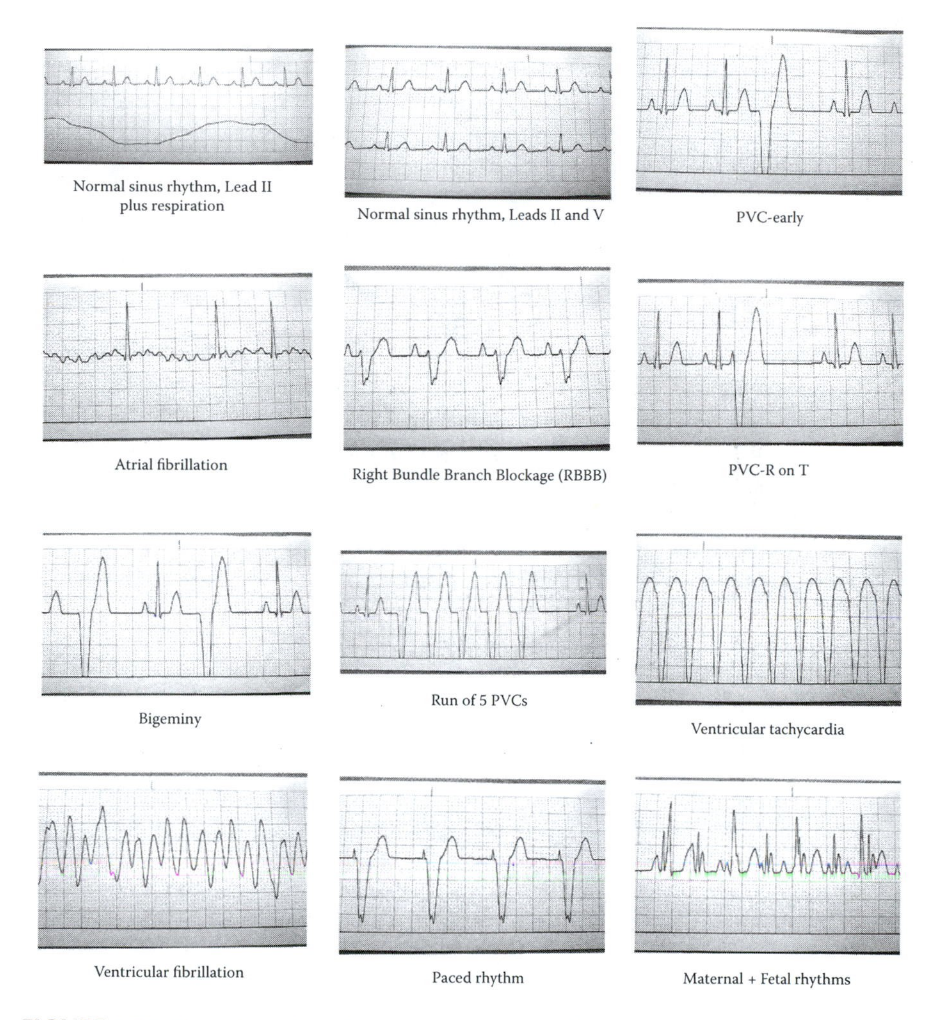

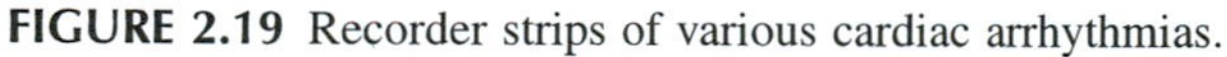

FIGURE 2.19 Recorder strips of various cardiac arrhythmias.

- Premature atrial contractions (PACs): Occasional extra contractions of the atria. These can give the patient the sensation of a missed beat, while actually the opposite is occurring. This is a very common condition, especially in younger people. It is not harmful and often disappears in time without any treatment.
- Right bundle branch block (RBBB): The right ventricle is not triggered to contract as normal (through the right bundle branch), but instead is triggered from the left ventricle contraction.
- Sinus tachycardia: A rapid, but otherwise normal, rhythm, usually as a result of exertion or stress.
- Sick sinus syndrome: An abnormality in the generation of signals from the cardiac sinus, resulting in bradycardia or sometimes alternating bradycardia and tachycardia.

- Supraventricular tachycardia (SVT): If a number of PACs occur sequentially, they can induce an increase in overall heart rate, called SVT. This is generally not serious, and while it is commonly seen in children, it usually disappears as the patient ages.
- Ventricular fibrillation (V Fib): Discussed above. This is an immediately life-threatening condition, which must be treated within minutes.
- Ventricular tachycardia (VT or V Tach): A rapid heart rate that is initiated within the ventricles, usually caused by serious heart disease. V Tach is potentially life-threatening and must be treated promptly. Usually considered as five or more consecutive PVCs.
- Premature ventricular contractions (PVCs): These extra beats originate spontaneously within the ventricles and, like PACs, can give the sensation of the heart "skipping" a beat. Also like PACs, PVCs are relatively common, especially in younger people, and often disappear with time.
- Ventricular couplet: Two PVCs, preceded and followed by normal beats. May also occur in other multiples.
- Bigeminy: Alternating normal beats and PVCs.
- Trigeminy: Two normal beats followed by a PVC, in a repeating pattern.

B. Stress Testing

Many ECG abnormalities that indicate heart disease do not show up when the patient is resting, and so systems were designed to allow monitoring while the patient exercises (Figure 2.20).

Such systems require an exercise device, usually a treadmill or stationary bicycle, an interface that allows the exercise device to be closely controlled, a controller, and an ECG monitoring and recording component (Figure 2.21).

Some systems may incorporate noninvasive blood pressure monitors or pulse oximeters, though these functions may be performed by stand-alone units.

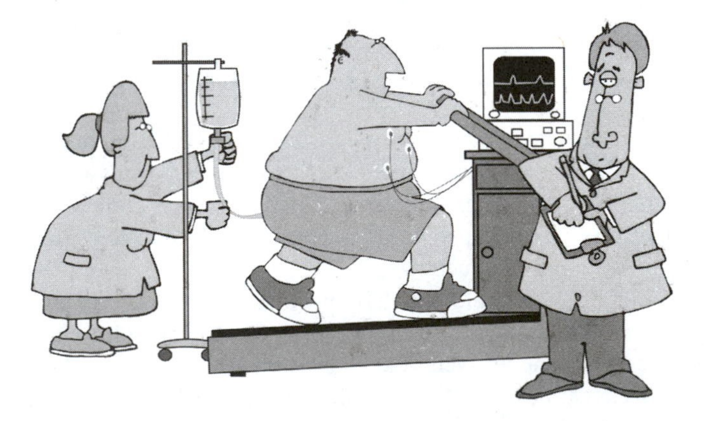

FIGURE 2.20 Back on the treadmill again. (Modified from Inmagine Corp, www.123rf.com, with permission.)

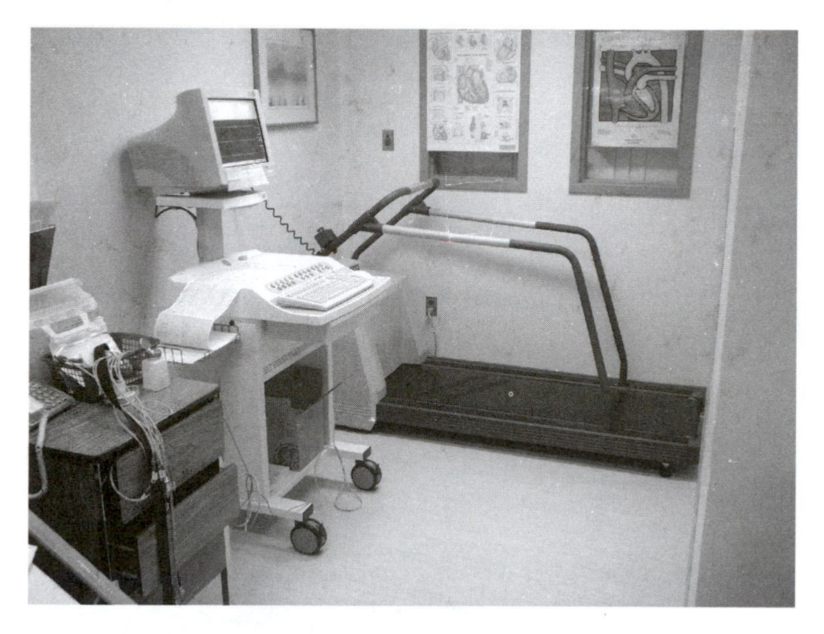

FIGURE 2.21 Stress test system.

Breathing analyzers and other metabolic measurement devices may also be used in conjunction with cardiac stress testing, or independent of it utilizing the same exercise equipment.

1. Exercise Component

This equipment must be robust and reliable enough to be used frequently, often by heavy patients. It must be capable of providing a wide range of exercise loads, and these loads must be accurate and repeatable. It must also have an accessible, easy to operate cutoff switch should the patient or staff determine that the exercise session has to end immediately. The device must stop quickly but in a controlled manner when the cutoff is activated. Finally, the device must have an interface to allow command of its operation by the controller.

Treadmills provide a better means of controlling patient effort than do bicycles, but they are bulkier and harder to stop safely. Both types must have adequate means of preventing patient falls should they lose their balance.

Treadmills (Figure 2.22) have a range of speeds, typically up to about 15 mph (25 km/h), as well as a range of elevation, from level up to about 15 degrees. Speed is controlled by varying the speed of the electric motor that drives the treadmill belt, while elevation is controlled by a smaller motor that drives a geared vertical shaft mechanism, moving the front of the treadmill up or down. Speed is measured by a tachometer, and this information is fed back to the controller; usually, the controller sends a signal to the main motor to change speeds, and when the tachometer reports that this speed has been attained, the change speed signal is cancelled. Elevation

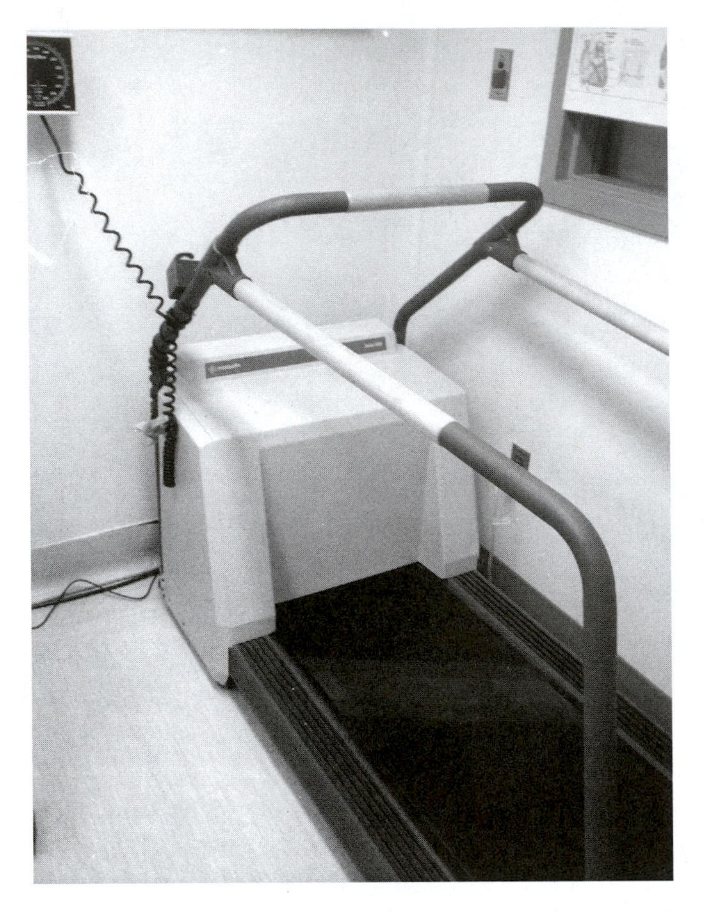

FIGURE 2.22 Stress test treadmill.

may be monitored and change requests handled in a similar manner, or a simple potentiometer may be used to determine angle.

Both speed and elevation components must have reliable safety mechanisms to prevent overactivation.

Exercise stationary bicycles may be upright or supine, and their load is usually controlled by means of a magnetic brake. As with a treadmill, speed is measured using a tachometer.

2. Interface

Signals originating in the controller are digital (D), and feedback from the exercise unit must be digital as well, but analog (A) signals are present in the exercise unit, both as control and feedback. D/A and A/D conversions may take place in the exercise unit or in the controller.

The interface between the exercise component and the controller is a shielded cable that has to be sturdy and reliable. It may carry analog or digital signals, depending on which end the conversions take place. Electric motors produce con-

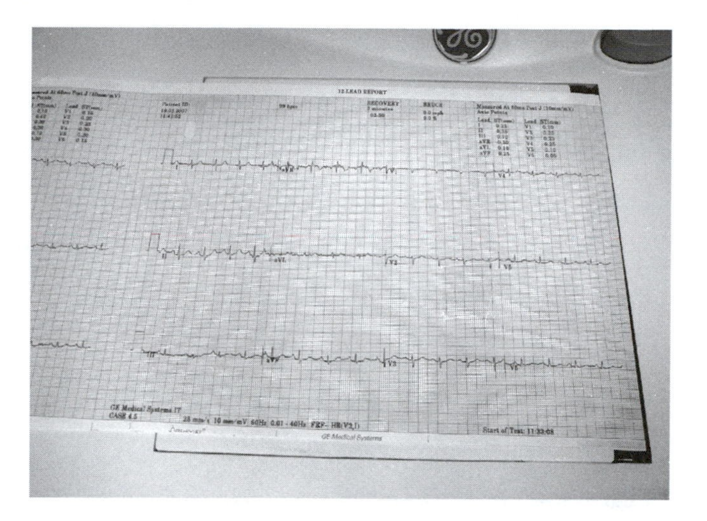

FIGURE 2.23 Bruce protocol ECG printout.

siderable electrical noise, and so both shielding and suppression components must be effective and reliable.

3. Controller

In order to get the most useful information from a cardiac stress test, the exercise program followed must bring the patient's heart rate up to certain predetermined levels for specific time intervals. These programs have been refined and defined as protocols, the most common of which is the Bruce protocol, named after its developer, Robert A. Bruce, and published in 1963. There are a number of other protocols available for use, but the Bruce protocol remains at the forefront.

The Bruce protocol involves seven steps of three minutes each. At each step, the exercise intensity is increased by increasing both speed and slope of the treadmill. The first step has the treadmill inclined slightly. The protocol is designed so that only those who are exceptionally fit can complete all seven steps. All patients are closely monitored, and when their heart rate reaches a specific level (or if problems start to become apparent), the test is ended, usually with a low intensity cool-down period (Figure 2.23).

Some other common protocols:

- **Modified Bruce:** Similar to the original Bruce protocol except the treadmill is level on the first step, and only slope, not speed, increases for the first few steps; both are increased in subsequent steps.
- **Balke or Balke-Ware:** The treadmill runs at a constant speed, and the slope is increased in very small, very close steps, so that the increase is almost linear.
- **Ellestad:** A six-stage protocol; speed is increased in five of the steps, and slope is increased in one.
- **Naughton:** A protocol with two-minute steps. Speed stays constant throughout, but slope is increased in each step.

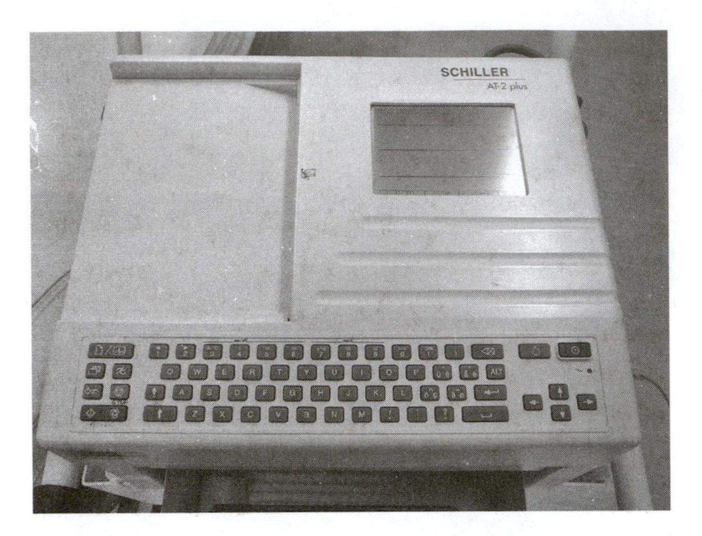

FIGURE 2.24 The recorder section of the GE Medical stress test.

Most controllers have a number of different protocols preprogrammed and can usually accommodate user-designed protocols as well. Protocol selection and treadmill override controls may be via hard keys on the front panel, or through menus on the display screen.

4. ECG Monitor

The ECG monitor of a stress test system is similar to other ECG monitors as discussed previously. A cable, usually 12 lead, attaches to electrodes on the patient. The electrodes may be somewhat different than those used for long-term monitoring. Skin sensitivity issues are not as important, but good adhesion on a moving, perspiring patient is critical. Skin preparation is just as important for obtaining a good signal as for any ECG monitoring situation, but with patient motion and the need for the best possible data, accurate electrode placement is required.

A display screen presents ECG waveforms as well as information about protocols, treadmill status, and patient information. Since target heart rates vary with age and gender, this information and more can be entered into the system and used both to help set up testing and in interpretation of results.

The system prints on a large-format chart recorder (8½ by 11-inch perforated sheets), in a variety of arrangements including 12-lead interval pages, with a few seconds of each of the twelve leads, continuous ECG, or (if so equipped) summary and analysis (Figure 2.24).

C. Ambulatory ECG Recorders/Analysis Systems

Some cardiac problems occur only occasionally, but are critical indicators of further, more serious difficulties that may develop if treatment is not initiated. Some of these initial problems can be triggered by exercise, as in cardiac stress testing, but others

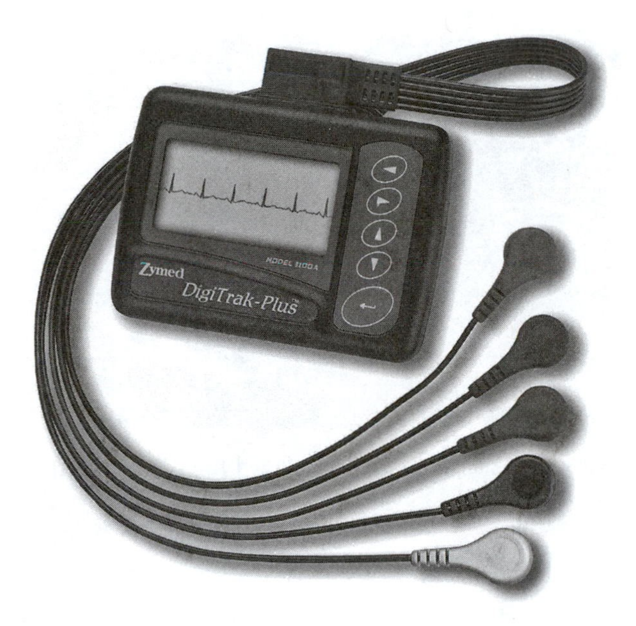

FIGURE 2.25 A modern Holter multiparameter recorder. (Modified from Philips Medical, CD provided directly, with permission. © 2006 Koninidijke Philips Electronics N.V. All rights reserved. Reproduction in whole or in part is prohibited without prior written permission of the copyright owner.)

may appear more or less randomly. If they are serious enough to require treatment, they will usually show up one or more times within a 24-hour period.

A physician in Montana, USA, named Jeff Holter developed, in 1949, a device to record ECG signals over a long time span. The unit worked, but at 75 pounds it was not something for an elderly person (or anyone, for that matter) to carry around with them for 24 hours. The 24-hour ECG recorder was named for its inventor (Figure 2.25).

The first units in use were capable of 24 hours of recording, but weight prevented them from being widely used. Advances in both electronics and battery technology allowed the units to shrink in size while expanding in capabilities.

Mid-generation recorders used standard audiocassette tapes running at a very slow speed to record the ECG signals in an analog format. Current devices digitize signals and record them in flash memory.

Most systems record two leads of information, partly to provide more complete information but also as a backup in case an electrode comes off or develops inadequate contact, or a lead wire breaks. Some record in multilead formats (Figure 2.26).

A button allows patients to insert a signal into the recording when they perceive unusual cardiac events (possible arrhythmias), and they also keep a diary that records physical activities, meal times and medication times, as well as a further indication of perceived arrhythmias.

The ECG signal is handled in much the same way as in other ECG systems, but of course no display or printout mechanism is required to be built into the recorder.

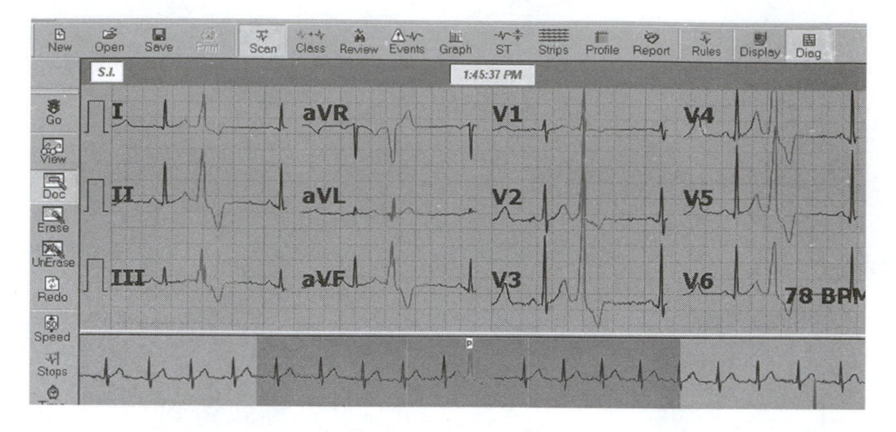

FIGURE 2.26 Multilead Holter ECG trace. (Modified from Philips Medical, CD provided directly, with permission. © 2006 Koninidijke Philips Electronics N.V. All rights reserved. Reproduction in whole or in part is prohibited without prior written permission of the copyright owner.)

When the recorder is first connected to the patient, it is also connected to a display that allows the operator to make sure an adequate signal is being picked up.

After the prescribed interval (usually 24 hours but sometimes less, and sometimes as long as 48 or 72 hours), the recorder and electrodes are removed from the patient. The recorder itself, or perhaps just the flash memory card, is then plugged into an analyzer, which copies all the data into internal memory. Data is run through a program that measures and tabulates overall and instantaneous beat rates. It also analyzes the waveforms for arrhythmias and counts the numbers of different types, highlighting them in the waveform tracing to enable staff to examine episodes in more detail (Figure 2.27). Analyzers are generally personal computers with good specifications and a card-reader interface, loaded with the analysis software.

Analysis systems include a high-resolution monitor for waveform examination and display of other data, as well as patient information, archiving parameters, and more. A printer is available for hard-copy information, and a high-capacity storage system allows archiving of information from many patients.

D. Cardiac Output

When a normal heart beats, the volume of blood pumped is predictable. Damage to any part of the heart, whether it be from ischemia, infarction, or valvular dysfunction, can cause a reduction of blood output, and measurement of this parameter can provide valuable clinical information.

There are various means of performing such measurements; until recently, the methods were invasive and uncomfortable, but newer techniques can accomplish the same goal noninvasively.

The invasive techniques involve inserting a catheter into the heart circulation (usually the pulmonary artery) and releasing a material at one point in the artery and then measuring its concentration at a point downstream. Applying a formula

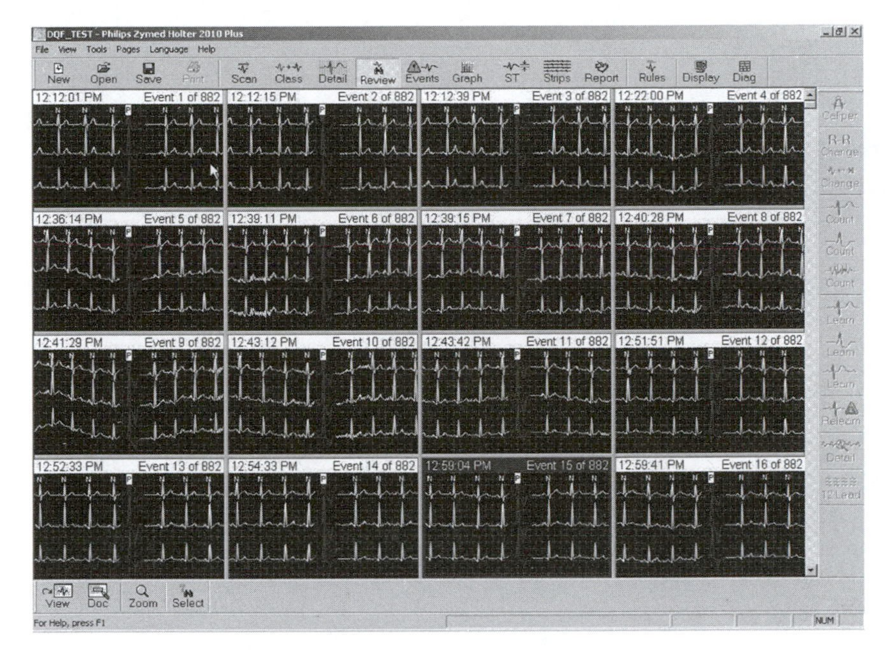

FIGURE 2.27 Sample Holter analyzer output. (Modified from Philips Medical, CD provided directly, with permission. © 2006 Koninidijke Philips Electronics N.V. All rights reserved. Reproduction in whole or in part is prohibited without prior written permission of the copyright owner.)

using the initial and final concentrations as well as the time and distance involved can yield an accurate value for cardiac output. Some systems used a dye, with an optical sensor to measure downstream concentration; others used a bolus of cold saline with a temperature sensor; still others used a radioactive isotope.

These methods all had drawbacks, primarily the discomfort for the patient and the potential for dangerous side effects. Some patients had negative reactions to the dye in use; there is a possibility of physical damage to cardiac structures; and infection at the catheter insertion site could occur.

Newer technology has made it possible to determine cardiac output accurately and noninvasively. Specialized devices using magnetic resonance imaging or ultrasound can develop images of the heart and major surrounding vessels as well as blood velocity at specific points. By calculating the area of the vessel being measure with the velocity measurement, cardiac output can be determined.

IV. CHAPTER SUMMARY

Chapter 2 includes descriptions of physiological monitors, central stations, details of cardiac function, some history of the ECG, a description of the various ECG lead systems, some discussion of digitizing ECG, arrhythmias, stress testing, Holter monitoring, and Cardiac Output testing.

3 Diagnostic Devices — Part Two

I. CIRCULATORY SYSTEM AND BLOOD

A. Introduction

Blood pressure is a vital sign that can give important information to medical staff and is thus one of the most commonly measured physical parameters.

Simply defined, blood pressure is the pressure exerted by blood on the walls of the circulatory system. Due to the structure and function of the system, pressure measurements vary both over time and from one location in the system to another.

The circulatory system is under the influence of gravity, so pressure tends to be lower in the highest parts of the body.

Due to the cyclic pumping of the heart, blood pressure varies correspondingly, with its highest (systolic) value at the point of maximal cardiac output, falling to a low (diastolic) value between contractions. A shoulder, called the dicrotic notch, occurs when the aortic valve closes. Both systolic and diastolic values, as well as the mean cycle pressure, can provide valuable information about the state of the individual.

Blood vessels have a degree of elasticity as well as mechanical resistance to flow. This means that pressure waveforms are reduced at points further away from the heart; both systolic and diastolic values are lower, as is the difference between the two. At the capillaries, pressure is almost constant.

Pressure in the venous portion of the circulatory system is also relatively constant at any given point, dropping in response to gravity at higher points in the body. Pressure must be adequate to allow blood to return to the heart.

Blood pressure in general is modified by various normal and abnormal physiological conditions.

1. Hypertension

Physical exertion increases pressure as the heart pumps harder and more rapidly in order to maintain adequate blood supply to muscles.

Various diseases, usually related to the renal system, can cause increases in blood volume, which in turn increases blood pressure (hypertension). Hypertension can also be produced by abnormal responses of the autonomic nervous system.

When deposits build up in blood vessel walls (arteriosclerosis), the vessels walls become thicker and less elastic, and the interior diameter of the vessels is reduced. Arteriosclerosis can be caused by prolonged periods of hypertension or by excess amounts of cholesterol in the blood, or a combination of these factors and others.

The changes of elasticity seen in arteriosclerosis also have an effect on blood pressure waveforms, with a greater difference between systolic and diastolic values. This, combined with the reduced blood flow resulting from narrowed arteries, means that cardiac muscle perfusion is reduced significantly, since cardiac muscle perfusion occurs mainly during diastole. This reduction in cardiac perfusion can produce angina (chest pains) and eventually lead to a heart attack.

Persistent hypertension can also cause strokes, aneurisms, and kidney failure.

2. Hypotension

Low blood pressure, or hypotension, can also be caused by faulty autonomic nervous system responses, or by blood loss. Some individuals are able to function normally with lower than "normal" blood pressure and actually may see some health benefits from this situation.

Abnormally low blood pressure leads to reduced perfusion of all organs, but most significantly the brain. Reduced cognitive function, dizziness, unconsciousness, and eventually death can result.

Some other causes of hypotension include severe infections, toxins, and hormonal imbalances.

B. Blood Pressure Measurement

1. Invasive Blood Pressure Monitors

The most accurate and timely method of measuring blood pressure is to insert a fine, saline-filled cannula (tube) into the blood vessel or structure of interest. The cannula is connected to a pressure transducer.

Alternatively, a small pressure transducer can be mounted on the tip of a catheter, which is then inserted into the target area. This provides a better response than the saline-filled cannula since the transducer is immediately at the site of the pressure being measured, but since it is a somewhat larger diameter, it cannot be used in the very small vessels that are accessible to a cannula.

In either case, the pressure transducer produces a signal that can be analyzed to provide a value for pressure. The pressure value can be given as a numeric readout, or charted on a recorder or video display. The response time of the system is faster than any significant temporal features of the actual pressure cycles, and when properly designed and calibrated, is completely adequate to represent the smallest significant amplitude features of the pressure cycle.

This technique has a number of disadvantages, however:

- It is invasive and thus somewhat difficult to set up and also uncomfortable for the patient.
- There is a possibility of infection developing at the insertion site.

- Some bleeding may occur at the site.
- A blood clot, or thrombus, may form in the vicinity of the cannula. If this breaks free it can cause a blockage in a smaller vessel. The cannula must be flushed regularly if used for an extended time, in order to reduce the formation of clots.

2. Pressure Transducers

Several different technologies can be used in the construction of a pressure transducer:

- Resistive elements, which change their impedance when under direct pressure
- Strain gauges, which change impedance when deformed
- Piezoelectric crystals, which produce an electrical potential when deformed; most medical applications use piezo transducers.

In order to provide medically useful results, pressure transducers must have adequate performance for a number of characteristics:

- Their sensitivity must be suitable for the range of pressures encountered in the human body. Sensitivity is defined as the amount of pressure change required to produce a specific amount of output variation. For example, a transducer might have a sensitivity specification of 20 mV/mm Hg, which means that, for each millimeter of mercury pressure applied, the transducer produces a potential change of 20 millivolts.
- They must have an adequate range, so that they can produce accurate outputs over the full range of pressures that they will be expected to measure.
- They must be sufficiently accurate to be able to measure the smallest pressure variations that are significant to the study.
- This accuracy must remain within specified limits over time. This factor also relates to resolution, or the smallest changes that the transducer can detect.
- Their output must be sufficiently linear over the expected range of values that accurate values can be obtained. Signals can be processed to provide linear outputs, but they must follow a smooth, mathematically predictable curve.
- Output must follow positive and negative pressure changes equally well. This parameter is called hysteresis.
- The response of the transducer must be rapid enough to capture significant fast changes in pressure.

3. Noninvasive Blood Pressure Monitors

Clinicians saw the need for an accurate, noninvasive method of measuring a patient's blood pressure.

It was known that, if a blood vessel within the arm (or other limb) was compressed, blood flow could be blocked completely. This in turn caused the pulse at the radial artery in the wrist to disappear. If the pulse and pressure were both monitored as pressure was released, the observer could detect when the pulse reappeared. This point corresponded to the systolic blood pressure.

Investigators found that, if the pressure applied was between the systolic and diastolic blood pressure, the vessel would open and close as blood pressure rose above the applied pressure and then dropped below it again. This opening and closing of the vessel produced a characteristic sound that could be detected at the brachial/cubital artery at the inner elbow using a stethoscope. When the applied pressure was above systolic or below diastolic, the vessel stayed open, and the sounds were not heard. These were named Korotkoff sounds, after one of the early researchers.

Around 1900 a technique was developed in which a cuff containing an air bladder was placed around the patient's arm just above the elbow. The cuff/bladder was connected to a manometer and to a mechanism for pumping up the pressure and then releasing it slowly (Figure 3.1). By reducing pressure slowly and noting its values when the Korotkoff sounds first started and when they ended, systolic and diastolic values could be determined.

This *auscultatory* method is still in common use, as it gives good results using inexpensive, reliable equipment. Its disadvantages are that it requires human attention, which can make frequent measurements very time consuming for staff, and that there is some variation in values obtained due to individual difference in technique.

Machines were soon developed to duplicate the technique mechanically. Systems used one of two methods to detect blood flow, though both used similar pumping and releasing mechanisms.

The first method placed a microphone at the brachial/cubital artery site, which simply picked up the Korotkoff sounds and analyzed the signals to determine systolic and diastolic values. This was more analogous to the manual method, but required precise placement of the microphone pickup. The microphone had to stay in place reliably over the time of monitoring. Microphones were sometimes external to the cuff, but more commonly built in to the cuff. Either location required wires to run from the cuff to the chassis along with the pneumatic tubes.

A more reliable and convenient method of mechanically detecting the variations in blood flow for pressure determination was developed, using the fact that pressure variations inside the arteries of the arm were transmitted to the skin, especially when constricted by a cuff. These pressure variations were also transferred into the cuff itself, and via the pneumatic tube to the inside of the device chassis. Here, the pressure variations could be measured, processed and analyzed, and used to determine systolic and diastolic values. This *oscillometric* technique provided reliable, repeatable results, which corresponded well with invasive pressure measurements. Since the technique is different from the auscultatory method, values obtained may be different, but not incorrect. Both techniques can give values slightly different from invasive measurements. Diastolic pressure is more difficult to determine than systolic, as the signals are at a lower level; this leads to greater variation in diastolic values between the various measuring techniques.

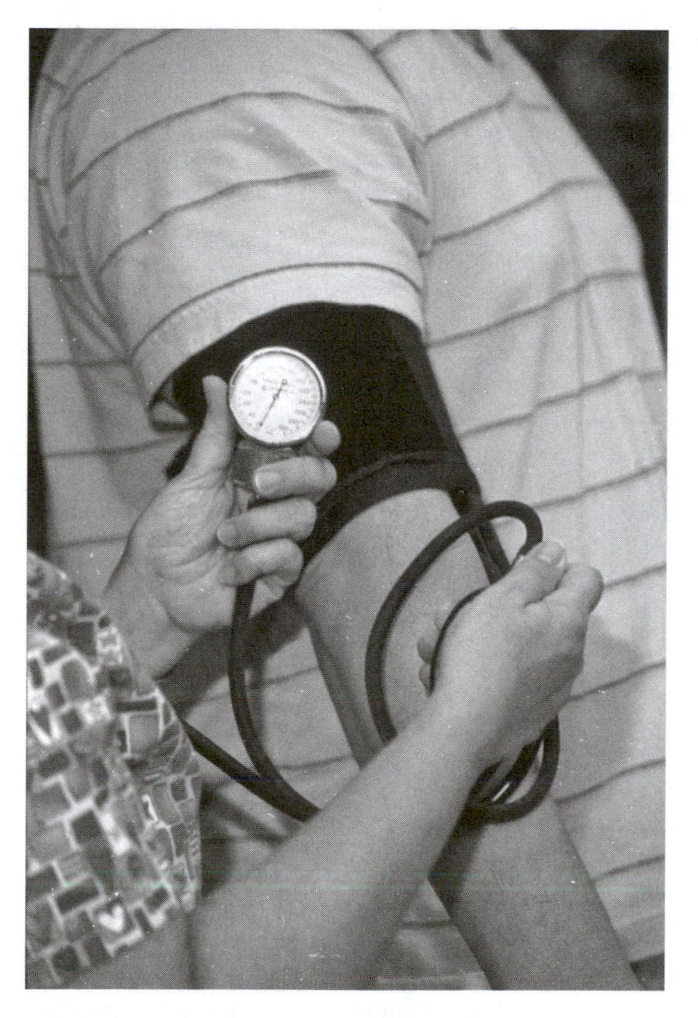

FIGURE 3.1 Blood pressure being taken manually. (Modified from Inmagine Corp, www.123rf.com, with permission.)

4. Pressure Measurement Cycle

Once placed in the correct position on the patient's limb (usually the arm, but measurements can be made on the leg), the cuff is pressurized to a specific value, which is above normal systolic. If oscillations are still detected, the pressure is increased in steps until oscillations are no longer detected. If the pressure required for this is above a threshold value, an alarm sounds and pressure is released, since there is either something wrong with the setup or the patient's blood pressure is dangerously high.

After stabilizing, pressure in the cuff is slowly released. This may be done in a linear manner, in which case the pressure value at the detection of systolic and diastolic points is assigned those values, or the pressure may be reduced in discrete steps. In the latter case, oscillations will likely start and stop at some point between steps, but an interpolation algorithm gives sufficiently accurate values.

Once the diastolic point has been passed, cuff pressure is released.

Note that, on the first measurement cycle especially, the cuff may "settle in," adjusting to the patient's arm and to the closure mechanism. This may affect measurements; therefore the second and subsequent readings taken are usually more accurate.

Systems may be set to take readings at specific intervals, or only when requested by the operator.

Alarm values may be set for systolic, diastolic, and mean readings.

Most systems are able to count pulses during the pressure measurement process and thus provide a heart rate value.

Values determined are usually displayed with separate numeric readouts or on a video screen. If a video screen in used, graphical trends may be available.

Some systems have a paper recorder that can print out values and graphs.

Noninvasive blood pressure (NIBP) units may be integrated into other devices, such as physiological monitors, defibrillators, or anesthetic machines. In these cases a shared display is used to present data.

5. Further Notes

For all blood pressure measurement systems, a formula is applied to the systolic and diastolic values to give a mean pressure value.

Also for all systems, the effect of gravity must be considered, in that standard blood pressure values are considered to be on the same horizontal plane as the heart. If the measurement site is above the heart, values will be lower; if the site is below the heart, values will be higher. The variation is about 3 to 4 mm Hg for every 5 cm change in vertical position relative to the heart.

Using the correct cuff size is important in obtaining the most accurate results. Most cuffs have either a recommended limb circumference or markings to indicate correct sizing, or both. Cuffs that are too large or too small will give incorrect readings; additionally, small cuffs will likely come undone as they are pumped up.

Systems may have a means of compensating for the maximum pressure applied. This may be adjusted depending on the previous value of systolic pressure, so that the cuff pumps up to an adequate level before readings begin.

Care must be taken when applying blood pressure cuffs to avoid a patient's arm on which other medical devices are being used, since the repeated occlusion of blood flow could affect the efficacy of the other devices. For example, intravenous therapy will be interrupted, and lines may lose patency when pressure is applied proximally to the insertion site. Pulse oximetry readings will also be altered if blood flow is blocked by the NIBP unit (Figure 3.2).

As a final note, some patients may suffer from "white coat hypertension," in that they become nervous or agitated when a doctor or nurse approaches or when undergoing any medical test. The reaction can cause an increase in blood pressure, which is usually temporary. Repeated measurements after the patient relaxes will give more realistic readings.

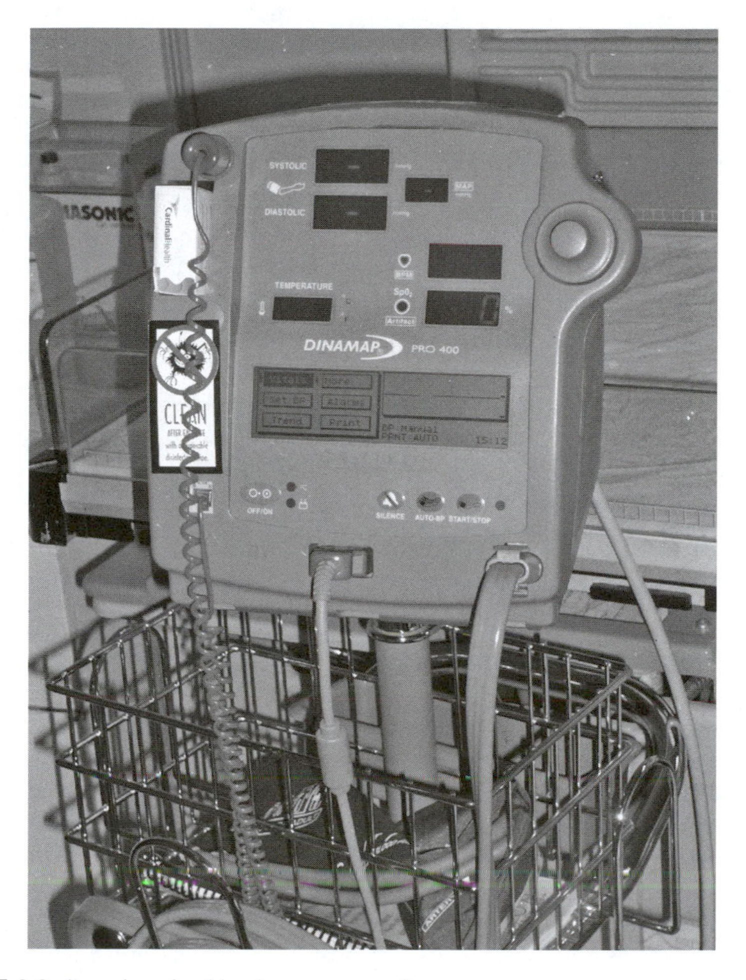

FIGURE 3.2 A noninvasive blood pressure monitor.

C. Pulse Oximeters

Traditional vital signs such as pulse, respiration, and temperature required only observation to gather information about a patient. Blood pressure was more difficult to measure, but simple mechanisms allowed reasonably accurate determinations to be made.

Another basic vital sign had to wait until sophisticated electronic equipment was available before it could be monitored effectively. While a patient may be breathing, and her heart beating, if sufficient oxygen isn't being transferred into the blood, she could be in critical medical difficulty. Skin tone may provide a small degree of insight into this parameter, but accurate values can only be obtained through blood sample analysis or by the use of a pulse oximeter.

Pulse oximetry takes advantage of the physics of hemoglobin, in that this molecule in red blood cells (Figure 3.3) absorbs specific wavelengths of light differently

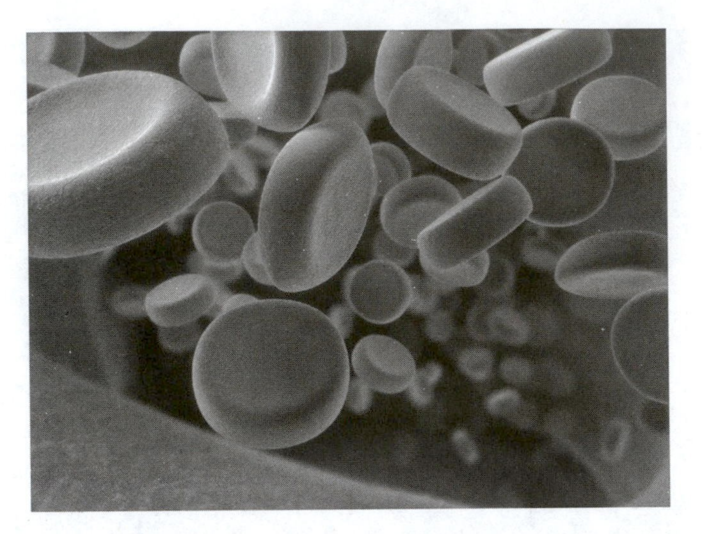

FIGURE 3.3 Red blood cells. (Modified from Inmagine Corp, www.123rf.com, with permission.)

depending on whether or not it is saturated with oxygen. The total amount of the saturated form of hemoglobin (oxyhemoglobin) compared to the nonsaturated form (hemoglobin) gives an indication of the effectiveness of ventilation and gas exchange in the lungs.

Two precise beams of light are used, with wavelengths of 650 nm (red) and 805 nm to 940 nm (infrared), as determined by lab experimentation. Oxyhemoglobin absorbs less red light than does hemoglobin, but it absorbs more infrared light than its unoxygenated counterpart.

By passing beams of both red and infrared light through an area of good blood flow (perfusion) but minimal thickness, such as a fingertip (Figure 3.4) or ear lobe — or toe or heel, especially in infants or neonates — and measuring how much light is received by a sensor on the other side, absorbance values can be measured.

By analyzing these signals with a computer algorithm that adjusts for calibration constants, nonlinearity, and other factors, a numeric value for oxygen concentration can be obtained. This value is shown as a percentage of maximum oxygen saturation.

Various factors can reduce the accuracy of oxygen saturation measurement:

- Some nail polishes absorb the two wavelengths differentially, introducing errors — sensors should not be used on fingers having nail polish, especially blue, green, or black (Figure 3.5).
- Carbon monoxide binds to hemoglobin, and can produce false readings.
- Some toxins or disease conditions can alter normal hemoglobin, producing methemoglobin, which greatly degrades pulse oximetry performance.
- Low perfusion reduces the accuracy of measurements; sensors should always be placed in areas of good perfusion. (Some units give a measure of perfusion, which in itself can be useful diagnostically).

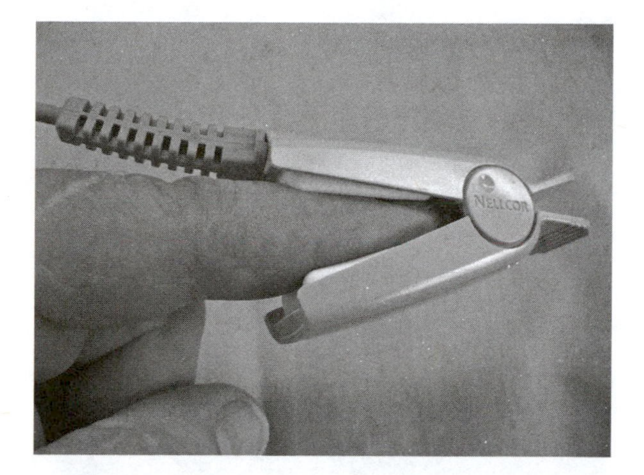

FIGURE 3.4 A pulse oximeter sensor in place on a finger.

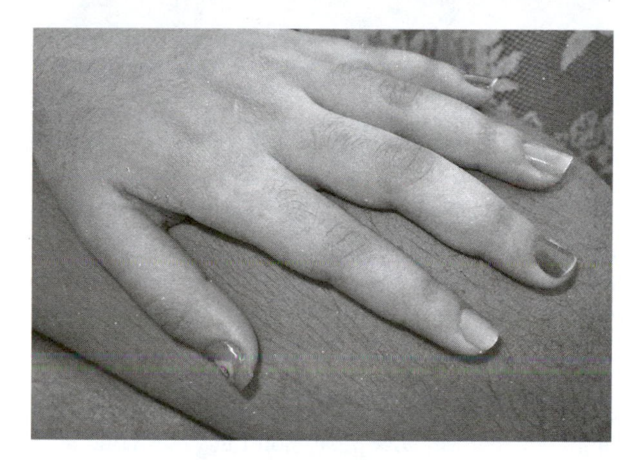

FIGURE 3.5 Fingernail polish can interfere with pulse oximeter measurements.

- Some medical dyes such as methylene blue can temporarily reduce displayed saturation values, without affecting actual values.
- High levels of ambient light can affect readings.

Most current pulse oximeters are accurate to within 1 or 2% at higher saturation levels, when compared to measurements made by drawing blood samples and measuring directly. At lower saturation levels, accuracy declines, but when patients are in such conditions they are usually being monitored very closely, and saturation is determined by direct blood sampling. Some systems display a value or a bar graph to indicate relative perfusion.

Some newer systems, such as those from the Masimo Corporation, use sophisticated algorithms to reduce noise interference and improve accuracy at low perfusion levels.

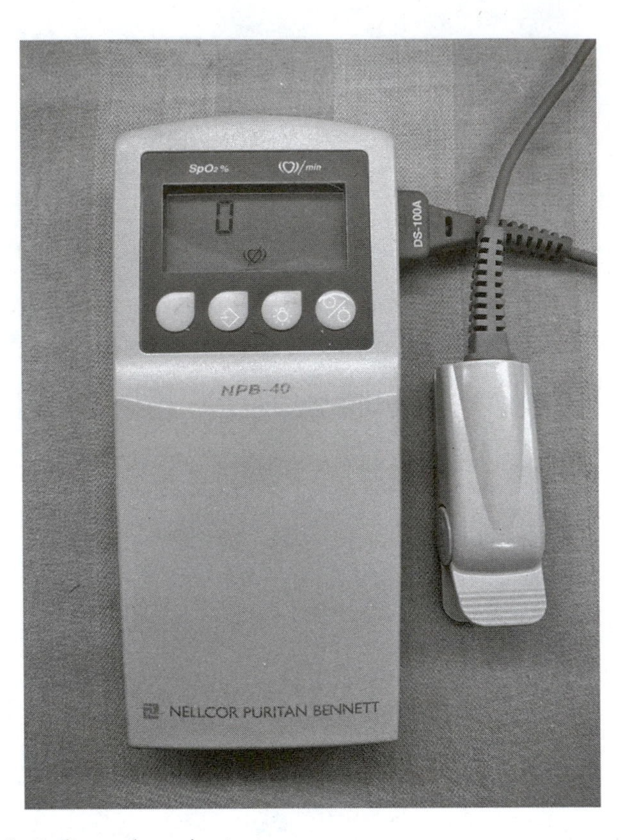

FIGURE 3.6 A modern pulse oximeter.

Pulse oximeters (Figure 3.6) may be small, handheld portable units, larger bench or pole-mounted devices, or they may be integrated into other devices such as physiological monitors, defibrillators, fetal monitors, anesthetic machines, or telemetry transmitters. The integrated oximetry circuitry may be proprietary to the main equipment manufacturer, or it may be licensed from another specialist manufacturer.

The pulsatile nature of blood flow through the oximetry monitoring site means that the absorption/transmission of the light beams will vary slightly over the cardiac cycle. At diastole, there will be more blood in the area, and less at diastole, so the instantaneous values of light intensity will approximately follow the blood pressure curve. This allows a pulse frequency value to be determined, and in systems so capable, a pulse waveform (plethysmograph) can be displayed. Typically, the displayed waveform amplitude is automatically adjusted to full scale, which means that it doesn't itself provide information about perfusion levels.

Various types of pulse oximetry sensors are available (Figure 3.7). In shorter-term monitoring situations, a finger-, toe-, or ear-clip unit is used, which is spring-loaded and can be applied and removed easily. For longer-term monitoring, or when the patient is too small for the normal clip type sensors, flexible wrap-around sensors can be used, held in place with an adhesive strip. Some manufacturers provide

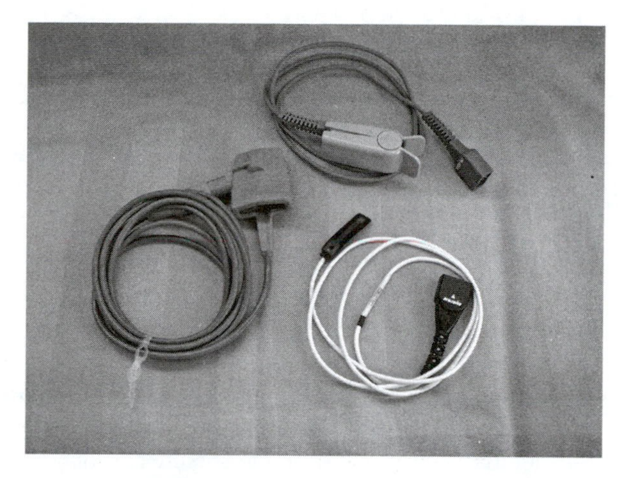

FIGURE 3.7 A variety of pulse oximeter sensors.

disposable sensors, intended for single-patient use, to help avoid the possibility of cross-contamination.

D. Transcutaneous CO_2 Analyzers

Blood oxygen levels can sometimes be normal, while inadequate carbon dioxide removal leads to elevated levels of that gas in the blood. This *hypercapnia* can cause acidosis, tachycardia, or even coma leading to death.

In order to monitor CO_2 levels in the blood, the patient's skin must be heated when in contact with an electrode. Heat increases perfusion and also increases the permeability of the skin, allowing some of the CO_2 in the blood to diffuse out through the skin. The electrode consists of an electrolyte-filled cell with a membrane covering. The membrane allows the CO_2 from the skin to enter the electrode cell, where chemical reactions with the electrolytes produce a voltage potential proportional to blood CO_2 concentration. This signal is processed to provide a numerical value, which can then be displayed and recorded.

E. Blood Chemistry Analyzers

Determining the balance of various chemicals in the blood is critical for both diagnosis and determining courses of treatment. Because imbalances can either cause or be a symptom of life-threatening medical conditions, quick and accurate analysis of blood chemistry is vital.

Most blood chemistry analysis is done by drawing a sample of the patient's blood, taking it to a laboratory, and passing it through one or more complex, computerized analyzers, and then reporting the results to staff at the patient's location. Lab analyzers are outside of the scope of this book and will not be examined.

This mode of testing requires careful documentation, special sample handling, and considerable travel, which when combined with the time taken by the analyzers, leads to significant delays between when the sample is taken and when results are reported.

A technology that is becoming more common is point-of-care (POC) blood analysis. With this type of device, much smaller samples of blood are required, and analysis is done, as the name implies, at the "point of care" — the patient's location. This means that results are obtained much more quickly. With an appropriate interface, measurement values may be able to be copied into the monitoring system being used, to form an integral part of the patient record.

Joe Biomed had just finished replacing a recorder module in the CICU central station when he noticed that staff at one of the bedsides was preparing to use their new point-of-care blood analysis unit. Since he had never seen it in operation before, Joe paused to look over the shoulder of one of the resident doctors who was also observing.

Normally, staff members could perform the test by themselves, but everyone wanted to play with the new toy, so there was a small crowd gathered around.

A nurse performed a finger-prick on the patient and drew a few drops into a capillary tube. He then transferred the blood to a small cartridge and sealed the cartridge.

"What can you measure with that one, Sam?" asked a GP who was watching the process with interest.

"This is one of the more basic ones," Sam replied, "It does sodium, potassium, hematocrit, and hemoglobin."

Sam inserted the cartridge into the analyzer, and within a few minutes, values for the four parameters appeared on the LCD screen of the analyzer (Figure 3.8).

Sam passed the unit around for everyone to take a quick look, and then pressed a few buttons to transfer the values to the patient monitor and from there to the central monitoring system. This made it available on the hospital intranet and, with proper clearance, to users from anywhere in the world through the Internet.

Sam removed the cartridge from the analyzer and disposed of it safely, and the test was complete.

Point-of-care analyzers have different features and technologies depending on manufacturer, and a wide range of parameters can be analyzed. An example of parameters available is given in Table 3.1.

As with any device used to determine treatment, accuracy of point-of-care analyzers is critical. This means that calibrations and cross-checks must be performed and documented as per manufacturer recommendations.

With such tools, clinicians can obtain vital information about their patient's condition quickly, allowing them to initiate or adjust treatments in a timely manner.

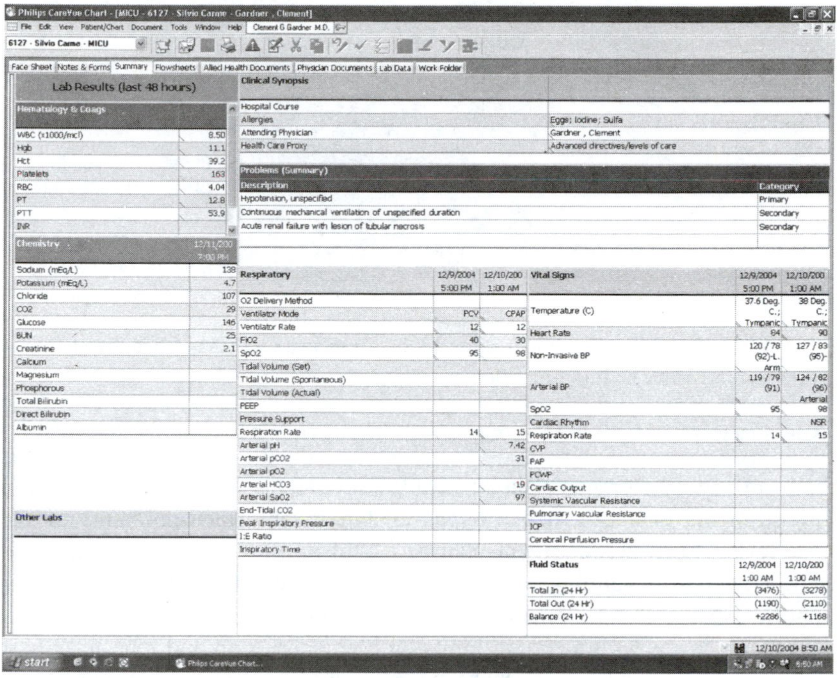

Philips CareVue Chart - [MICU - 6127 - Silvio Carme - Gardner , Clement]
File Edit View Patient/Chart Document Tools Window Help Clement G Gardner M.D.
6127 - Silvio Carme - MICU
Face Sheet | Notes & Forms | Summary | Flowsheets | Allied Health Documents | Physician Documents | Lab Data | Work Folder

Lab Results (last 48 hours)

Hematology & Coags	
WBC (x1000/mcl)	8.50
Hgb	11.1
Hct	39.2
Platelets	163
RBC	4.04
PT	12.8
PTT	53.9
INR	

Chemistry	12/11/200 7:00 PM
Sodium (mEq/L)	138
Potassium (mEq/L)	4.7
Chloride	107
CO2	29
Glucose	146
BUN	25
Creatinine	2.1
Calcium	
Magnesium	
Phosphorous	
Total Bilirubin	
Direct Bilirubin	
Albumin	

Other Labs

Clinical Synopsis	
Hospital Course	
Allergies	Eggs; Iodine; Sulfa
Attending Physician	Gardner , Clement
Health Care Proxy	Advanced directives/levels of care

Problems (Summary)

Description	Category
Hypotension, unspecified	Primary
Continuous mechanical ventilation of unspecified duration	Secondary
Acute renal failure with lesion of tubular necrosis	Secondary

Respiratory	12/9/2004 5:00 PM	12/10/200 1:00 AM
O2 Delivery Method		
Ventilator Mode	PCV	CPAP
Ventilator Rate	12	12
FiO2	40	30
SpO2	95	98
Tidal Volume (Set)		
Tidal Volume (Spontaneous)		
Tidal Volume (Actual)		
PEEP		
Pressure Support		
Respiration Rate	14	15
Arterial pH		7.42
Arterial pCO2		31
Arterial pO2		
Arterial HCO3		19
Arterial SaO2		97
End-Tidal CO2		
Peak Inspiratory Pressure		
I:E Ratio		
Inspiratory Time		

Vital Signs	12/9/2004 5:00 PM	12/10/200 1:00 AM
Temperature (C)	37.6 Deg. C.; Tympanic	38 Deg. C.; Tympanic
Heart Rate	84	90
Non-Invasive BP	120 / 78 (92)-L. Arm	127 / 83 (95)-
Arterial BP	119 / 79 (91)	124 / 82 (96) Arterial
SpO2	95	98
Cardiac Rhythm		NSR
Respiration Rate	14	15
CVP		
PAP		
PCWP		
Cardiac Output		
Systemic Vascular Resistance		
Pulmonary Vascular Resistance		
ICP		
Cerebral Perfusion Pressure		

Fluid Status	12/9/2004 1:00 AM	12/10/200 1:00 AM
Total In (24 Hr)	(3476)	(3278)
Total Out (24 Hr)	(1190)	(2110)
Balance (24 Hr)	+2286	+1168

12/10/2004 8:50 AM
start Philips CareVue Chart... 8:50 AM

FIGURE 3.8 Screen shot showing blood chemistry results.

TABLE 3.1

CHEM8+	pH
BNP	PCO2
CK-MB	PO2
Troponin I	TCO2**
Creatinine	HCO3*
Urea Nitrogen (BUN)	BEecf*
Glucose (Glu)	sO2*
Chloride (Cl)	Lactate
Sodium (Na)	Anion Gap*
Potassium (K)	ACT (Celite)®
Ionized Calcium (iCa)	ACT (Kaolin)
Hematocrit (Hct)	PT/INR
Hemoglobin (Hgb)*	

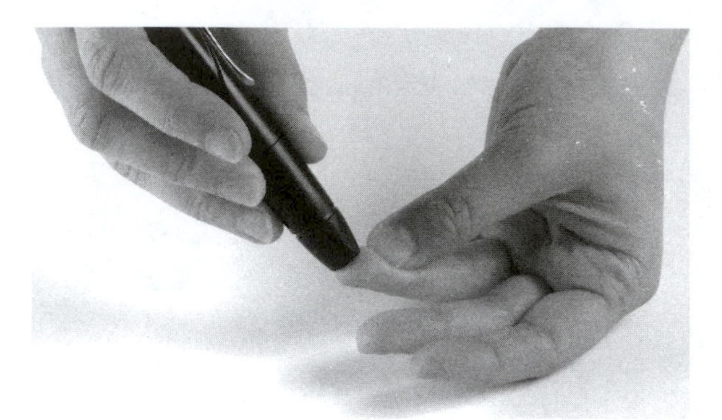

FIGURE 3.9 A stylet being used to draw blood from a finger. (Modified from Inmagine Corp, www.123rf.com, with permission.)

F. Glucometers

Diabetes in various forms is a major health issue, and a large part of successfully dealing with the condition depends on regular, reliable measurements of blood glucose levels. Such measurements can be useful in other situations than diabetes as well, but the overwhelming majority of such tests are done with diabetic patients.

The well-being of diabetic patients is greatly enhanced if they can maintain their blood glucose levels within certain limits on both short-term and long-term bases.

Laboratory and point-of-care analyzers can measure blood glucose, but of course this is inconvenient for patients, especially if they need to perform tests several times a day. Such tests also involve the time of healthcare professionals and are quite expensive.

To deal with this situation, small, handheld glucometers were developed. These units can easily be operated by patients or family members and provide quick, accurate results.

A typical glucometer "kit" consists of:

- A set of clean stylets, use to puncture the skin (Figure 3.9). Most stylets are spring-loaded and are designed to provide an optimum skin puncture, neither too shallow nor too deep, with maximum ease of use.
- A set of test strips, onto which a droplet of blood is placed. The blood sample reacts with chemicals in the strip for a specific time, and then the strip is inserted into the reader.
- A calibration strip for each batch of test strips. These are used regularly to ensure that the reader is calibrated internally and adjusted to the specifics of the batch of test strips that it came with.
- A strip reader, which takes the test strips that have been exposed to blood and performs measurements in order to produce a display of blood glucose level. The reader may also have a timer to prompt the user to insert the strip after the correct reaction time has passed (Figure 3.10).

Blood glucose levels are measured in milligrams of glucose per deciliter of blood (mg/dl; used mainly in the United States) or millimoles per liter (mmol/l; used in

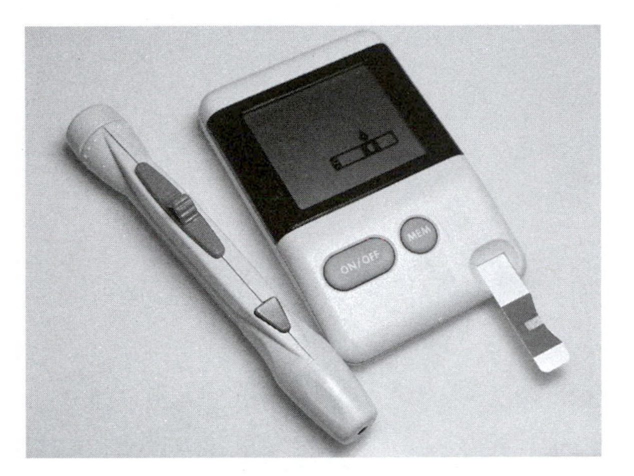

FIGURE 3.10 A typical home glucometer. (Modified from Inmagine Corp, www.123rf.com, with permission.)

most other countries, including Canada). The two different standards mean the great care must be taken with new or unfamiliar glucometers to be sure the user knows which units are in use.

To convert from mg/dl to mmol/l, readings are multiplied by 0.0555. For example, 100 mg/dl equals 5.55 mmol/l. To perform the reverse calculation, multiply by 18.02.

Glucometers may have extra functions such as storage of recent readings, or a "diary" function to allow patients to note when insulin was taken and/or when meals were eaten. They may provide an alarm to remind patients to test at specific times of day or at a specific time after meals. Some glucometers may be able to communicate with equipment such as computers or PDAs, and some may interface with insulin pumps, so that insulin administration can be triggered when blood glucose levels rise above a set level.

Normal blood glucose levels can fluctuate considerably, depending on when and what the subject has eaten, when and how much exercise has been done, and the time of day. To obtain some kind of standard measurement, patients are asked to avoid food and drinks other than water for a specific time, usually 8 to 13 hours. This allows levels to stabilize before measurements are taken.

Normal fasting blood glucose levels are below 110 mg/dl or 6.105 mmol/l. If fasting readings are over 126 mg/dl (6.993 mmol/l), the patient is considered to be diabetic, according to the American Diabetes Association.

Low blood glucose levels (hypoglycemia) can produce symptoms such as unsteadiness, perspiration, dizziness, rapid heart rate, and confusion. Below 50 mg/dl (2.775 mmol/l) unconsciousness usually ensues, a condition called insulin shock. This occurs almost only in patients with diabetes.

High blood glucose levels (hyperglycemia) are any readings over about 180 mg/dl (9.99 mmol/l). Symptoms of hyperglycemia include excess thirst, headache, blurred vision, and fatigue. Chronic hyperglycemia can lead to impaired nerve

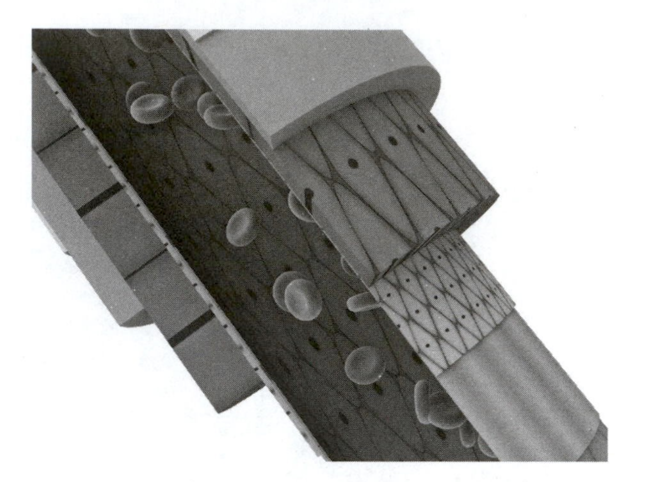

FIGURE 3.11 Blood cells moving in a vessel. (Modified from Inmagine Corp, www.123rf.com, with permission.)

function in the lower legs and feet, decreased healing ability, vision problems including possible blindness, and stomach and intestinal malfunctions.

Most glucometers have no field-serviceable parts; if they fail to operate correctly, they must be replaced.

G. Doppler Blood Flow Detectors

Tissue health throughout the body depends on adequate blood circulation. Circulation can be impaired by various disease conditions or by trauma including surgery. If impaired circulation can be detected before damage occurs, preventive measures can be taken.

Blood behaves like an ideal fluid in some ways, but not in others, mainly because it contains particles in the form of red blood cells (Figure 3.11). (White blood cells and others make up an insignificant portion of blood from a hydrodynamic point of view).

Particles moving in flowing blood can provide a target for ultrasound signals, in that the frequency of ultrasound waves reflected back from them is subject to the Doppler effect (see Chapter 1). This Doppler frequency shift can be detected and analyzed in such a way as to provide information about blood flow with a noninvasive technique.

Ultrasound waves can be beamed into various parts of the body and positioned in such a way that they intersect with blood moving in a target vessel. Some of the ultrasound energy is reflected by the red blood cells, the frequency is altered according to the Doppler effect, and a transducer picks up the reflected waves. By filtering out non-Doppler-shifted signals and analyzing the degree of shift, a measure of the blood flow in the target vessel can be derived.

Such Doppler blood flow detectors (Figure 3.12) may be relatively simple handheld devices that provide feedback about blood flow via sound from a speaker or headset. Moving blood produces a rushing sound, which varies with the pulsatile flow. This provides a quick means of determining if there is circulation in various parts of the body, usually the limbs. (These devices are very similar to ultrasound fetal heart detectors — see Chapter 4.)

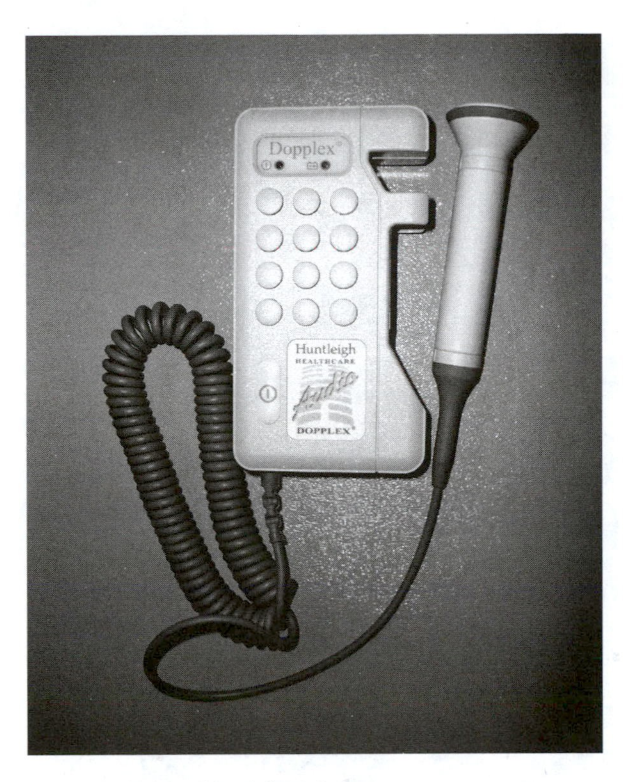

FIGURE 3.12 A simple Doppler blood flow detector.

Computerized blood flow systems (Figure 3.13) utilize the same principle as the simpler systems, but can provide quantitative and graphical data about blood flow that can be analyzed and stored, along with information about which blood vessels were being targeted, patient parameters, transducers in use, and more (Figure 3.14).

Ultrasound transducers consist of piezoelectric crystals mounted on a probe. When stimulated with an electrical signal, the crystals emit ultrasound waves. The crystals can be arranged in such a way that the beams from the different crystals intersect at a specific depth, or they may use a frequency that penetrates to a specific depth range.

Different transducers may be available for blood flow analyzers, since lower frequencies penetrate more deeply than higher frequencies.

As with all ultrasound technology, a gel is used to provide better coupling between the probe (Figure 3.15) and the patient, improving wave transmission in both directions and reducing noise.

II. RESPIRATORY SYSTEM

A. Pulmonary Function Analyzers

The respiratory cycle consists simply of breathing in and out; however there are a number of aspects to this cycle. In normal resting breathing, a relatively constant

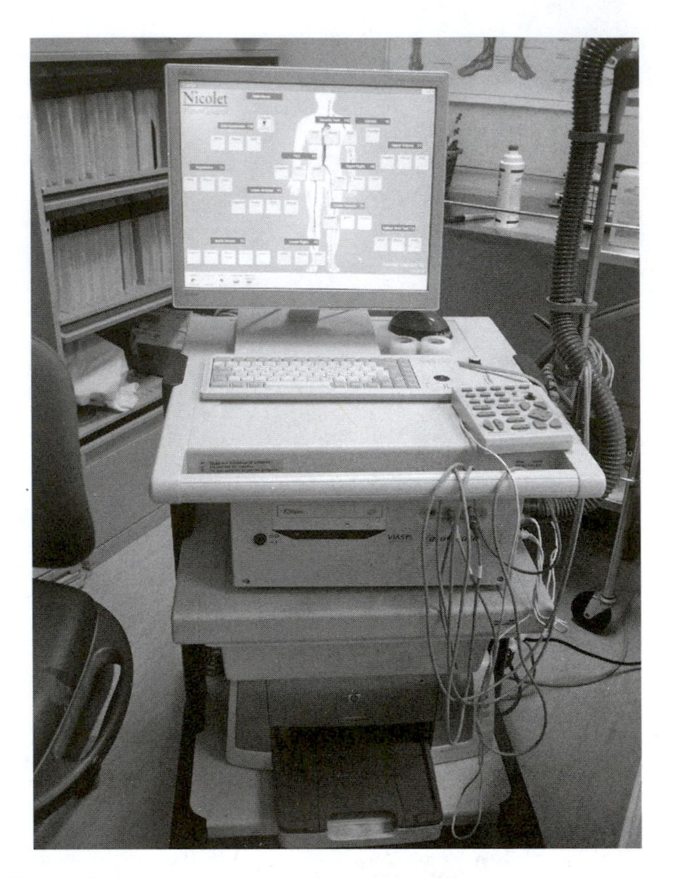

FIGURE 3.13 A full body vascular blood flow measurement system.

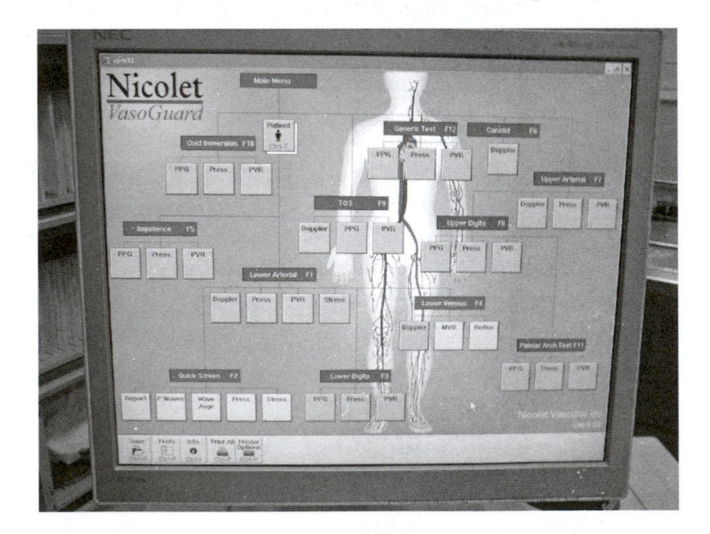

FIGURE 3.14 Vascular blood flow system screen shot.

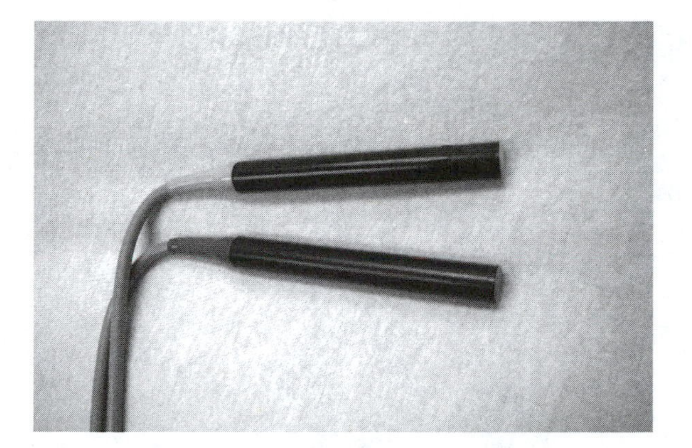

FIGURE 3.15 Two vascular blood flow probes.

volume of air is inhaled, with a consistent pattern of flow; exhalation removes the same volume, with somewhat different, but still consistent, flow patterns. An individual can take in a considerably larger breath than normal if necessary and can also exhale some of the air that normally remains in the lungs after a resting breath. Even after such a forced exhalation, there is some air remaining in the lungs that cannot be expelled (though of course, with mixing, it is not always the same air with each breath).

While simply listening to the chest may provide some important information regarding the general health of a patient's respiratory system, this doesn't provide any quantitative data, and many aspects of system function are not evaluated.

As the respiratory or pulmonary system (Figure 3.16) was studied in more detail, different parameters were noted, all of which gave important information about the patient's condition.

Some of the parameters of interest are (note that specific terms and abbreviations may vary):

- ERV — Expiratory Reserve Volume — the maximum amount of air that can be exhaled starting from the low point of the normal breathing cycle
- FEV_1 — Forced Expiratory Volume in one second — the volume of air exhaled in the first second of an FVC test
- FEV_{1}/FVC — the ratio of these two values, as a percentage
- FRC — Functional Residual Capacity — the amount of air left in the lungs at the end of normal resting breath
- FVC — Forced Vital Capacity — the maximum amount of air that can be exhaled in a single breath, with full effort
- IC — Inspiratory Capacity — the maximum volume of air that can be taken into the lungs in a full inhalation, starting from the low point of the breathing cycle; IC is equal to the tidal volume plus the inspiratory reserve volume
- IRV — Inspiratory Reserve Volume — the maximum amount of air that can be inhaled from the end-inspiratory position, starting from the high point of the breathing cycle

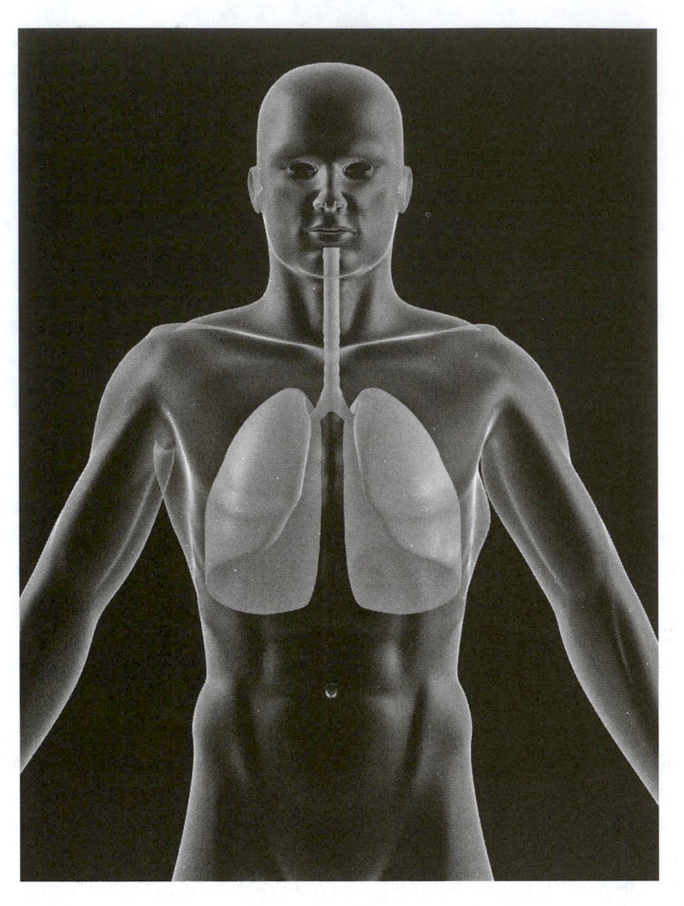

FIGURE 3.16 Human respiratory system. (Modified from Inmagine Corp, www.123rf.com, with permission.)

- MV — Minute Ventilation (also called Total Volume) — the total volume of air exhaled from the lungs per minute
- MVV — Maximum Voluntary Ventilation — maximum breathing capacity; the greatest volume of air that can be breathed per minute by voluntary effort
- RV — Residual Volume — the amount of air remaining in the lungs at the end of a maximal exhalation
- TLC — Total Lung Capacity — the amount of air contained in the lung at the end of a maximal inhalation
- VC — Vital Capacity — the volume of air that can be expelled from the lungs after a maximal inhalation; equal to inspiratory capacity plus expiratory reserve volume
- VT — Tidal Volume — the volume of gas inhaled and exhaled during one breathing cycle

Respiration or pulmonary function analyzers range from simple devices that simply measure volumes, to complex computerized systems that measure every aspect of respiration and produce charts and tables as well as providing analysis, comparisons with previous tests, archiving, and full information about each patient including medications.

1. Incentive Spirometer

The simplest devices for evaluating respiratory function are tubes containing a ball meter or vane. The patient breathes through the tube, causing a deflection in the measuring component that is proportional to breathing effort. These units are sometimes called incentive spirometers as they are often used to help patients keep up breathing exercises after surgery or recovery from some respiratory diseases.

2. Graphing Spirometer

Simple spirometers consist of a breathing tube for the patient and a bellows or piston mechanism that can move when air from the patient's breathing enters or leaves the system. The movement can be indicated by a pointer and calibrated strip, or by a pen moving against a chart recorder or drum recorder.

The spirometer graph may plot volume against time, pressure against time, or pressure against volume.

More complex spirometers may have flow transducers that can provide direct rather than calculated flow rates. Some may have digital readouts, built-in printers, or memory for storing past results.

3. Pulmonary Function Analyzer

Complete pulmonary function analyzers (Figure 3.17) utilize flow transducers similar to those in spirometers, but the data generated is handled differently. A computer system analyzes the data to provide values for most or all of the parameters described above. Values and flow and volume charts can be displayed on a video screen or printed, and there is extensive analysis and documentation for all relevant information.

Exercise equipment may be used to provide physical stress while the patient is being tested. Oxygen and carbon dioxide levels may be measured within the patient breathing circuit, and pulse oximetry may be integrated into the device.

B. Respiration Monitors

Respiration being one of the basic vital signs, it is important to be able to monitor this parameter automatically. More common mechanisms may detect the variations in impedance of the chest directly, or by placing a band with a sensor around the chest, or by having an air-flow sensor near the patient's nose or mouth. Some systems apply a magnetic field to the chest; variations in intensity of the field on the opposite side of the chest are indicative of lung volume.

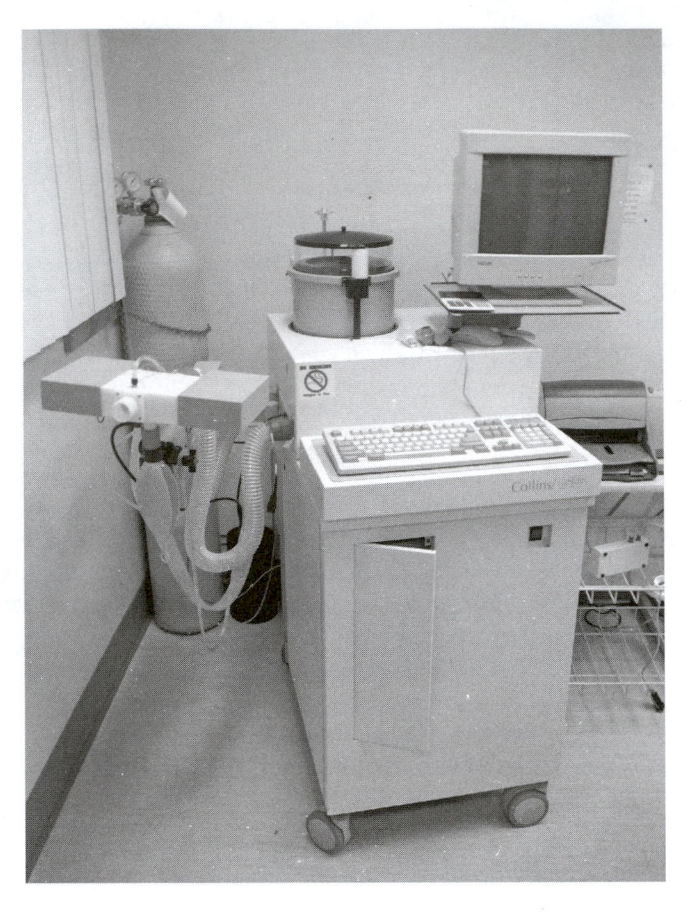

FIGURE 3.17 Pulmonary function analysis system.

ECG monitors have electrodes paced on the patient's chest already, so it is relatively easy to derive impedance-based respiration data.

In impedance pneumography, a constant electrical current is passed through the patient's chest. By measuring changes in voltage between the contact points (for example, the ECG electrodes), impedance can be inferred, with increased impedance corresponding to an increased volume of air in the lungs. These values can be analyzed to produce a respiration tracing, usually along with an ECG tracing, as well as a numeric value of breaths per minute (Figure 3.18).

C. Capnography Monitors

As described previously (see section on transcutaneous CO_2 analyzers), carbon dioxide levels can be critical in determining the state of a patient's health and in planning a course of treatment. High carbon dioxide levels are a strong indicator of hypoxia, which if left untreated, can lead to brain damage or death. Blood CO_2 measurements are important, but determining the amount of CO_2 in exhaled breaths

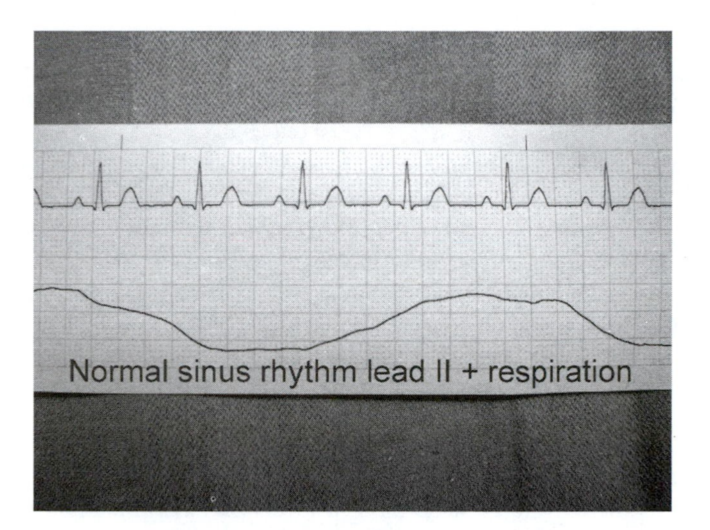

FIGURE 3.18 Respiration (and ECG) waveform.

provides additional information. Capnographs are designed to measure this parameter, and some designs use the fact that carbon dioxide absorbs certain frequencies of infrared light differently than does room air. Passing a sample of exhaled air from the patient through a sensor with an infrared emitter and receiver and then analyzing the variations in absorbance can provide accurate values of CO_2 levels.

This type of sensor requires regular user calibration, usually by placing the sensor on a closed cell that contains a known concentration of carbon dioxide (Figure 3.19). The sensor has to warm up to a certain temperature since measurements vary with temperature. Also, most such systems need to have the infrared signal modulated (turned on and off rapidly) in order to perform analysis; a motor driving a rotating shutter may be used.

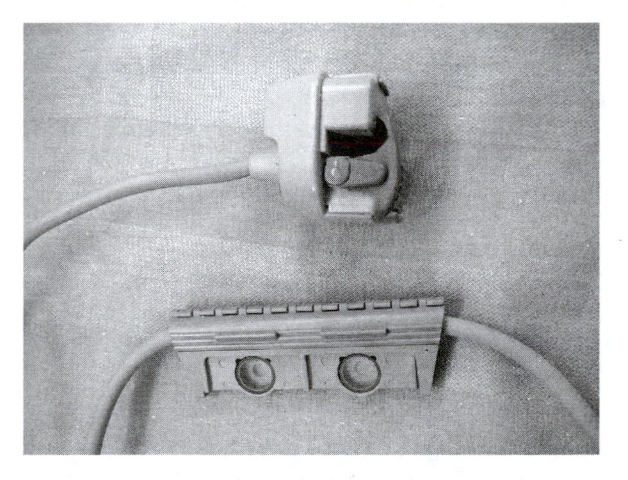

FIGURE 3.19 A capnography sensor and calibration window.

Newer sensors use spectroscopy or nanotubes coated with special chemicals for CO_2 measurements. These systems allow faster sampling with shorter (or eliminated) warm-up times and smaller sample volumes, and most alleviate the need for user calibration.

Most patients for whom capnography is beneficial will be on a ventilator, either during anesthesia or in an intensive care situation.

Some systems use a sensor mounted directly in the breathing circuit (mainstream sampling), while others draw off a sample from the circuit to an external sensor (sidestream sampling). Mainstream sampling provides more reliable results, but the sensor and attachment apparatus is more bulky that that of sidestream sampling systems.

D. Oxygen Analyzers

Although adults can tolerate high oxygen concentrations for breathing, the same is not true for infants. While elevated oxygen levels may be important in caring for neonates, if the levels are too high, blood vessel formation can be significantly altered, especially in the retina and lens. This can result in vision impairment or blindness, and so oxygen must be monitored carefully with these small patients to keep it below 40%.

Even with adults, however, oxygen concentrations close to 100% can cause problems such as pulmonary edema, reduced gas exchange in the lungs, and oxidation of some substances within the body.

Maintaining delivered oxygen levels at specific values is important in many other situations as well, since levels that are too low may not provide adequate oxygenation in patients with impaired pulmonary or circulatory function, or when undergoing anesthesia.

Oxygen analyzers (Figure 3.20) utilize a chemical reaction that occurs between certain chemicals (such as potassium hydroxide) and oxygen that produces an electrical potential. When oxygen comes in contact with the chemical in a cell with electrodes, the potential developed will be proportional to the oxygen concentration. This type of device is called an electrogalvanic fuel cell, since oxygen is consumed as the material within the cell oxidizes.

Obviously since the supply of "fuel" in the cell is limited, the chemical reaction will eventually cease, and the generated electrical potential will drop to zero. This means that cells must be kept in very well-sealed containers until they are put into use, and also that they must be replaced when depleted.

The exact potential produced within the cell will also vary somewhat over time, as the reactant in the cell is used up, so the system must be calibrated whenever a cell is replaced, and regularly while in use. Most systems will provide an indication when calibration is necessary.

Calibration consists of exposing the cell to two known concentrations of oxygen and taking voltage readings at each point. These values can then be used to adjust the compensation required to produce linear results. Room air consists of 20.95% oxygen with almost no significant variation except at high elevations. Room air can thus be used as a convenient calibration point, with the other being 100% oxygen.

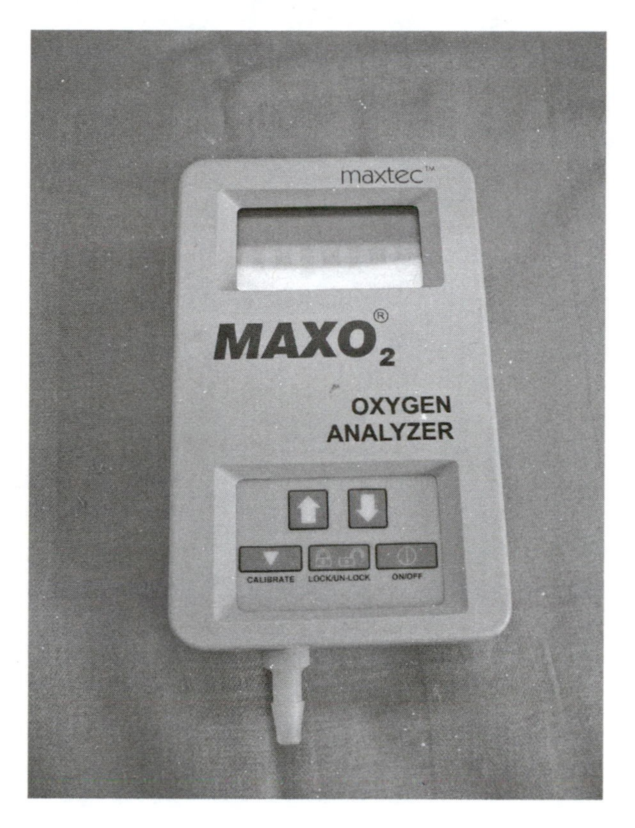

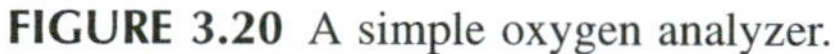
FIGURE 3.20 A simple oxygen analyzer.

E. Bronchoscopy Systems

Bronchoscopy systems allow health professionals to see within the upper part of a patient's respiratory system in order to look for damage, restrictions, or abnormal tissues. The systems consist of tubes (the actual bronchoscope) that can be inserted via the mouth or nose, past the larynx and through the epiglottis to the trachea and the left or right bronchi; a light source; a camera; one or more video monitors; possibly a video recorder and/or printer; possibly a mechanism for flushing and suctioning the area being observed; and various associated apparatus (Figure 3.21).

Bronchoscopy systems are similar in many ways to other endoscopic systems, the common components of which are described in detail in Chapter 4.

The bronchoscope tube (or "scope") has optical channels that can deliver light to the end of the scope and also send an image from the end of the scope back to the viewer. Some scopes have one or more hollow sections that can admit instruments or be used for irrigation, suction, and insufflation.

Bronchoscopes may be flexible or rigid. Flexible scopes can be made thinner and can thus reach further into the bronchial passages, but rigid scopes can allow certain instruments or lasers to be introduced through the tube to perform procedures such as biopsies, dilations, or burning of small growths.

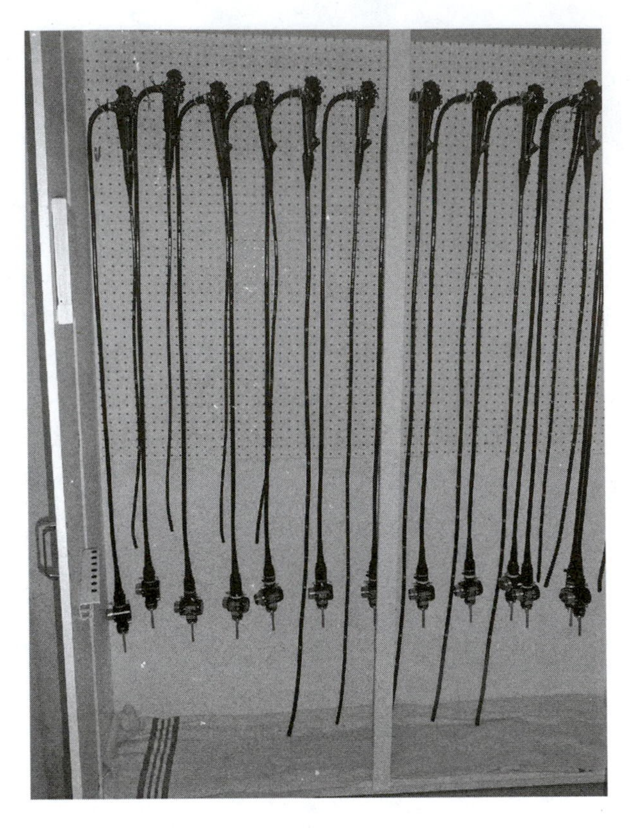

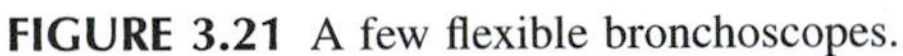

FIGURE 3.21 A few flexible bronchoscopes.

Rigid bronchoscopes are usually used only with general anesthesia and are only introduced through the mouth. Rigid scopes generally use lenses within the tube to transmit illumination and images, while flexible scopes use fiber optics.

Cracked or otherwise damaged lenses in rigid scopes and broken optical fibers in flexible scopes will reduce illumination and image quality.

Most scopes until recently have used camera sensors at the proximal end, to pick up the visual images transmitted by the fiber optic channels, but with advances in miniaturization, some newer scopes have imaging chips mounted on the distal end, which can eliminate some transmission problems, since wires can be made smaller and more flexible than optical components.

III. NERVOUS SYSTEM

Nerve signals are conducted through the body via two processes. Within nerve cells (Figure 3.22), the signal is transmitted in long cell extensions called axons. This is not as simple as an electrical signal in a wire, as the cell membrane along the axon must be polarized and then depolarized as the signal passes along. There is a time lag, or refractory period, that must pass before another signal can be handled in this way. Overall conduction speed within an axon is in the range of 50 to 200 meters

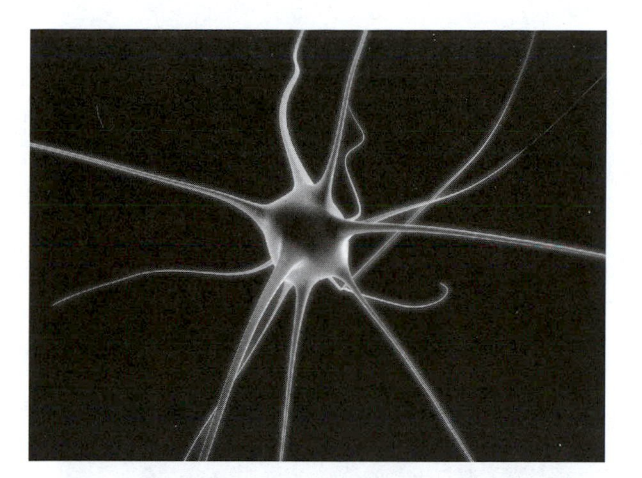

FIGURE 3.22 A neuron, or nerve cell. (Modified from Inmagine Corp, www.123rf.com, with permission.)

per second, far slower than the near-speed-of-light conduction of electrical signals in wires.

At various points within the nervous system, signals must be passed from one cell to another through a connection called a synapse. A synapse can connect two nerve cells to simply pass a signal along. Other synapses can actually inhibit signal transmission within the target axon, while some are an interface between nerve axons and muscle cells. This last type, called a neuromuscular junction, uses a chemical called acetylcholine to transmit signals. Acetylcholine must be broken down by an enzyme (acetylcholinesterase) in order for the muscle to relax.

Various drugs affect the nervous system in specific ways. Generally, they can either excite the system (agonists) or inhibit it (antagonists.) Commonly known agonists include caffeine, cocaine, ecstasy, and amphetamines. Antagonists are such drugs as alcohol, Valium, barbiturates, marijuana, and heroin and its derivatives.

Some nerve gases (e.g., sarin) as well as pesticides (e.g., DDT and parathion) inhibit the action of acetylcholinesterase. This causes muscles to remain contracted for prolonged periods in spasms, which can lead to a painful death.

Local anesthetics like procaine, xylocaine, and benzocaine act by blocking motor and sensory synapses in the area of application.

General anesthetics such as isoflurane, sevoflurane, and desflurane act by blocking ion channels in the nervous system, thus blocking pain and producing unconsciousness. Anesthetic machines are described in Chapter 7.

Various devices are used to test for the effectiveness of anesthetics, such as nerve stimulators (see the section on nerve/muscle stimulators later in this chapter) and BiSpectral Index monitors (see the section on BIS monitors later in this chapter).

A. EEG Monitors and Machines

Structural abnormalities within the brain (Figure 3.23) can cause many harmful effects, including epilepsy and other seizures, aphasia, hallucinations, and comas.

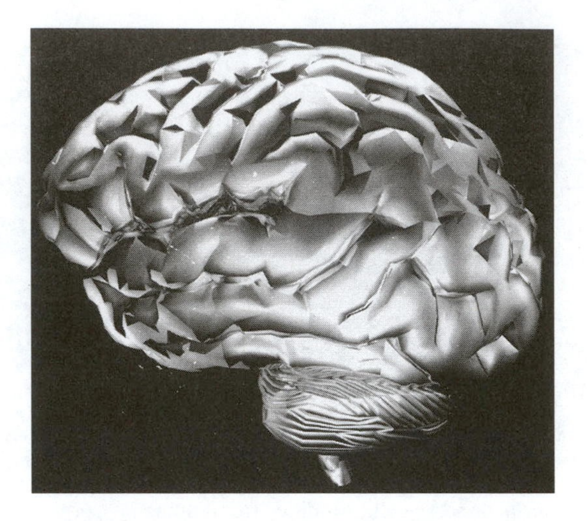

FIGURE 3.23 The human brain. (Modified from Inmagine Corp, www.123rf.com, with permission.)

Various disease processes such as tumors, Parkinson's disease, and cerebral palsy can lead to extreme difficulties for patients.

In the past, an EEG was almost the only tool available, but now diagnosing such problems can involve imaging equipment such as CT, MRI, or PET scanners (see Chapter 5). Still, measurement of the electrical activity of the brain in real time can provide information that other sources cannot, and it can also confirm or expand on the results of other tests.

An electroencephalogram (EEG) machine consists of a set of a dozen or more electrodes that are placed in specific locations on the scalp and are connected to an amplifier/digitizer/analyzer/display/recorder unit that has some similarity to ECG systems. The signals are stored and can be analyzed later and/or printed out on a recorder strip.

Some special studies use electrodes that are inserted through the skull and directly into brain tissue, allowing precise determination of the location of anomalies.

The signals recorded from brain electrical activity form recognizable waves that are divided into groups according to their characteristics.

Alpha waves range from 9 to 14 Hz and are of relatively high amplitude. They are seen in EEG records when the subject is awake but relaxed.

Beta waves are lower in amplitude than alpha waves, but higher in frequency, about 15 to 40 Hz. They indicate that the subject is aroused in some way, angry, or frightened, or closely involved in a conversation or activity.

Theta waves show a variation in amplitude, though usually greater than beta waves, at a low frequency of about 4 to 8 Hz. Theta waves correspond to periods of inattentive consciousness such as daydreaming.

Delta waves are the highest in amplitude but lowest in frequency, about 1.5 to 4 Hz. Periods of sleep show delta wave activity, with frequency corresponding to depth of sleep — deeper sleep means lower frequencies. Delta waves can be analyzed to indicate depth of unconsciousness during general anesthesia.

An absence of brain wave activity can be a legal indication of brain death in some jurisdictions.

EEG activity changes in characteristic ways when various stimuli are applied to the subject, such as flashing and/or colored lights or various sounds. Abnormal responses to these stimuli can indicate various brain abnormalities.

Also, in studying epilepsy, it is sometimes useful to be able to induce seizures under controlled conditions. This is often done using flashing lights of controlled frequency (usually around 16 to 25 Hz) and intensity. Only about 5% of patients with epilepsy have such photosensitivity.

It has been found that subjects can learn to control some aspects of their brain waves, by using biofeedback training. This can be useful in stress or pain reduction and in focusing concentration. Some experiments have found that subjects can control external devices by altering their brain waves in a particular manner, with suitable analysis and interface circuitry.

B. BIS Monitors

A special application of EEG technology allows clinicians to evaluate the depth of unconsciousness of patients. This can be useful during general anesthesia or when patients are being kept in an induced coma.

Under general anesthesia, if the level of consciousness is too high, patients can experience awareness during surgery, which can be very distressing. If the level is too low, recovery from the anesthetic can be prolonged, or in extreme cases physiological damage can occur.

Comas may be induced to help keep a patient immobile when recovering from various traumas, and as with general anesthesia, a balance must be struck between too high and too low depths of unconsciousness.

A BiSpectral index monitor (BIS) takes EEG signals from a few specifically placed EEG electrodes and analyzes them with a complex algorithm to produce a “BIS” value, a unitless number that corresponds to level of consciousness. A BIS value of zero would correspond to brain death, while a value of 100 corresponds to full consciousness and awareness.

C. Muscle/Nerve Stimulators

Under certain circumstances it is necessary to greatly relax or paralyze a patient’s muscles. During surgical procedures when electrosurgery machines (ESUs) are in use, the signals produced by the ESU action could cause muscle contractions in various areas of the body. Also, some surgeries involving muscles are much easier when the muscles being worked on are relaxed. Patients on ventilators may fight the action of the machine if their breathing muscles are active. Finally, when electroconvulsive therapy (see Chapter 7) is being administered, the ECT pulse can cause extreme contractions in many muscle groups, which can result in injuries to patient or staff.

As described earlier in this chapter, nerve signals are transmitted to muscles across the neuromuscular junction via acetylcholine. Muscle-relaxing agents actually block the action of acetylcholine so that muscle activity is reduced. The degree of

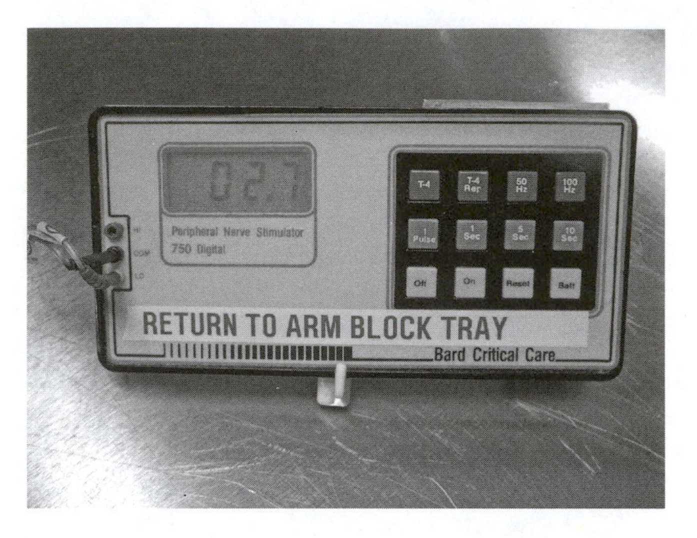

FIGURE 3.24 A nerve stimulator.

inhibition must be sufficient to prevent unwanted muscle activity, but excess dosages are to be avoided.

Nerve/muscle stimulators apply calibrated signals to a patient's skin in a convenient location near a muscle group, for example the thumb or big toe. Normally, once over a certain threshold, the signals will cause muscle contractions to a degree corresponding to the signal amplitude. Once the stimulus reaches a certain high value, muscle contraction is the greatest that is possible. By adding about 10% to this stimulus level (a supramaximal stimulus), maximal muscle contraction is ensured.

When muscle relaxants are administered to the patient, supramaximal stimuli can be delivered until such time that muscle action is reduced to a certain percentage of maximum, for example 20%. At this point, relaxant administration can be leveled or reduced in order to maintain the desired reduction in muscle response.

Nerve stimulators (Figure 3.24) can be set to deliver pulses of various amplitudes and durations and may have settings where pulses are delivered in continuous trains or in bursts of a specific number of pulses.

IV. CHAPTER SUMMARY

Chapter 3 continues descriptions of diagnostic devices, covering equipment used with the circulatory system and blood, the respiratory system, and the nervous system.

Theories of invasive and noninvasive blood pressure measurement are discussed, along with pulse oximetry, capnography, and blood glucose analysis.

The anatomy and physiology of the respiratory system is described, along with methods of analyzing these systems.

Nervous system function is examined, and EEG and BIS monitors plus nerve stimulators are described.

4 Diagnostic Devices — Part Three

I. DIGESTIVE SYSTEM

A. Endoscopes

1. General

"Endoscope" literally means "inside looking," and these systems are designed for just that. The general term "endoscope" describes any device that has a tube that can be inserted into an opening in the body, either natural or surgical, for the purpose of viewing structures inside the body (Figure 4.1). This means that they must have channels both to provide lighting and to transmit visual images back out to the user. Endoscopes may also have the capacity to supply fluids such as saline solutions for irrigating sites to provide a clearer view, suction to remove the irrigation and other fluids, an air channel for insufflation, and a channel that can allow the entry of special instruments for doing various procedures inside the body.

Newer scopes have video camera chips mounted on the distal end, which means that images are carried back along the scope as electronic signals rather than light. This results in better images and more durable scopes.

2. Types of Endoscopes

Some types of endoscopes, with their target areas and insertion points, include:

- Arthroscope — joints such as knees; surgical incision
- Bronchoscopes — trachea and upper bronchial passages; mouth or nose
- Colonoscopes — colon; anus
- Colposcope — vagina and uterus; vagina
- Cystoscope — bladder and urinary tract; urethra
- Gastroscope — esophagus, stomach and sometimes upper small intestine (duodenum); mouth
- Laparoscope — various abdominal organs; surgical incision
- Proctoscope — rectum and lower (sigmoid) colon; anus
- Sigmoidoscope — sigmoid colon; anus
- Thoracoscope — organs of the thorax, including the pleura (outer covering of the lungs) and pericardium (outer covering of the heart); surgical incision

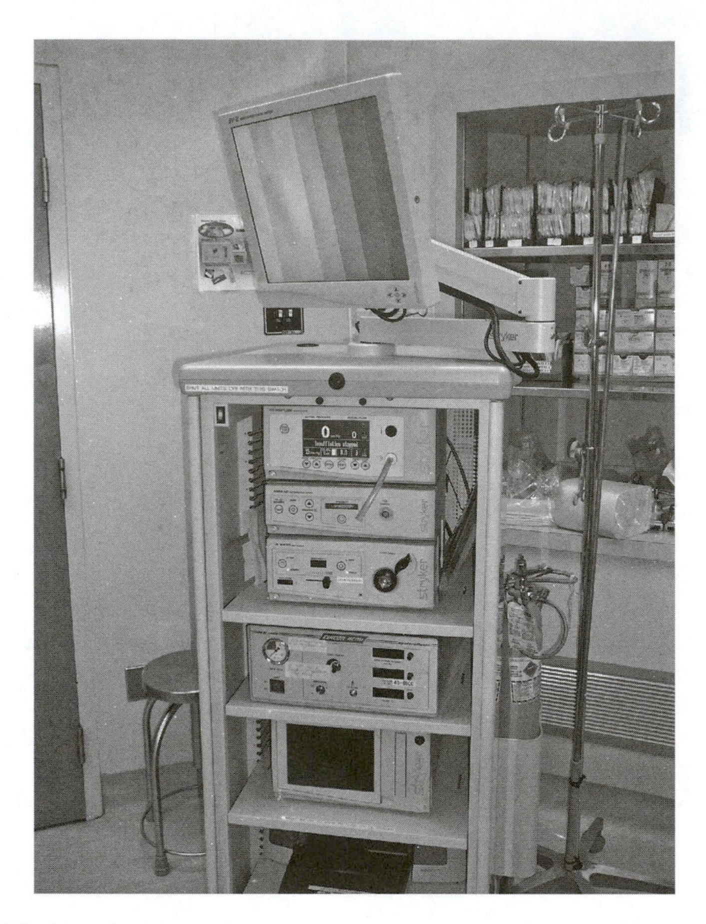

FIGURE 4.1 An endoscopy system.

Arthroscopes (see section titled "Arthroscopy Systems") and bronchoscopes (Chapter 2) are described separately.

Endoscopy is less invasive and less traumatic than exploratory surgery, and while laparoscopic procedures require one or two small incisions, these are much smaller than open abdominal or thoracic surgery; recovery times are much shorter, and the incidence of complications much lower.

Endoscopes are divided into rigid or flexible types, the difference being self-explanatory.

3. Rigid Endoscopes

Rigid endoscopes consist of a tube, usually made of stainless steel, which contains fiber optics, a series of lenses, and one or more open passages (Figure 4.2).

At the distal end of the scope, an objective lens receives light from the object and directs it into the tube. The angle at which the objective lens is set determines the viewing angle of each individual scope, from straight ahead to various angles to the side, to partially in reverse.

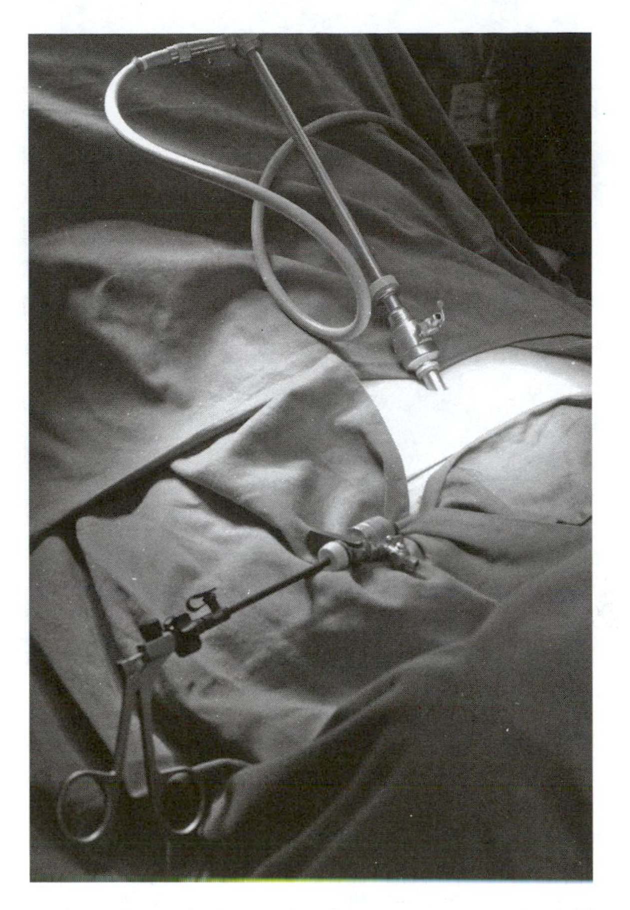

FIGURE 4.2 An endoscopic surgical procedure in progress — note the rigid scope. (Modified from Inmagine Corp, www.123rf.com, with permission.)

The other lenses, commonly referred to as the telescope, are separated by spacers. They take the light through the tube from the objective lens to the eyepiece.

Fiber optic strands are installed around the lenses to carry illumination light to the subject, and a fitting near the eyepiece allows a light cable to attach to the scope.

The open passages in the scope allow for irrigation and suction of the observation site to remove obscuring material such as blood. Also, pieces of tissue that have been cut or otherwise separated from structures such as tumors or polyps can be withdrawn for disposal or examination. The passages can also be used to fill the area around the object of observation with either clear fluid or air in order to allow a clearer view. Finally, the passages can allow the entry of special tools used for such purposes as excising tissue or cauterizing structures.

4. Flexible Endoscopes

Flexible endoscopes (Figures 4.3 through 4.5) carry both illumination and visualization light through fiber optics, which allows the flexibility in their name. Flexi-

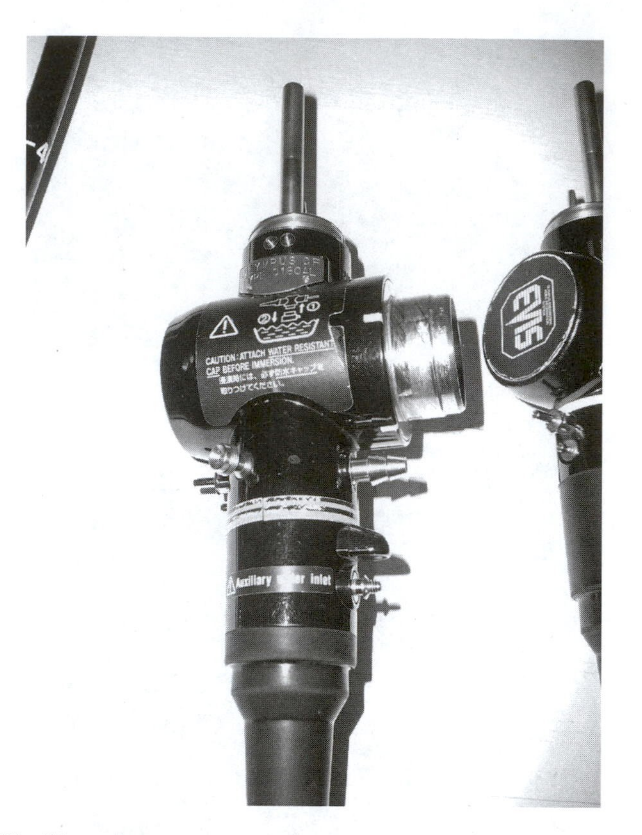

FIGURE 4.3 Flexible endoscope — connector end.

bility allows the scopes to pass around corners to reach the object of observation; it also means that flexible scopes can be much longer than rigid scopes. They generally carry markings on the outside to indicate depth of insertion. Some models have special mechanisms operated by cables that allow the operator to turn the end portion of the scope in different directions. Otherwise, flexible scope function is similar to that of rigid scopes.

Some flexible scopes mount directly onto the light source, which makes video and other connections simpler and more effective. Viewing images from such scopes is done via video monitors rather than direct eyepieces.

5. Other System Components

a. Light Source

Accurate recognition of normal and abnormal tissues during an endoscopic procedure requires bright illumination with light having a specific spectrum and color temperature. The light also must not impart any significant amount of heat to the tissues in the target area.

Most endoscopy light sources (Figure 4.6 and Figure 4.7) use quartz halogen bulbs that run in a controlled environment to avoid overheating, with accurate power

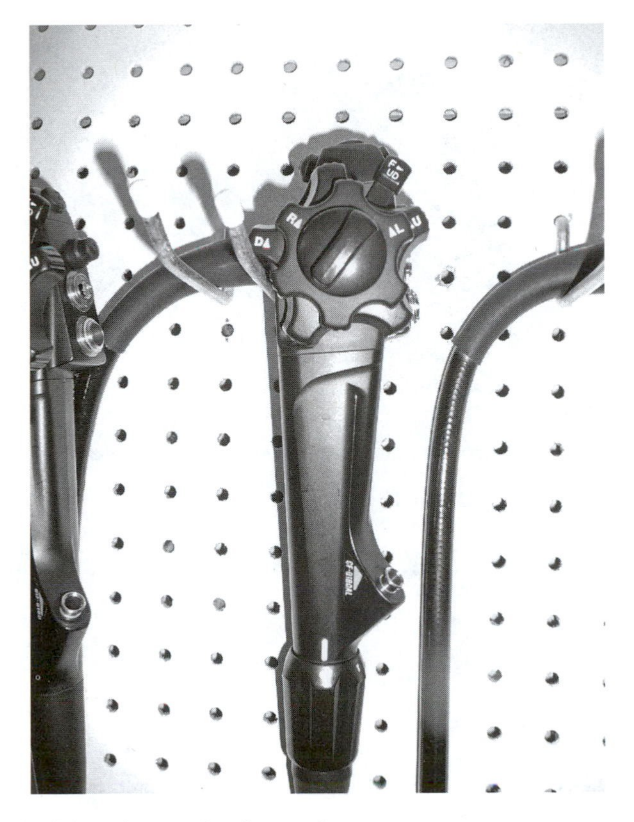

FIGURE 4.4 Flexible endoscope hand controls.

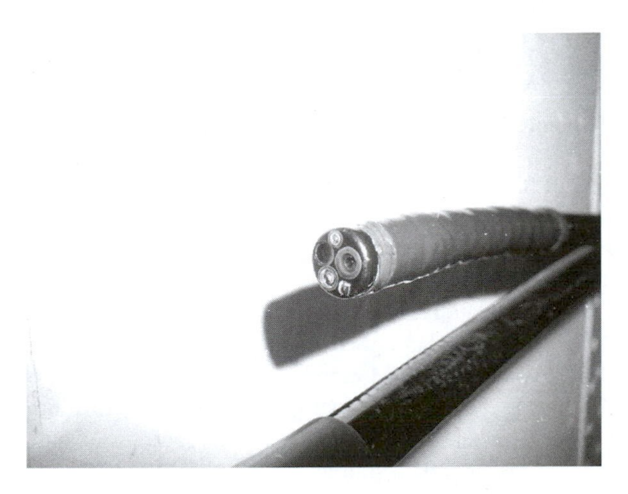

FIGURE 4.5 Distal end of endoscope — note various channels.

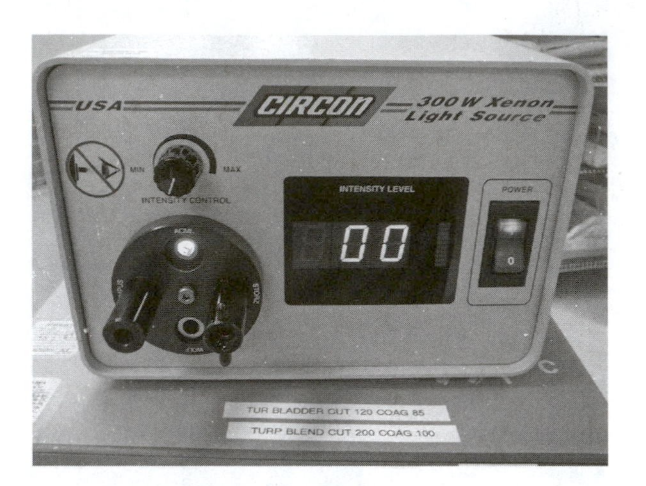

FIGURE 4.6 An older endoscopy light source.

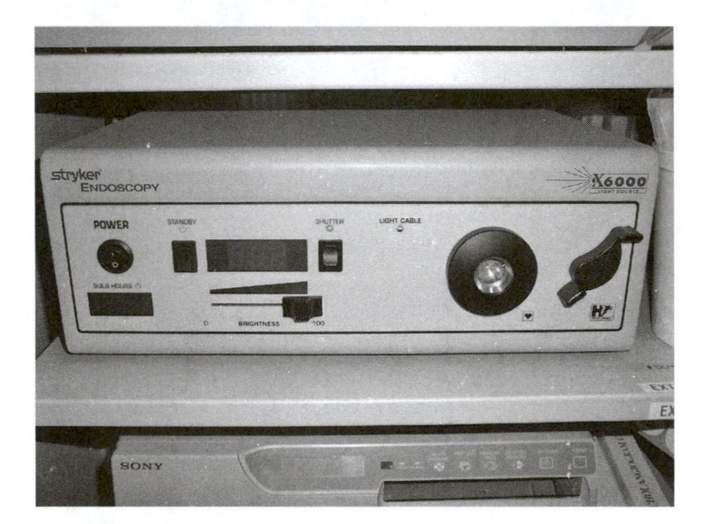

FIGURE 4.7 A current endoscopy light source.

supplies, since both temperature changes and supply voltage variation can change light characteristics.

Higher intensity bulbs are fitted with heat sinks and fans to help keep them in the correct temperature range.

In order to accommodate requirements for different light intensities, a mechanical device is used to block some portion of the light. Simpler light sources have manual controls for intensity, while more sophisticated units can be controlled by the video portion of the system in order to maintain optimum illumination.

Light source units have a connector on the front panel to accommodate the fiber optics for the scope; this may be a simple, single-purpose plug, or it may be a more complex connector that can carry optical or electronic images and control signals, as well as air, irrigation, and suction.

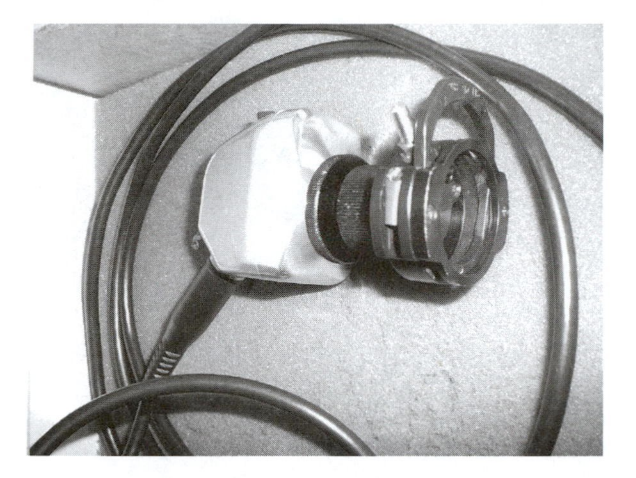

FIGURE 4.8 Endoscopy camera head.

By using fiber optics to carry light from the source (bulb) to the viewing area, an adequate amount of light is delivered with very little heat.

b. Camera

Video cameras used in endoscopy systems must be able to generate high-resolution images with accurate color reproduction. In most systems the camera is in two parts: the image sensor portion and the video-processing portion. Some systems have the image sensor on a head that attaches to the proximal part of the scope (Figure 4.8), while newer systems mount the sensors at the distal tip of the scope.

Image sensors may consist of a single-chip array, or three-chip arrays. With the single-chip arrangement colors are differentiated electronically, while with three-chip systems each chip responds to a single primary color. Single-chip systems tend to be smaller and less expensive, while three-chip systems tend to provide higher image quality. Both single-chip and three-chip cameras are available with high-definition resolution (Figure 4.9); again, higher resolution means higher costs.

In each system, video signals are taken from the sensors to a processing component, usually cabinet mounted (Figure 4.10). This part of the camera handles the video signals to adjust for light intensities and can perform such tasks as white balancing to help ensure color accuracy.

The video processor interfaces with light sources as well as video image recorders, printers, and video displays.

c. Video Recorder/Storage

Systems may record video as either motion or still pictures, or both, so that clinicians can later examine the images for specific details, or use them for teaching purposes. Recorded images from one test on an individual patient may be compared to those from a later test in order to see if changes in tissues or structures have taken place.

In the past, endoscopy systems recorded video on videocassette recorders, but new systems use recordable optical disks and/or hard drives, which provide much quicker access to images (Figure 4.11).

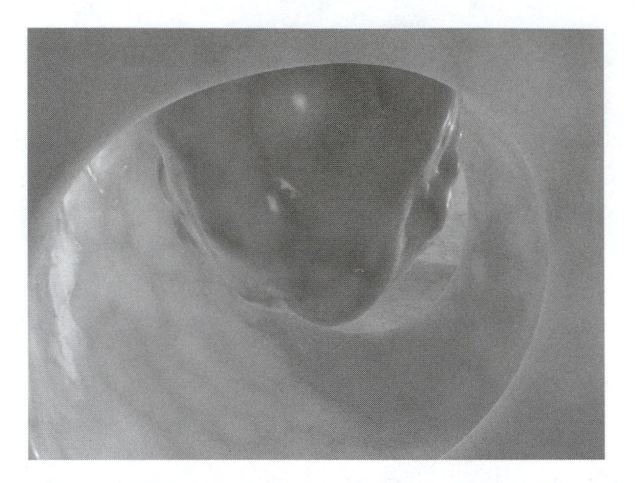

FIGURE 4.9 Endoscopy image showing a colon tumor. (Modified from Inmagine Corp, www.123rf.com, with permission.)

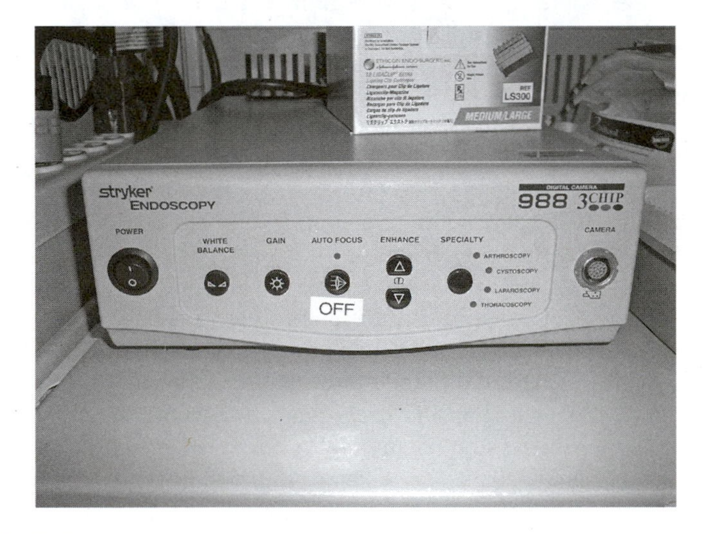

FIGURE 4.10 Endoscopy camera/video processing unit.

d. Video Monitor

As part of the system, video monitors must have equal capabilities to other links in the imaging chain in terms of resolution and color reproduction. Both CRT and LCD monitors are used, with the size and weight advantages of LCD making them increasingly common.

Monitors are mounted to give the person performing the test a clear view, and secondary displays are often used to provide a good view to other staff or students.

e. Insufflator

Obtaining a clear view of many internal structures can be difficult when other organs or tissues get in the way; there is normally very little open space inside the body.

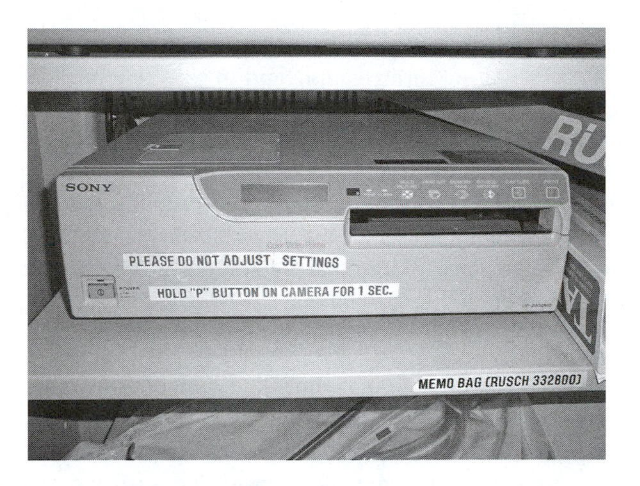

FIGURE 4.11 Endoscopy video recorder.

To alleviate this problem, an inert gas such as carbon dioxide may be introduced to the target area. Obviously such insufflatory pressures must be carefully limited to avoid damage, and so systems are equipped with regulators and over-pressure alarms. Insufflating gas usually comes from pressurized tanks, since most facilities don't have carbon dioxide wall outlets.

Room air is not used for insufflation because it is not absorbed by tissues as well as carbon dioxide. Excess nonintestinal gas remaining in body cavities after scope procedures can cause pain and discomfort for the patient.

Insufflators typically have controls and displays (usually digital) for patient pressure, gas flow rate, and total volume delivered (Figure 4.12). Since there may be some leakage of gas from the scope, and also since carbon dioxide can be absorbed quite easily by internal body tissues, some level of continuous flow must be maintained after adequate insufflation is achieved.

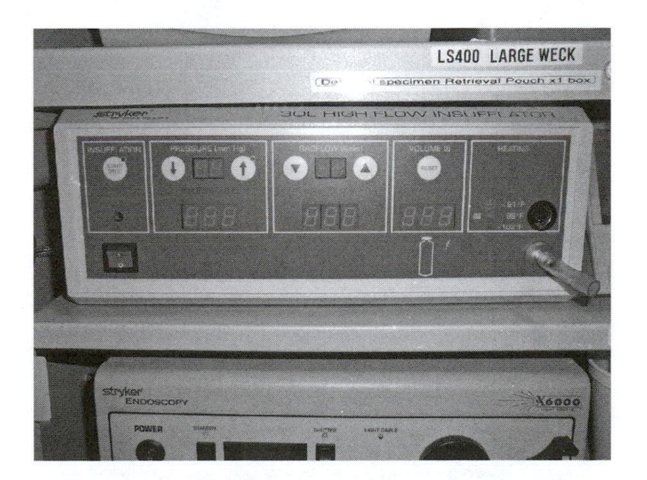

FIGURE 4.12 An insufflator front panel.

f. Irrigation and Suction

Isotonic saline is usually used for irrigation, and in some circumstances it is used to distend the viewing area to provide more clearance, when gas insufflation would not work, such as in the confined spaces of joints when performing arthroscopic procedures. The saline is pumped in through the scope lumen using a low-pressure pump.

Removing blood, tissue particles, or the debris from surgical procedures is necessary to maintain good visibility, but as with any body fluid, the evacuated material must be handled using appropriate precautions. A low-suction vacuum pump or line suction is used via the scope lumen.

g. Tools

A wide range of procedures can be accomplished with endoscopy, using an equally wide range of tools.

For some laparoscopic or thoracoscopic procedures that might require bulkier or multiple tools, a separate tube may be inserted into a second small incision.

A common goal of endoscopy, in addition to simple observation, is the removal of small samples of suspect tissue in order to examine the sample in detail to help diagnose or eliminate conditions such as cancer. Special fine grasping and cutting tools allow such biopsies to be performed quickly and accurately.

Larger amounts of tissue can be excised and removed as well, for example in the removal of tumors or polyps. Since the suction lumen of an endoscope is limited in size, such tissue must be reduced to relatively small pieces before suction is applied. Gall bladder removal is commonly performed in this manner, a procedure called a laparoscopic cholecystectomy.

Electrosurgery (see Chapter 8) can be performed laparoscopically, using long, thin electrode probes that are well insulated except for the tips (Figure 4.13). These tips can be snares or pincers, and can be used for such things as polyp ligation or fallopian tube sealing. The inner conductor must be insulated from the outer sleeve. A flat electrode may be used to cauterize highly vascularized tissue that is causing blood loss, such as in the liver or uterus.

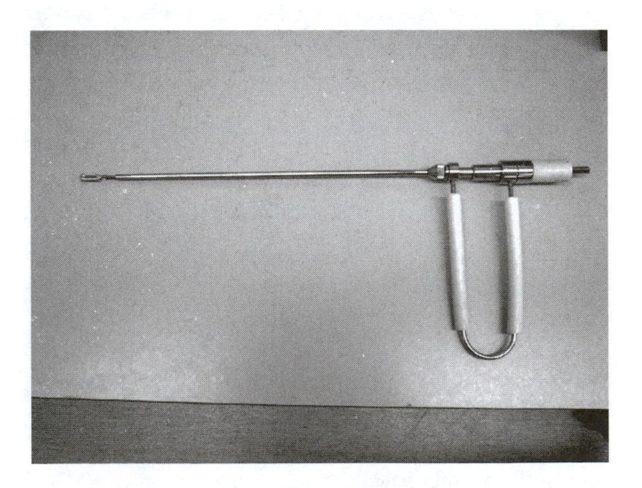

FIGURE 4.13 A laparoscopic electrosurgery probe (bipolar).

In arthroscopy (see section titled "Arthroscopy Systems"), harder material such as cartilage or bone may need to be removed, in which case rotating grinding tools can be used through the scope.

II. SENSORY ORGANS

Of the various human senses, only sight and hearing have a significant amount of medical technology devoted to their study and treatment.

Visualization is the primary method of diagnosing problems with the eyes or ears, and specialized devices have been developed to provide effective means of seeing into those organs. Included in this section are tools used to examine the mouth and throat, even though they are not particularly concerned with the mouth as a sensory organ.

A. Oto/Laryngo/Ophthalmoscopes

The eyes, ears, and throat are readily available for examination, but each presents certain difficulties to direct observation. Much of the critical structures of the eye are located behind the iris and can only be seen through the small opening of the pupil (Figure 4.14). The tympanic membrane of the ear is at the end of a narrow passageway, and the tongue and uvula can block the view any further into the throat.

A set of tools for looking into the eyes, ears, and throat are often grouped together, utilizing the same power source and handle. The device used to examine the eyes is called an ophthalmoscope; for the ears, an otoscope; and for the throat, a laryngoscope.

Most of these devices derive power from a battery (rechargeable or disposable) in the handle, though in locations where patients come and many examinations will be performed, the scopes may be line powered.

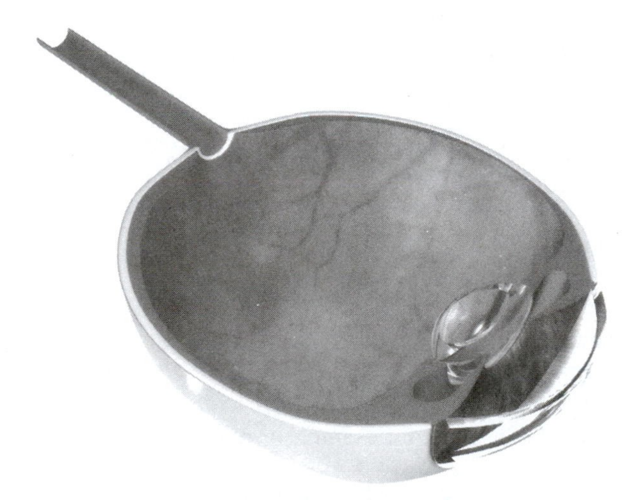

FIGURE 4.14 Structure of the eye. (Modified from Inmagine Corp, www.123rf.com, with permission.)

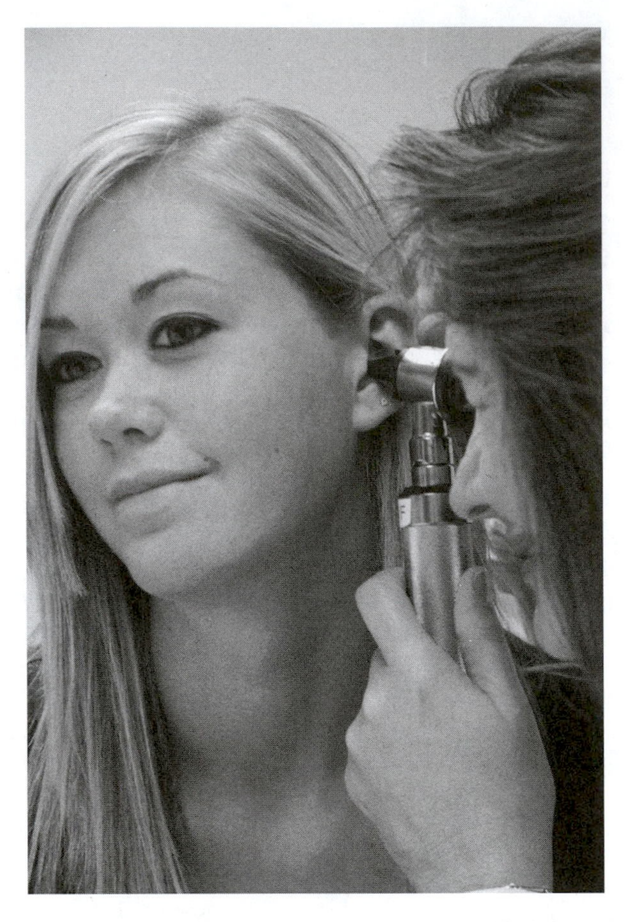

FIGURE 4.15 An ear examination using an otoscope. (Modified from Inmagine Corp, www.123rf.com, with permission.)

1. Otoscope

The main difficulty in looking into the ear canal is that most light sources that might be used to illuminate the area will also block the view. Otoscopes use fiber optics in a ring around an observing tube to overcome this problem; a low-power lens aids in visualization (Figure 4.15). Different tubes may be attached for various depths, and a disposable cover is used to prevent cross infection between patients. The intensity of the light source can be varied for different conditions.

The lens of the otoscope may be designed to move out of the way to allow small instruments to be inserted, for example to remove foreign objects or buildups of ear wax.

Some units may have an air channel that allows small bursts of air to be directed toward the tympanic membrane, to help evaluate its tension.

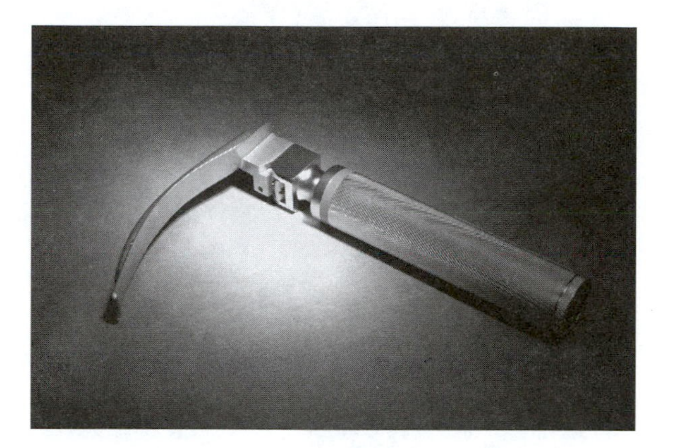

FIGURE 4.16 A laryngoscope. (Modified from Inmagine Corp, www.123rf.com, with permission.)

2. Laryngoscope

Keeping the tongue, and to a lesser extent the uvula, out of the way while providing illumination is the main goal of a laryngoscope (Figure 4.16). Most consist of a metal or plastic blade that has a very small light bulb or a fiber optic outlet near the tip.

Blades are designed to accommodate different depths of observation and different throat sizes. Some have a mechanism to spread the throat passage open, which can be necessary for some visualizations, or for performing minor surgical procedures, or in the process of intubating a patient.

A specialized type of laryngoscope uses fiber optics for both illumination and visualization. The very thin, flexible line is passed though the nose in order to have a better viewing angle in the throat.

3. Ophthalmoscope

First developed by Welch and Allyn in 1915, the handheld ophthalmoscope has evolved into a powerful device for performing eye examinations; the Welch-Allyn name is still commonly seen on this type of equipment (Figure 4.17).

Ophthalmoscopes have a number of lenses of different magnifications and a light source that can be adjusted in intensity, shape, and color. This arrangement allows the clinician to examine the outer surface of the eye and also the inner structures, via the pupil (Figure 4.18). Eye drops to cause pupil dilation are often used to allow a larger opening for observation.

The lens and vitreous humor can be examined, but the most important structure viewed by an ophthalmoscope is the retina. By utilizing the different patterns of illumination (including full, slit, and small circle) along with certain color filters, the condition of the retina can be determined. This can aid in the diagnosis of such conditions as increased intracranial pressure, glaucoma, macular degeneration, detached retina, brain tumors, diabetic retinopathy, and hypertension.

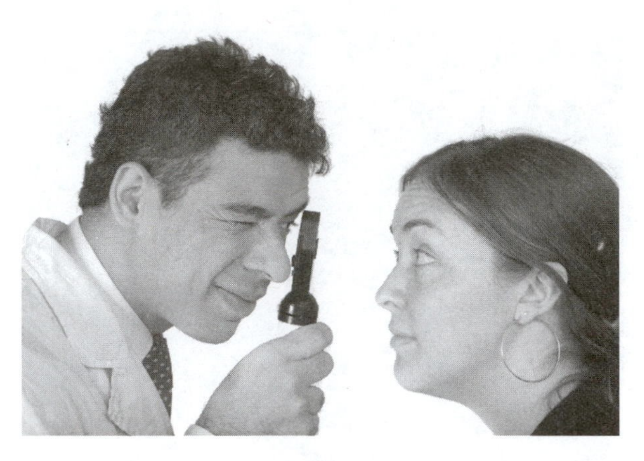

FIGURE 4.17 An ophthalmoscope in use. (Modified from Inmagine Corp, www.123rf.com, with permission.)

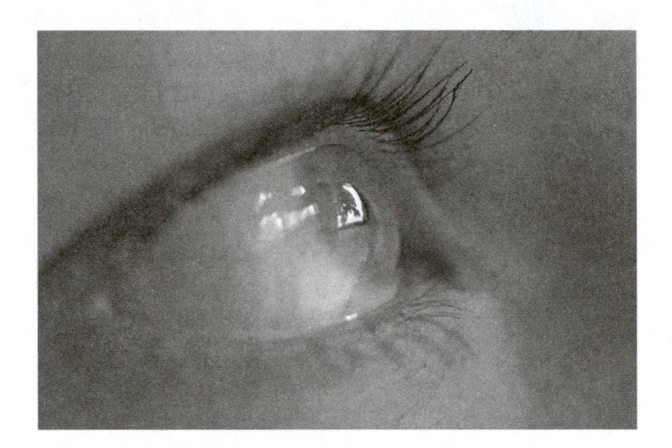

FIGURE 4.18 A close up view of an eye. (Modified from Inmagine Corp, www.123rf.com, with permission.)

B. Slit Lamps

A slit lamp is a tool commonly used in eye examinations (Figure 4.19). It provides a stable, adjustable platform for the patient to rest their head, keeping it comfortably but reliably in place during the examination.

Binocular eyepieces with multiple objective lenses of different magnification allow for a wide variety of examinations.

A high intensity lamp provides illumination, with the light focused into a narrow line, or slit, which can be turned to various angles and adjusted in position. Various filters can add color to the light, which can aid in identifying certain structures or tissue characteristics.

As with ophthalmoscopes (of which the slit lamp is really just a complex version), eye drops may be administered to the patient to produce pupil dilation, allowing a better view inside the eye.

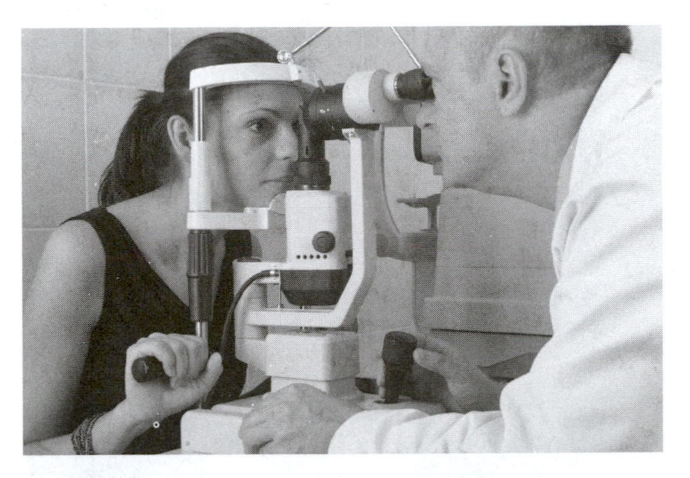

FIGURE 4.19 A slit lamp being used to examine a patient's eyes. (Modified from Inmagine Corp, www.123rf.com, with permission.)

III. REPRODUCTION

A. Fetal Heart Detectors

In utero, a fetus has a rapid heart beat from a very early stage of development (Figure 4.20). The rate and strength of the heart beat can give important information about the health of the fetus, and so a simple means of detecting it is very useful. A stethoscope can sometimes pick up the sounds of the fetal heart, but this can be

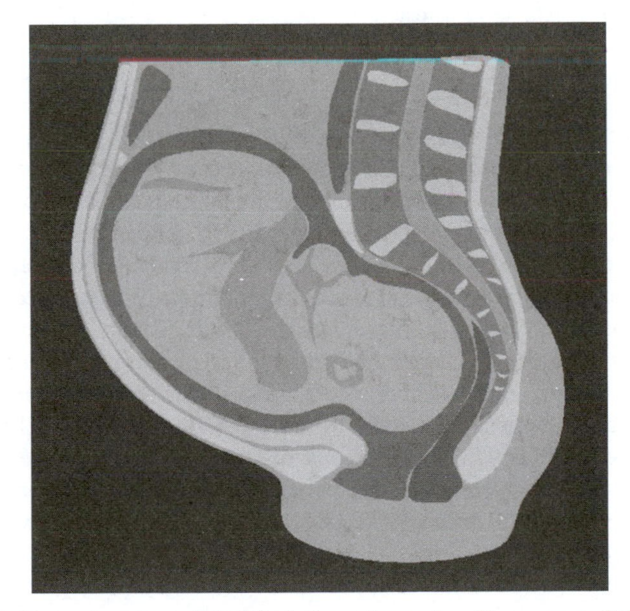

FIGURE 4.20 Fetus in utero. (Modified from Inmagine Corp, www.123rf.com, with permission.)

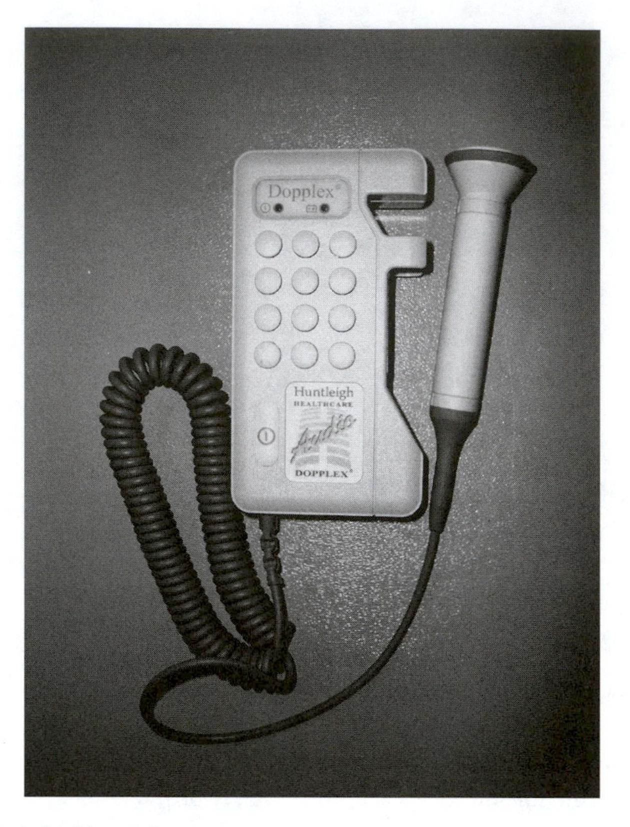

FIGURE 4.21 A fetal heart detector.

difficult, especially early in pregnancy, since the heart is small and usually quite deep within the mother's body.

Fetal heart detectors (Figure 4.21) utilize the Doppler effect in much the same way as blood flow detectors (Chapter 3), sending a beam of ultrasound in the direction of the fetus and listening for the fluctuations in sound resulting from the ultrasound being reflected by the moving parts of the fetal heart. Fetal heart beats can be detected in this manner as early as 7 or 8 weeks gestation.

Ultrasound gel provides good sonic coupling between the detector head and the mother's abdomen. Some experience is necessary for accurate determination of fetal heart detection, since the pulsing of the mother's aorta can give a similar signal. Maternal aortic pulse is much slower than the fetal rate, however, and the slower motion produces a distinctive sound. Fetal heart rate is typically between 120 and 160 beats per minute, while resting adult rates are usually around 60 to 80 beats per minute. In some circumstances the maternal rate may be high, and in these cases care must be taken to differentiate between the two, perhaps by trying different angles to try to avoid the aorta.

Because Doppler fetal heat detectors are relatively inexpensive, very portable, and easy to use, they can serve as a vital "early warning system" to potential fetal

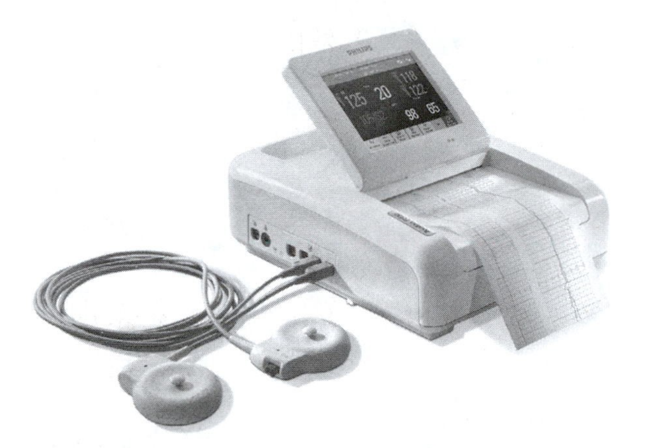

FIGURE 4.22 Overview of a fetal monitor. (Modified from Philips Medical, CD provided directly, with permission. © 2006 Koninidijke Philips Electronics N.V. All rights reserved. Reproduction in whole or in part is prohibited without prior written permission of the copyright owner.)

difficulties. If a problem is suspected, further examination using sophisticated ultrasound machines can be performed.

Ultrasound crystals are fragile and can be cracked by a blow. Cracked crystals can sometimes still work, but performance is greatly reduced. Damaged wires for the earpieces, if used, can result in noisy or intermittent signals.

B. Fetal Monitors

As mentioned above, fetal heart rate and strength can be a good indicator of fetal health. It may be advantageous to monitor the heart rate for a longer period of time than is convenient with a fetal heart detector.

It is also valuable to be able to determine the correlation of fetal heart rate and uterine contractions, and so a means of quantifying contractions is necessary.

Fetal heart monitors, sometimes called antepartum fetal monitors or cardiotocographs, provide these functions (Figure 4.22).

Fetal heart detection in these units uses the same principle as the simpler fetal heart detectors described above. However, an array of ultrasound crystals is used, which provides a better signal. The crystals are arranged in such a way that the beams from each intersect at a point roughly corresponding to the normal position of the fetus in the mother's abdomen. This improves the signal and also helps to eliminate signals from other sources, such as the mother's aorta or the heartbeat of a twin.

These ultrasound transducers (Figure 4.23) are positioned (using ultrasound gel) on the mother's abdomen to obtain the best possible signal, and a strap is then used to hold the transducer in place. Some monitors have two transducer inputs and are capable of monitoring twins simultaneously. The transducers may have to be adjusted occasionally due to slippage or to the movement of the fetus.

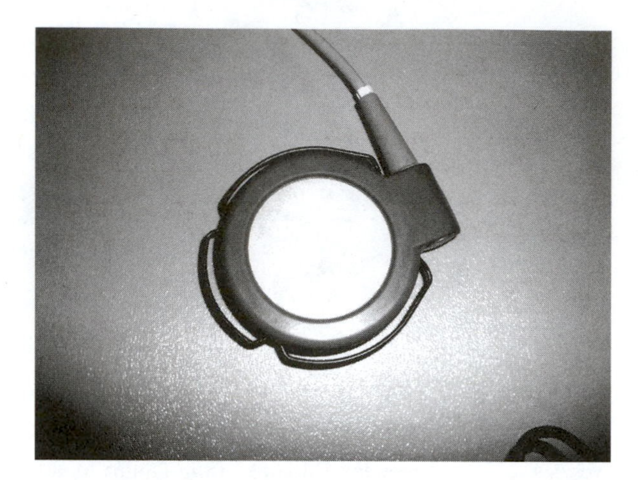

FIGURE 4.23 Fetal monitor ultrasound transducer.

Fetal heart signals are amplified, and three outputs are derived: a sound signal, much like that of the simple fetal heart detectors; a numeric rate value, displayed on the front panel; and a signal fed to a chart recorder that produces a trace indicating rate. Some systems also can send heart rate data to a central monitoring system.

The second part of a fetal monitor is the uterine contraction detector, called a tocograph (Figure 4.24). This sensor is simply a pressure transducer mounted in a housing and strapped against the mother's abdomen. When a uterine contraction occurs, the abdominal wall becomes more rigid, and this causes the transducer to be compressed. The amount of deflection is translated into a relative, unitless value.

The contraction value is displayed on the front panel of the monitor (Figure 4.25) and also produces a recording on the same chart recorder as the fetal heart rate, which allows easy visual correlation.

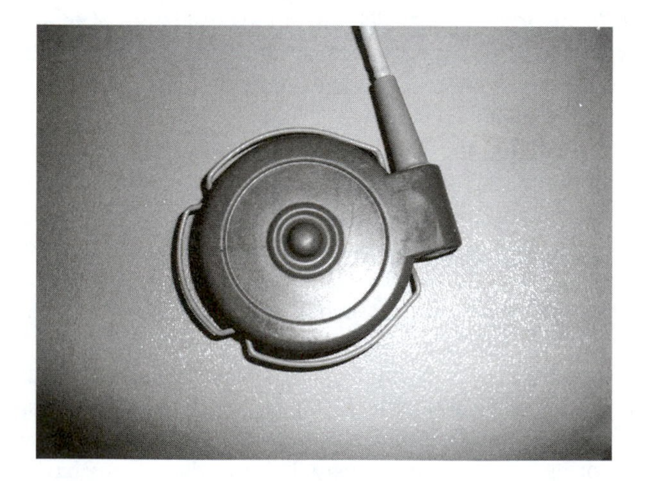

FIGURE 4.24 Fetal monitor toco transducer.

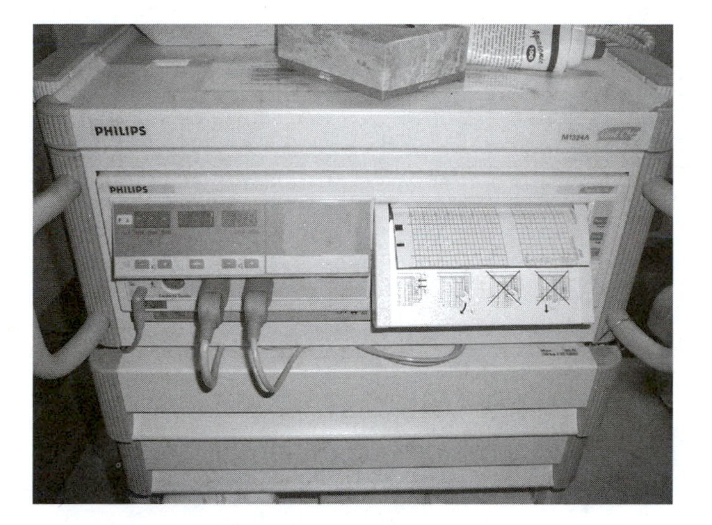

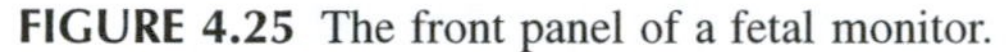

FIGURE 4.25 The front panel of a fetal monitor.

Most monitors have a button switch that can be pressed by the mother to indicate particular events, such as felt fetal movement. This can help in evaluating changes in fetal heart rate. Pressing the button makes a mark on the chart recording (Figure 4.26).

Chart recorders print the time and date at regular intervals along the edge of the paper, which can serve as both a medical and a legal notation.

C. Infant Scales

Infant weight is important in determining growth, fluid balance, and other values, but since babies tend to be quite active at times, the scales (Figure 4.27) used to weigh them must have a means of averaging readings over a short time period in order to give a stable weight reading. Scales have a "tare" function that allows staff to compensate for the weight of objects other than the baby that may have to be on the scale, such as a diaper or blanket.

Scales typically use strain gauges for weight determination. The signals from these units are amplified, digitized, and averaged, and a numeric value is then displayed.

D. APGAR Timers

A quick, standardized means of evaluating the health of a neonate is important, and to that end Dr. Virginia Apgar developed the Apgar scoring system in 1952. The scale evaluates five criteria, giving each a score of zero, one, or two (Table 4.1). The scores are totaled, and the resulting value gives a good indication of condition.

Acronyms for each criterion have been used as a memory aid, but the name for the test is derived from its originator.

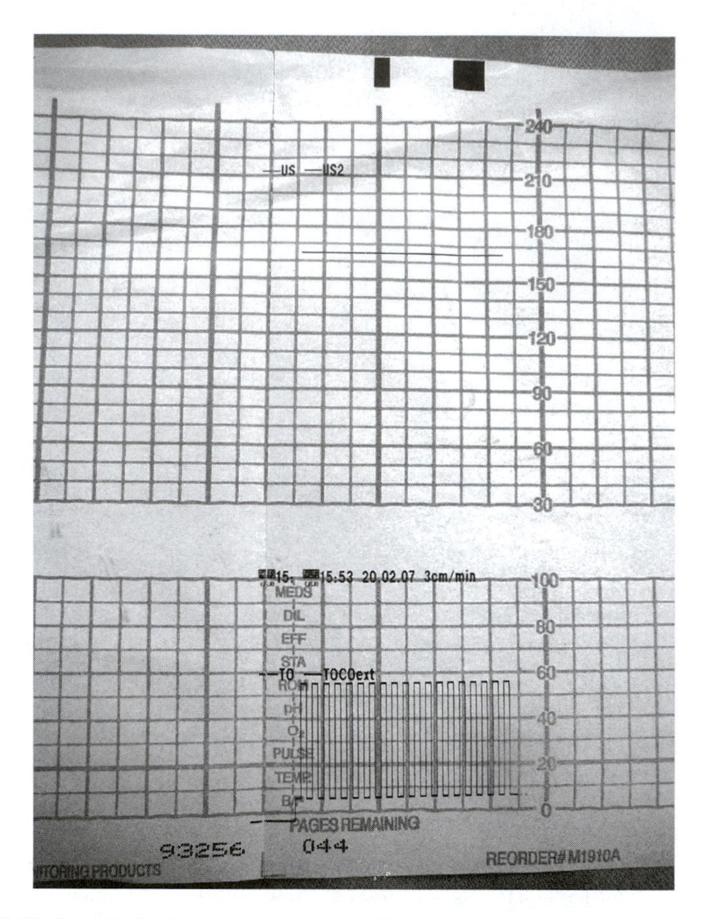

FIGURE 4.26 Sample fetal monitor chart recording — test patterns.

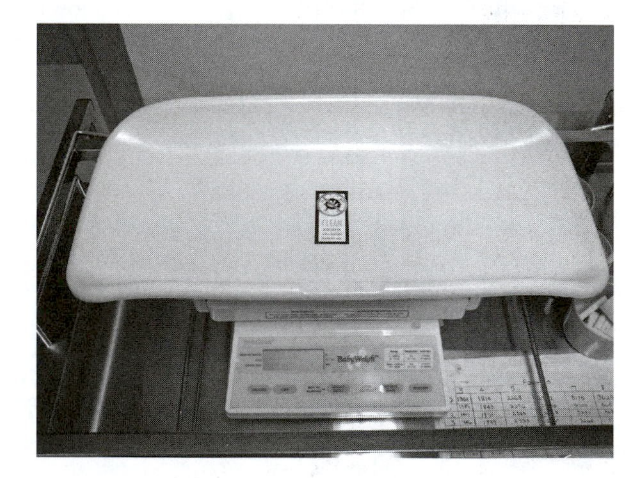

FIGURE 4.27 An infant scale.

TABLE 4.1
Apgar Test Terms

Criterion	Acronym	Score 0	Score 1	Score 2
Skin color	Appearance	Blue all over	Blue at extremities	Normal
Heart rate	Pulse	Absent	Less than 100	Greater than or equal to 100
Reflex	Grimace	No response	Grimace/feeble cry	Sneeze/cough/pulls away
Muscle tone	Activity	None	Some flexion	Active movement
Respiration	Respiration	Absent	Weak or irregular	Strong

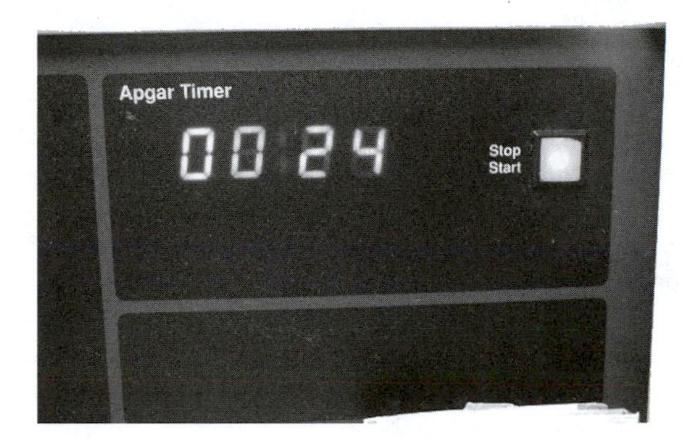

FIGURE 4.28 An Apgar timer built in to an infant resuscitator.

The tests are normally done at one minute and five minutes after birth, and possibly later if scores are below normal. Generally, total scores under 3 are considered to be critically low, and 7 or above normal.

Low scores at the one-minute mark are cause for extra attention but may not indicate major problems, especially if scores improve with time. If the scores are 3 or less for longer times, up to 30 minutes, it may indicate that the infant is at significant risk of long-term neurological impairment.

A variety of timers are available to signal when to perform the one-minute and five-minute tests, since this is usually a busy time for staff who may not be able to watch a clock (Figure 4.28). Timers may be stand-alone or built into equipment such as infant resuscitators (Chapter 8).

IV. SKIN, BONE, MUSCLE, MISCELLANEOUS

A. Thermometers

Humans are homeothermic organisms, with most individuals maintaining a core temperature very close to 37°C. Variations from this normal value indicate problems, and so measuring temperature at regular intervals is an important diagnostic procedure.

While core temperature is normally maintained within very narrow limits, temperatures of other parts of the body, especially the extremities, can vary considerably.

Finding an accessible place to measure temperature that will accurately reflect the core value is vital.

Oral (sublingual) temperature, as long as the patient has not consumed food or drink recently, or been breathing through their mouth, is a reasonably good measure of core temperature and is the most commonly used determination point. It is inconvenient for long-term monitoring, however, and is impractical for patients who are unable or unwilling to hold the measuring device under their tongue for the prescribed time.

Axillary temperature can be close to core, but significant variations are possible.

Rectal temperatures provide very good correlation to core, but can be uncomfortable for the patient and inconvenient for staff.

The temperature of the tympanic membrane in the ear is close to core temperature, but measurement is very technique dependent.

Long-term temperature monitoring is most easily done with a probe attached to the patient's skin, but since this value often does not correspond to core temperature, it is mainly a relative value: if it goes up or down significantly from a previously steady value, it can indicate problems that need further attention.

Overall, there is no one method of temperature measurement that will suit all situations, so various methods may have to be employed.

The original method of determining temperature was to simply feel the patient's skin. This method requires no tools and, with experience, can be a reliable indicator of significant variations in the patient's temperature. However, it is subjective and does not provide a numerical measurement.

Glass tube thermometers were invented in the fifteenth century and used mercury or colored alcohol to indicate temperature (Figure 4.29). These devices continue to

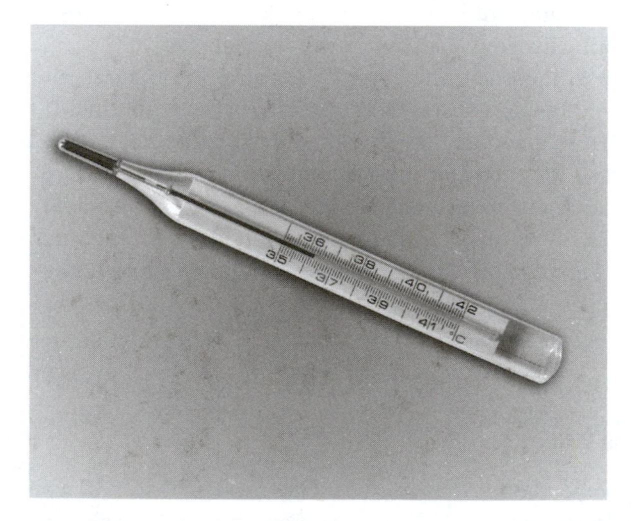

FIGURE 4.29 Old-style glass tube thermometer. (Modified from Inmagine Corp, www.123rf.com, with permission.)

be used today, though their use with patients has essentially ceased, due to the possibility of injury and the danger of mercury contamination if the tube was broken.

Most hospitals use electronic thermometers, which can be of two basic types.

1. Electronic Probe Thermometers

Electronic probe thermometers (Figure 4.30) use a resistive element (thermistor) that changes its resistance according to temperature. By passing a constant current through the device and measuring voltage drop, and then applying the results to a curve-correcting algorithm, a value for temperature can be determined.

Probes can be various shapes, depending on application, but most used in hospitals are either slender rods or flat buttons.

Rod-type probes are used for oral or rectal, or less commonly, axillary measurements, while button probes are used for skin measurements.

Rod probes are used with a disposable cover, replaced for each patient to help prevent cross infection. Systems are designed to make it difficult to take a temperature reading without using a cover, and then will not take a subsequent reading without replacing the cover.

Some models come with two different probes, one for oral and one for rectal measurements; probes are color-coded, usually blue for oral and red for rectal. Single-probe units usually use this same color code.

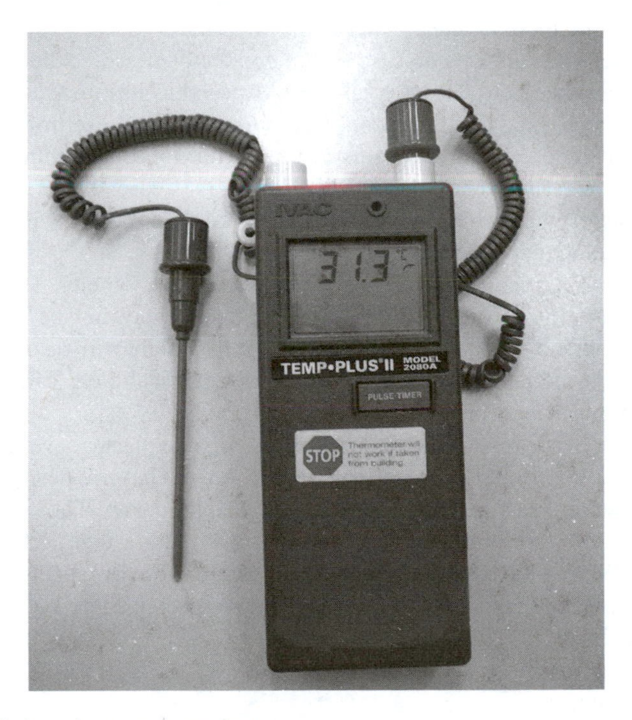

FIGURE 4.30 A probe type thermometer.

Probes are generally replaceable, and often are available with various cord lengths.

The body of these units has a battery compartment, a probe holder, a holder for a supply of covers, and a display that gives the temperature reading as well as other indicators such as low battery, probe fault, low or high temperature alarms, and possibly a timer to indicate when temperature readings should be stable.

Generally there is a switch in the probe holder that turns the device off when the probe is inserted and on when it is removed, for battery conservation.

Some may have an internal mechanism such as a magnetic relay or Hall effect switch that is activated when the unit is placed in a wall or desk holster; if the unit doesn't get reset by this mechanism after a certain number of readings, the unit becomes inoperative to deter theft.

Units can usually be changed from Celsius to Fahrenheit, depending on application. The control for this is usually hidden, often inside the battery compartment.

2. Tympanic Thermometers

The tympanic membrane is almost always at core temperature, being well inside the skull at the end of a narrow passage, so in that way it makes an ideal candidate for temperature measurement. Because of its delicate nature, however, direct contact with a temperature probe could be harmful. Methods were developed in industrial applications to measure temperature remotely by measuring the infrared radiation emitted by an object. This method was refined and miniaturized to produce the infrared tympanic thermometer.

Infrared temperature sensors use a semiconductor device called a thermopile, which generates an electrical potential when exposed to infrared radiation.

Because there is a delay in response time for thermopile sensors, they must be kept shielded behind a shutter mechanism until the time of temperature measurement. When the unit is pointed in the right direction (in this case, at the tympanic membrane) the shutter is triggered to open for a specific time, during which the temperature of the membrane is determined.

Technique is critical when using a tympanic thermometer. If the unit isn't adjusted and inserted correctly into the ear canal, it may not be pointing at the tympanic membrane when measurement is taken, which will result in erroneous values. Also, the body of the probe should seal against the ear canal, because air currents entering the ear past the unit can cause errors.

These devices are designed to use a thin, deformable plastic cover over the probe portion in order to avoid cross infections (Figure 4.31). They are designed so that the cover has to be replaced before another reading can be taken. The cover forms part of the optical path, and therefore accurate readings require that probe covers be in place. Similarly, any dirt or foreign material on the lens or cover will affect readings.

IR thermometers tend to drift with time, and so they must be calibrated on a regular basis.

B. Densitometers

In the movie, *The Pursuit of Happyness,* the protagonist tried to make a living in the early 1980s by selling bone densitometers to doctor's offices and clinics. He had

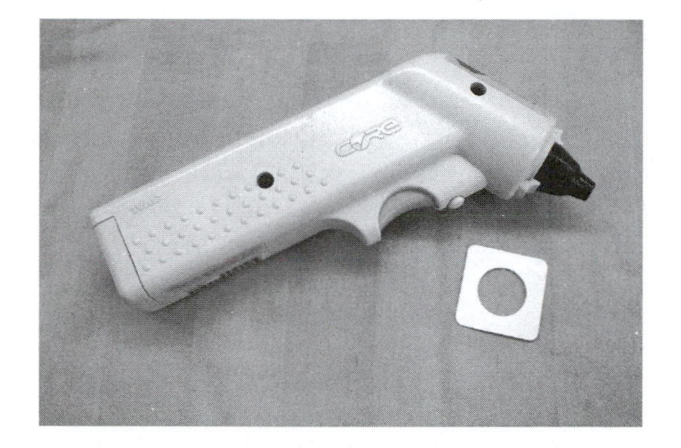

FIGURE 4.31 Tympanic thermometer with lens cover.

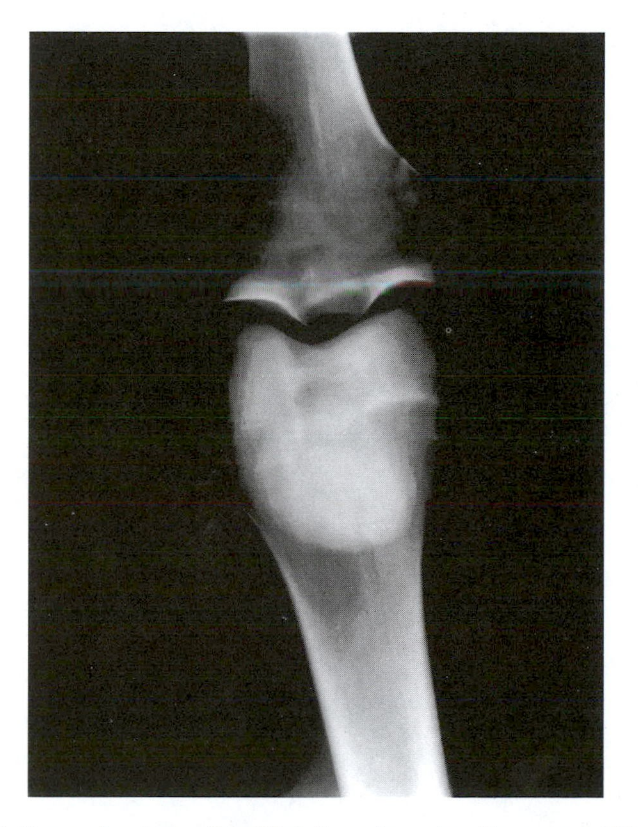

FIGURE 4.32 X-ray of a knee. (Modified from Inmagine Corp, www.123rf.com, with permission.)

a hard time convincing some of his potential customers of the value of the devices, but now, with the prevalence and awareness of conditions such as osteoporosis, he may have had an easier time.

Densitometers use low-level x-rays or ultrasound beams to produce a density reading of the bone tissue through which the exposure in made. Some units are as portable as the ones that Will Smith's character lugged around in the movie, but most are larger, fixed devices that scan a prone patient from above.

C. Arthroscopy Systems

Arthroscopy systems share a number of characteristics with other endoscopy systems, but because they are working in the confined spaces of joints (Figure 4.32), some of the hardware is designed differently. Scopes are smaller and shorter and always rigid. Instruments are passed into the joint via a second (or sometimes third) tube, which also handles irrigation and suction. Instead of gas to expand the target area for improved viewing, a clear fluid is used.

Since repair of injured joints often involves the removal of torn or damaged cartilage or sometimes calcareous growths on bone, rotating cutting and grinding instruments are used in arthroscopy.

Some procedures, such as the repair of tears in the meniscus (the membrane that hold lubricating synovial fluid in the joint) or the repair of torn ligaments, may involve suturing through the tubes.

V. CHAPTER SUMMARY

Chapter 4 is concerned with the digestive, sensory, and reproductive systems, as well as miscellaneous topics such as the skin, muscles, and bones.

Function and application of gastroscopes is covered, as well as equipment used to examine the eyes, ears, and throat.

Perinatal monitoring and care are examined, along with various types of thermometers and the principles of thermoregulation.

Arthroscopy is briefly discussed.

5 Diagnostic Imaging

I. INTRODUCTION

As discussed in the preface to this book, diagnostic imaging (DI) is a large, specialized field with mostly very complex, manufacturer-specific equipment. Most DI equipment requires factory training before BioMedical Engineering Technologists (BMETs) can provide effective service. Therefore, it will not be dealt with in depth in this book, but an outline of the various technologies involved is included.

For further reading, please refer to the bibliography.

A. X-Rays

1. History

Being able to look inside the living human body without cutting it open was a dream of medical workers for most of history. Visible light, no matter how bright, could not provide any significant information about structures beneath the skin. The sense of touch could be used to help diagnose some conditions, but it too was limited.

In 1895, Wilhelm Roentgen, in Germany, discovered some previously unknown rays that were emitted from a vacuum tube across which a high voltage was applied. The rays, which Roentgen named "x-rays," passed through some materials that were completely opaque to visible light, though not others. Dense materials such as bone or metal blocked the rays, and so he used them to make an image of his wife's hand, passing the rays through her hand and onto a photographic plate.

For some time, the rays were called Roentgen rays in honor of their discoverer, but the x-ray term has prevailed (Figure 5.1).

2. Physics

Eventual research showed that x-rays were simply very short-wavelength emissions in the same spectrum as light and radio waves (see Chapter 11), with wavelengths from 0.01 nm to 10 nm. X-rays with wavelengths greater than 0.1 nm are called "soft" x-rays, while those of less than 0.1 nm are "hard" x-rays.

The means of producing x-rays were refined, and most current x-ray tubes utilize a beam of electrons accelerated to extreme velocity by high voltage. The beam then collides with a metal target (typically tungsten), and the collision produces x-rays. By angling the target, the x-rays can be directed as desired.

Copper is often used as a substrate for the metal target in an x-ray tube because of its high heat conductivity; heat buildup is reduced in the target contact area. With

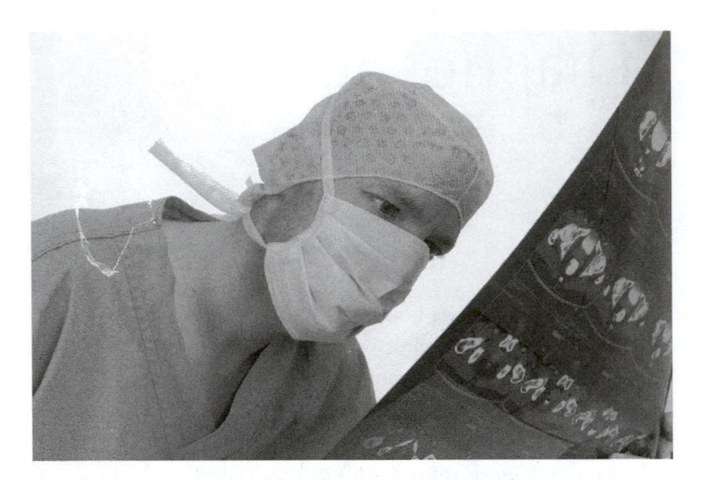

FIGURE 5.1 A physician examining an x-ray film. (Modified from Inmagine Corp, www.123rf.com, with permission.)

this same heat-reducing end in mind, many modern tubes have a spinning target, first developed by the Philips Company in 1929.

X-ray characteristics are determined by the voltage and current used to produce them. Voltages are in the thousands of volts range, and their values are given as the peak voltage, or kVp. Current is in milliamps (mA), but the duration of the current is a factor as well, so the two components are often combined as milliamp-seconds, or mAs.

Typical values for voltage, current, exposure time, and radiation dose (in microsieverts or millisieverts, μSv or mSv, respectively) for different types of x-ray procedures are given below.

Dental x-rays: 70–90 kVp, 3–10 mA, 0.05–4 s, 20 μSv
Mammograms: 25–26 kVp, 70–126 mAs, 0.7–1.5 s, up to 2.50 mSv
Chest/abdominal/extremity x-rays: 60–120 kVp, 1–100 mAs, 0.1–3 mSv
Fluoroscopy: 40–120 kVp, 1–20 mA, up to a few minutes duration, 20 mSv/min

3. Definitions of Units

- A rad is an older unit; rad stands for Radiation Absorbed Dose and is defined as 1 watt of x-ray power entering 100 kg of tissue.
- The rem is also an older unit; rem stands for Roentgen-Equivalent-Man; that is, 1 rem is the amount of radiation required to produce the same biological effect as 1 rad (1 rem = 0.01 Sv).
- Gray (Gy) — 1 joule of x-ray energy entering 1 kilogram of tissue (1 Gray = 100 rad).
- Sievert (Sv) — The amount of radiation required to produce the same biological effect as 1 Gray (1 Sv = 100 rad).

4. Detectors

1. Originally x-rays were detected by exposing them to a standard (at the time) glass photographic plate. The x-rays caused chemical changes in the silver compounds in much the same way as light did. Since x-rays are blocked to a greater or lesser degree by the tissues they pass through, an x-ray image on a plate is a negative; that is, the lighter areas on the plate correspond to more dense tissue, while the darker areas correspond to less dense tissue.
2. Glass plates were replaced by sheets of photographic film, which, since they would be ruined if exposed to light, were held in cassettes that blocked visible light but were transparent to x-rays. The cassettes could be unloaded manually or automatically for processing.
3. Certain materials glow, or fluoresce, when struck by x-rays, so if a sheet of such material is used in place of x-ray film, a continuous (moving) image can be seen. This process is called fluoroscopy and can be very useful when examining situations that involve movement, such as swallowing, or the injection of a radiopaque dye into the patient.
4. Scintillation counters are devices that convert x-ray photons into visible light photons and then use a photomultiplier section to amplify the visible light. This means that acceptable x-ray images can be obtained with lower doses of x-rays.
5. Digital detectors using CCDs (charge coupled devices) similar to those found in digital cameras (but larger) can be designed to detect x-rays. Due to the sensitivity of these devices, lower x-ray doses can be used to produce adequate results, and resolutions are available that can rival that of x-ray film. Because CCDs produce digital signals, the x-ray images are then available for digital manipulation, storage, or transmission to other areas.

5. Effects and Dosage Limits

X-radiation is ionizing radiation; that is, it can remove electrons from the atoms of the material it strikes. This has significant effects on living tissue, in that it can cause burns as an immediate effect, or it can cause damage to the chromosomes of some cells, possibly causing or allowing them to become cancerous. For these reasons, dosage limits have been set for x-ray exposure. Some values relating to x-ray exposure (U.S. values; most other jurisdictions are similar):

- 1 mSv — the recommended maximum annual dose for individuals in the general public
- 20 mSv — the recommended maximum five-year-averaged annual dose for workers in radiation industries
- 50 mSv — the recommended maximum single-year dose for workers in radiation industries

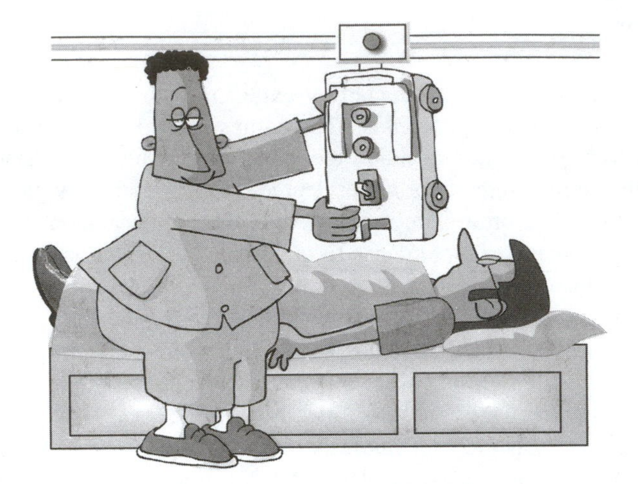

FIGURE 5.2 Fun with x-rays. (Modified from Inmagine Corp, www.123rf.com, with permission.)

- 100 mSv — the dose that gives a 0.5% chance of causing cancer later in life
- 1 Sv — the dose that gives a 5% chance of causing cancer later in life
- 10 Sv — the dose that may cause death within days or weeks

People who work in radiation environments, such as x-ray technologists, wear exposure badges that must be read regularly to ensure dose limits are not exceeded.

6. X-Ray Safety

Great efforts are made to reduce exposures to patients and staff, including the use of lead shields and lead aprons to protect the areas of patient's bodies that are not being x-rayed; lead aprons for staff when they are in the immediate vicinity of x-rays; leaded glass and walls for staff observation areas; and lead shielding in the outside walls, doors, and windows of x-ray rooms.

7. X-Ray Procedures

X-rays are used in a wide variety of situations in health care, with machines that range from simple, inexpensive dental x-ray units to room-filling, multimillion-dollar computed tomography (CT) scanners (Figure 5.2).

a. *Dental X-Rays*

Dentists are only concerned with teeth, and dental x-ray units are specialized for taking x-rays of teeth, to show root structure, filling, and crown placement, locations of decay, and other conditions. The machines are limited to relatively low voltages and currents, often having only a few preset exposures available (Figure 5.3).

They are relatively small and light and can be mounted on wheeled stands so they can be moved to different areas. They generally operate on power from wall outlets.

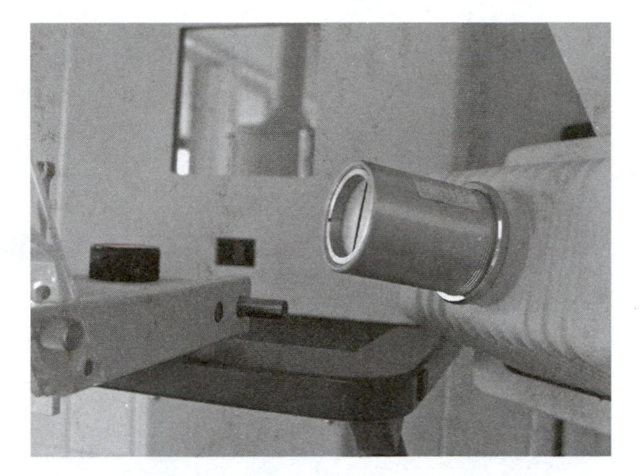

FIGURE 5.3 Dental x-ray unit. (Modified from Inmagine Corp, www.123rf.com, with permission.)

b. General-Purpose X-Ray Rooms

These are the most common x-ray units in hospitals, and can be used for a variety of applications, from taking x-rays of small structures like hands or feet, to chest and abdomen x-rays, to studies of larger skeletal components. They usually have a table that can be moved in three dimensions, as well as a head that can move in three dimensions plus rotate around two axes (Figure 5.4).

The table can also tilt, and it contains slots for film cassettes or digital detectors.

Some units have a second detector section mounted vertically on a wall, for doing studies in which the subject must be standing.

X-ray heads contain the x-ray tube as well as a collimator, a device that can open or close to limit the area of exposure (Figure 5.5). Collimators usually have lights in them that illuminate the same area that the x-ray exposure will cover, with grids to aid in placement (Figure 5.6).

Standard x-ray rooms can be used for procedures using radiopaque liquids and dyes. The liquids, usually a barium suspension, can be given to the patient as a drink, for studying the upper digestive system, or as an enema, for studying the lower system (Figure 5.7).

Dyes may be injected into the blood stream to follow cardiac arteries; some dyes are rapidly excreted by the kidneys and can be used to obtain more details of the renal system.

c. Mammography

Mammograms are x-rays specifically designed to detect breast cancer and other breast disorders. Since the tissues involved are soft, only low levels of x-rays are needed, with doses only around 0.7 mSv.

Mammography is most effective when the x-rays pass though a wide but thin area, and so the units include a mechanism to compress the breasts horizontally and then vertically while images are taken (Figures 5.8 and 5.9).

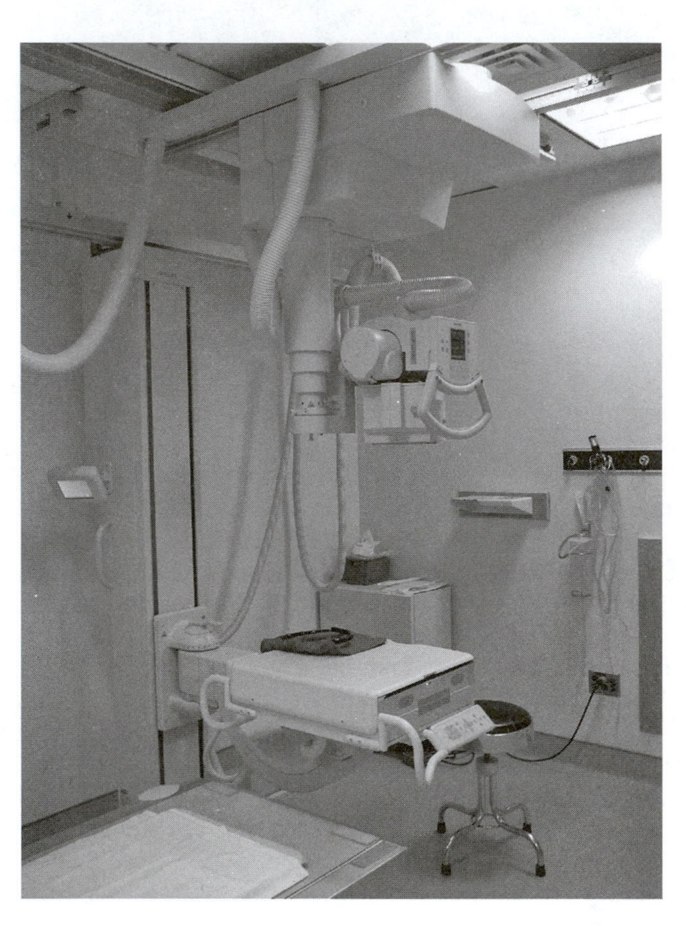

FIGURE 5.4 A typical room x-ray system.

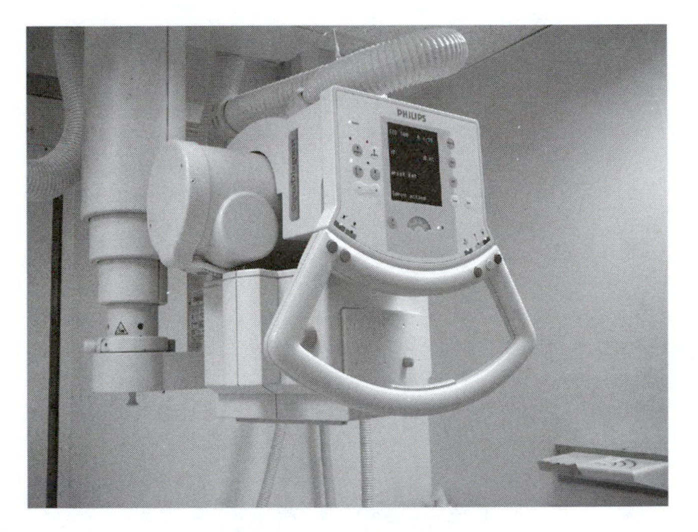

FIGURE 5.5 X-ray head containing the tube and collimator.

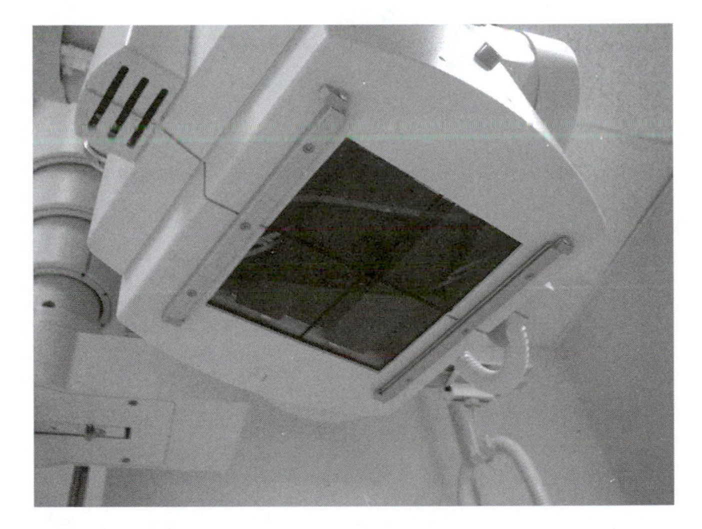

FIGURE 5.6 View of a collimator from below.

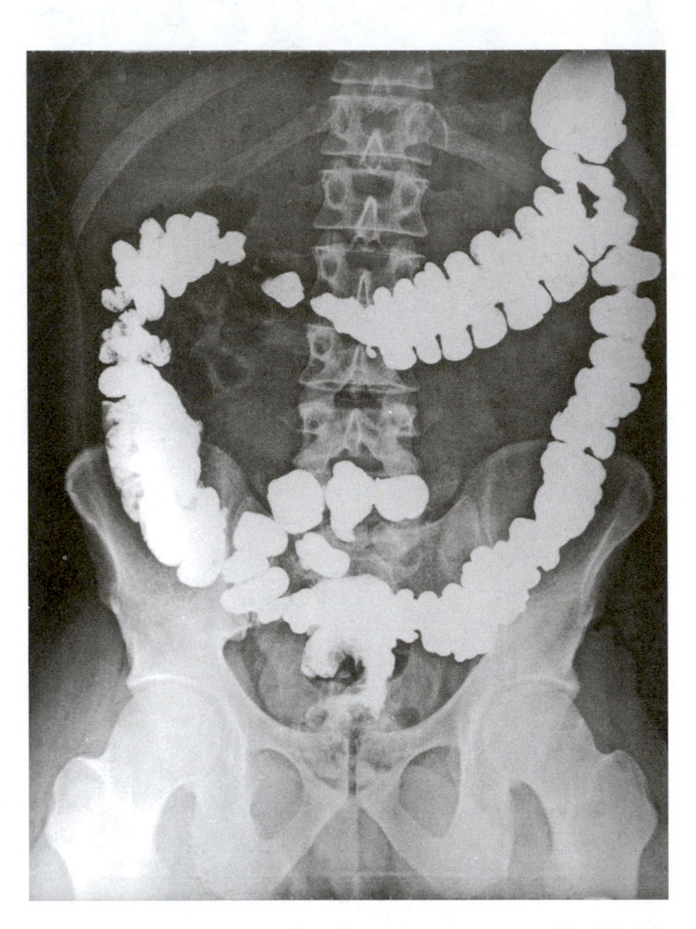

FIGURE 5.7 X-ray image of a colon with barium contrast agent. (Modified from Inmagine Corp, www.123rf.com, with permission.)

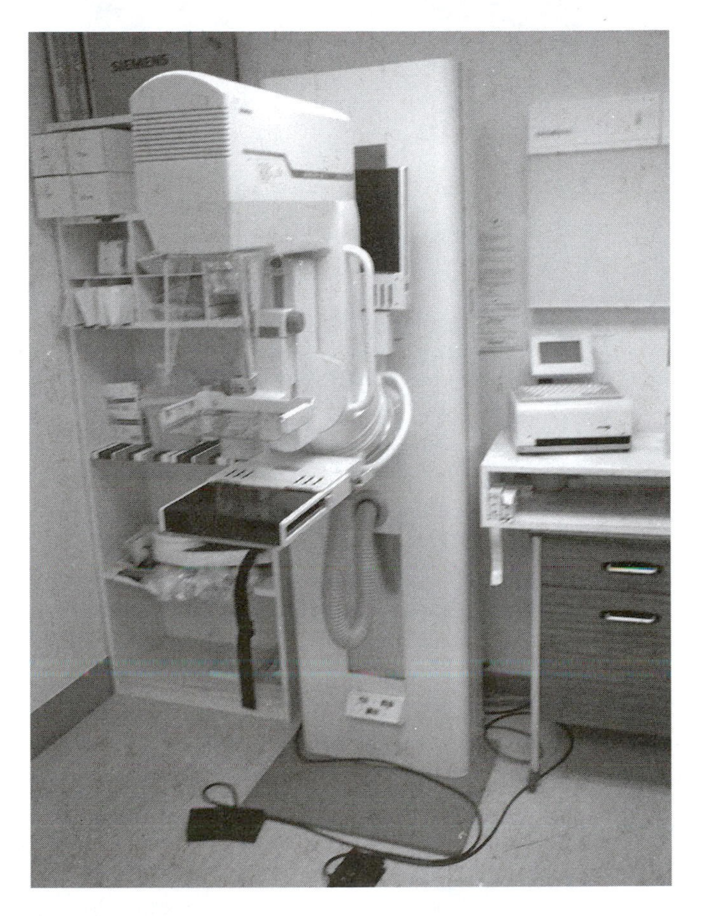

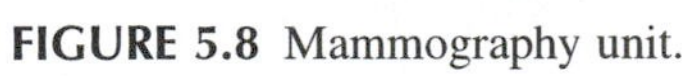
FIGURE 5.8 Mammography unit.

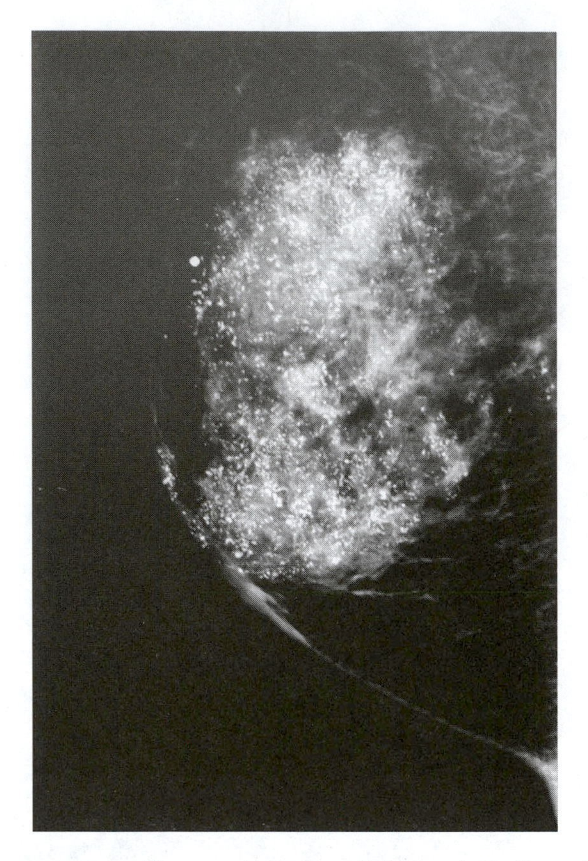

FIGURE 5.9 A mammogram film — note the large light area indicating a tumor. (Modified from Inmagine Corp, www.123rf.com, with permission.)

d. Computerized (Axial) Tomography Scanners

CT or CAT scanners evolved from simpler tomography units, which moved the x-ray head in circles while exposures were made to produce a "slice" of image, rather than a "shadow" as do normal x-rays (Figure 5.10).

CT units take this several steps further, with an x-ray tube that can produce a "fan" of x-rays and a large number of detectors arranged in a large ring. Each detector picks up part of the x-ray fan that passes through one axis. Some systems have many detectors (up to 64 sets) that can process image data separately, producing multiple slices at once.

The patient lies on a table that can move in and out of the ring, stopping at locations where imaging is needed. An exposure is made, and each detector feeds its information into a computer, which combines the data from all detectors and constructs a "slice" that represents the structures found transversely through the patient at that location.

Slices are repeated through the area of interest and can be studied individually, or as a "movie" of a cross-section passing through the body.

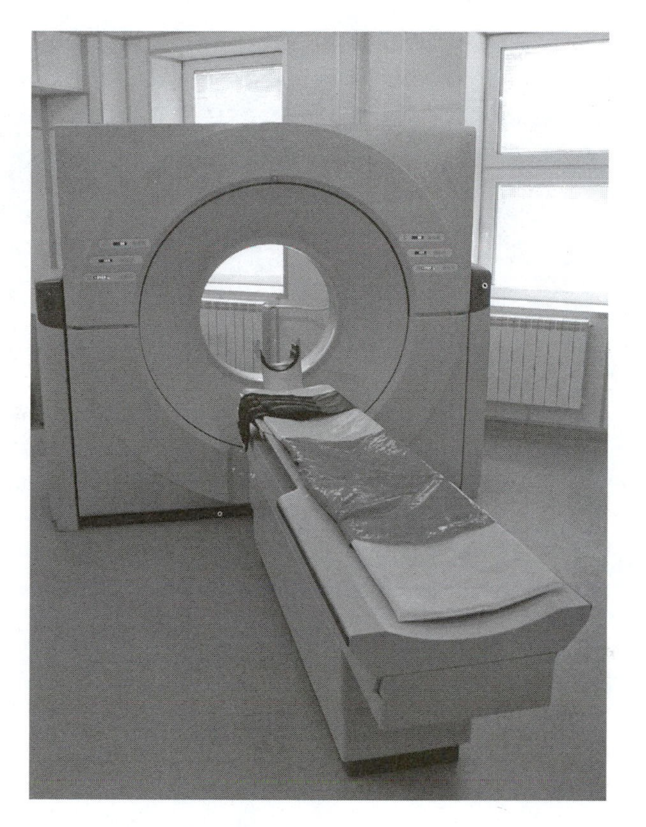

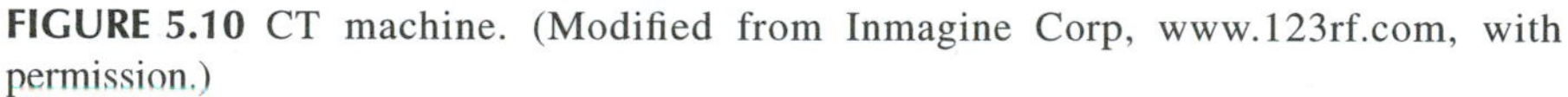

FIGURE 5.10 CT machine. (Modified from Inmagine Corp, www.123rf.com, with permission.)

Newer systems with more computing power can complete more slices, more quickly, and can also combine the data from multiple slices to create a three-dimensional model of specific structures (Figure 5.11). The 3-D data can also be used to perform virtual dissections, with the operator "removing" different sections or layers of tissue to expose something of interest, such as a tumor.

B. Magnetic Resonance Imaging Scanners

Though images produced by MRI scanners (Figure 5.12) may look similar to those from a CT machine, the principles of operation are quite different. Originally called nuclear magnetic resonance imaging (NMRI) scanners, they operate on the basis of atoms having magnetic properties. The "nuclear" part of the name was dropped because patients were fearful of anthing nuclear.

The details of MRI theory involve complex nuclear physics and a lot of esoteric math, but for our purposes a few basic ideas will hopefully make the technology somewhat understandable.

"Spin" is a fundamental property of matter, in the same way as mass or electrical charge are fundamental properties, though not as apparent in everyday experience.

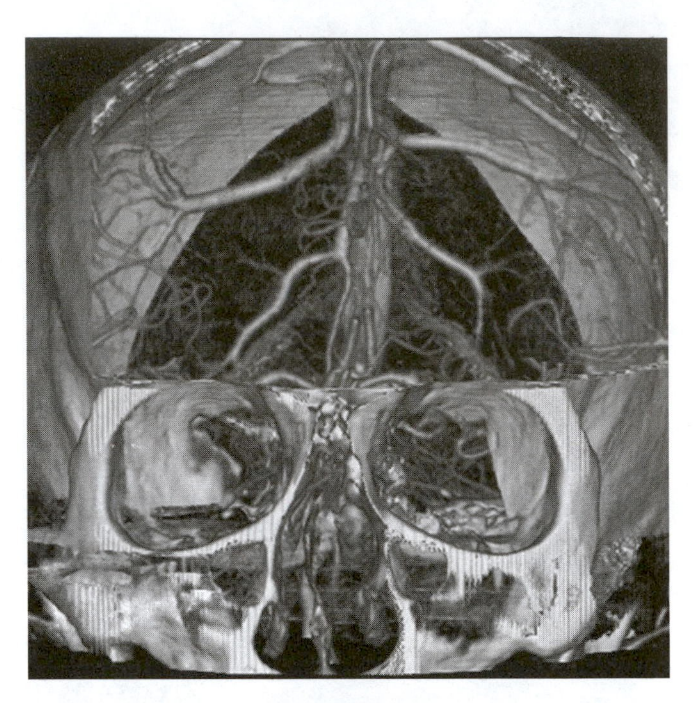

FIGURE 5.11 Three-dimensional CT image of brain and skull. (Modified from Inmagine Corp, www.123rf.com, with permission.)

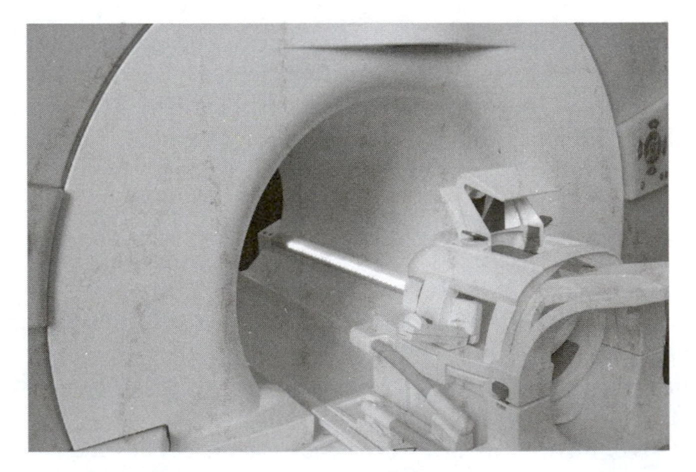

FIGURE 5.12 MRI scanner. (Modified from Inmagine Corp, www.123rf.com, with permission.)

Electrons, protons, and neutrons when on their own each have a spin value of $^1/_2$, and this can be either positive or negative.

When particles combine to form atoms or molecules, the spin values of each particle sum together. Thus the total spin value of an atom or molecule can be various positive or negative multiples of one half, or if the positive and negative spin particles balance out, the sum can be zero.

Atoms or molecules with a nonzero spin sum can be affected by a magnetic field. They act something like tiny magnets themselves and align with the applied magnetic field. Hydrogen atoms are an example of a nonzero spin sum material.

The magnetic fields in MRI units are generated by superconducting electromagnets. Field strength is usually about 2 to 4 teslas. (By comparison, the Earth's magnetic field has a strength of about 50 microteslas).

Molecules aligned in a magnetic field can be in a high-energy state, as if the north poles of both the magnetic field and the molecule point in the same direction (as do the south poles), or a low-energy state, in which the field and molecular north poles point in opposite directions.

If the various aligned molecules in the magnetic field are hit with a pulse of electromagnetic radiation (EMR; radio waves), some of the low-energy state molecules will absorb the EMR energy and jump up to the high-energy state. Afterward, some of the high-energy-state molecules will fall back to the low-energy state and emit electromagnetic radiation of their own. The frequency of radiation is typical of the particle absorbing or emitting it, so hydrogen atoms will absorb/emit a different frequency of radiation than, for example, atoms of sodium-23, another nonzero-sum particle that is relatively abundant in the human body.

By detecting, measuring, and analyzing the radiation emitted in this manner, an image can be developed of the nonzero-sum materials in the magnetic field (Figure 5.13).

Since hydrogen atoms constitute a large proportion of the nonzero-sum particles in the human body, a map or model of hydrogen distribution can be produced. Further, since different tissues have different amounts of hydrogen in them, tissue structures can be determined.

Using a different EMR frequency to pulse the particles in the magnetic field will produce maps of different particles, each of which can provide its own set of useful information. The resonant frequency of the particles to be examined must be known; this is the frequency used to study that particle's distribution.

Other nonzero-spin particles include the isotopes carbon-13, oxygen-17, and phosphorus-31. Some of the useful isotopes can be administered to the patient to increase their numbers in the body. For example, water made up of oygen-17 atoms can be simply ingested and distributed throughout the body just like normal oxygen-16 water.

Special isotopes used in MRI studies are generated in research facilities with such equipment as linear accelerators.

The powerful magnetic fields used in MRI systems will attract any magnetic material in the vicinity, accelerating it toward the center of the field, sometimes with disastrous results. Such materials, therefore, must be completely absent from the imaging vicinity.

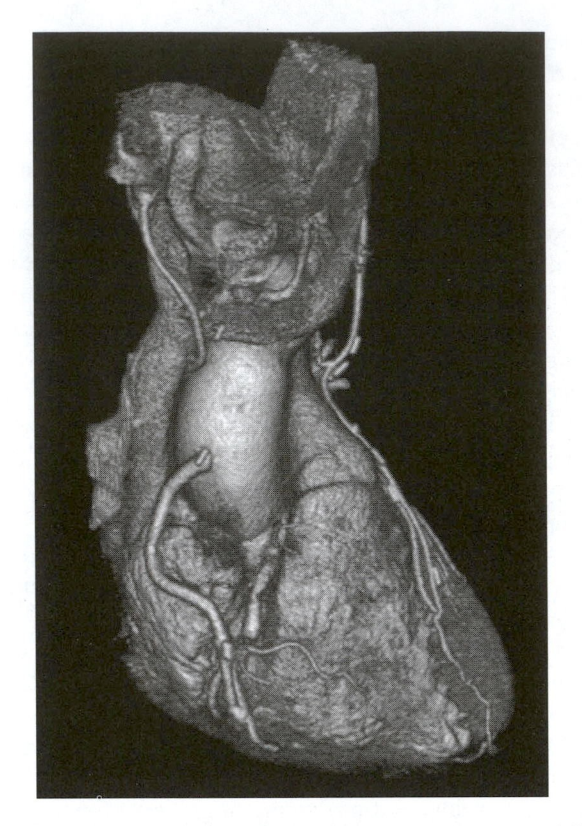

FIGURE 5.13 Three-dimensional MRI scan of a heart. (Modified from Philips Medical, CD provided directly, with permission. © 2006 Koninidijke Philips Electronics N.V. All rights reserved. Reproduction in whole or in part is prohibited without prior written permission of the copyright owner.)

The EMR signal is very powerful, as well, and can act like a microwave oven, overheating the patient.

Such devices as implanted pacemakers will react very negatively to MRI.

C. Positron Emission Tomography

When a radioactive isotope decays, it emits a positron (an antielectron, having the same mass as an electron but a positive charge) as radiation. The positron soon collides with an electron, and they are mutually annihilated, emitting two photons in exactly opposite directions in the process. These photons can be detected with two scintillation scanners placed opposite each other. If two photons are detected 180 degrees apart from each other and within a few nanoseconds of each other, they are from the same isotope decay event, and the axis of their travel can be determined.

By averaging thousands of such events, an image of the tissue structure containing the isotope can be formed.

Different isotopes are absorbed by different tissues, and so by choosing the appropriate isotope, images of these tissues can be made.

PET scanners can be integrated with other imaging equipment such as MRI or CT scanners, and when scans using the two different techniques are done simultaneously, the PET image can be placed in context with the more comprehensive but less specific MRI or CT image.

Isotopes may be taken up by tissues depending on their rate of metabolism, so PET scans can provide information about these rates. Cancer tumors, for example, often have much higher metabolic rates than other, surrounding tissues.

The radioactive isotopes, or radionuclides, have a very short half-life. For example, carbon-11 has a half-life of about 2 minutes, while fluorine-18 is relatively long-lived with a half-life of about 110 minutes. The short half-lives mean that the radionuclides must be produced very near the PET scanner, and delivered to the patient immediately after production.

The isotopes are produced in a huge device called a cyclotron.

D. Diagnostic Ultrasound

X-rays have the potential of causing tissue and genetic damage, especially in a developing fetus. Imaging of the fetus is important in monitoring development, however, so means were explored to accomplish this without using x-rays.

Ultrasound proved to be such a technology, and scanners were developed to produce two-dimensional slices of the fetus in utero (Figure 5.14).

Technological advances gave higher-quality images and also allowed the data from many two-dimensional scans to be combined to form a three-dimensional image.

Fetal ultrasound machines (Figure 5.15) use heads with multiple piezoelectric crystals, and different frequencies of heads are used to scan at different depths.

Similar machines have been optimized for cardiac imaging as well as for other specialized applications.

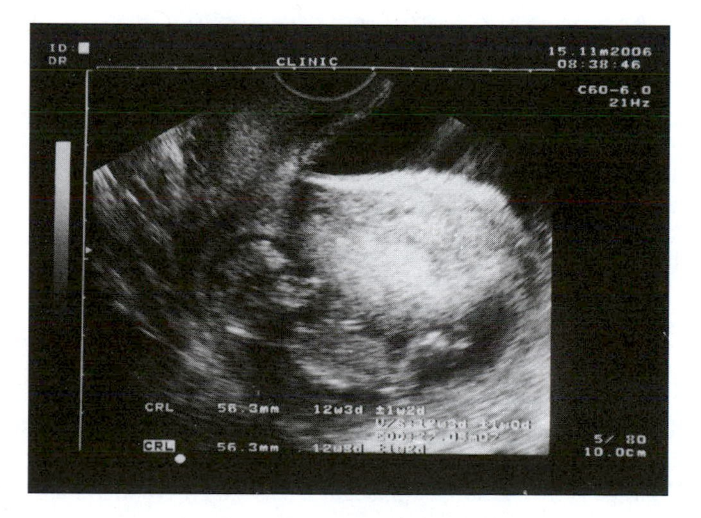

FIGURE 5.14 An early fetal ultrasound image — note indistinct images. (Modified from Inmagine Corp, www.123rf.com, with permission.)

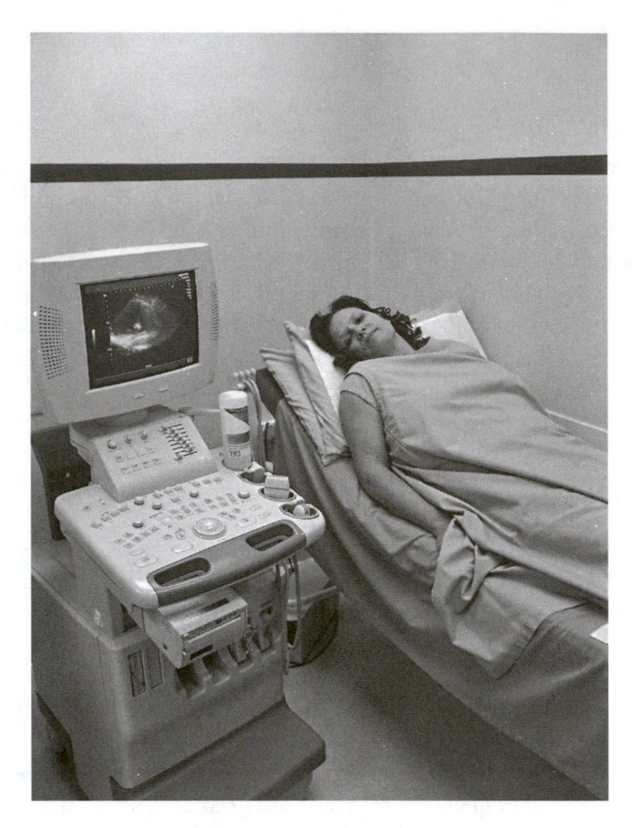

FIGURE 5.15 Woman awaiting an ultrasound exam. (Modified from Inmagine Corp, www.123rf.com, with permission.)

E. Picture Archiving and Communication System

With the advent of digital image techniques, powerful and relatively inexpensive computers, and high-speed data networks, it became possible to handle diagnostic images in a coordinated manner. Images could be stored, distributed, and presented in a consistent format, allowing various medical personnel to have access to high-quality images from many different locations.

Such systems came to be called picture archiving and communication systems, or PACS.

Any digital image can be handled with a PACS system, including x-rays and CT, MRI, PET and ultrasound scans, as well as endoscopy or microsurgery images.

Specialists can evaluate images from a distant location where such expertise may not be available, without the delays and inconvenience of having to ship hard-copy images from place to place. Various people can look at the same image simultaneously for collaborative or educational purposes.

Digital storage is much more compact and less expensive than the huge archives used in keeping traditional film images.

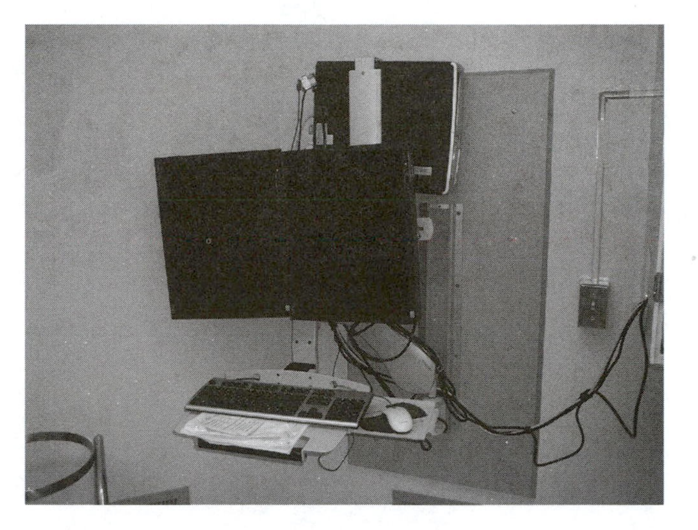

FIGURE 5.16 PACS terminal.

A PACS network consists of a central server connected to various client workstations though a local and/or wide area network. Several PACS systems can be connected together, and the Internet can also be used as a communications channel.

Because diagnostic images are large and of high resolution, system data rates must be high enough to allow image transfers in reasonable time periods.

Workstations must be capable of displaying images at diagnostic-quality levels and be able to handle them quickly. Two video displays are usually included to allow comparison of images (Figure 5.16).

The central server stores images in a database and handles requests for access to existing images or storage of new images. Functions such as database maintenance, including data backup and system upkeep, are performed as with any other database.

Since images can come from many sources, there must be a very effective means of naming and organizing them.

II. CHAPTER SUMMARY

Chapter 5 covers the field of diagnostic imaging. A history of x-rays is provided along with some of the physics involved. Various x-ray technologies, dose limits, and safety are examined.

Specialized scanners like CT, MRI, PET, and diagnostic ultrasound are described.

Finally, the picture archiving and communication system (PACS) is discussed.

6 Treatment Devices — Part One

I. HEART

As the heart is the most intensely monitored organ in the body, it is also the most intensively treated, with a variety of devices used to stabilize or improve the function of a patient's damaged or diseased heart.

A. Defibrillators

The defibrillator (or "defib") is perhaps the most recognized high-tech medical device, thanks to movies and television (Figure 6.1). A doctor holds paddles over a dying patient. She yells "clear" and then places the paddles on the patient's chest. The patient's body jerks spasmodically, and the steady beep–beep of monitor resumes — or perhaps a flat line on a screen changes to a familiar waveform.

The popular perception is that a defibrillator is used to "restart" a heart that has stopped beating, but its name implies something different. Though occasionally a "flatliner" can be revived with a defib, it is most commonly used to change the uncoordinated contractions of the heart (fibrillation) into a normal sinus rhythm — that is, to defibrillate the heart (Figure 6.2).

In this section, we will briefly review the history of defibrillators, and examine the theory of operation and application of a modern device. The various types of defibrillators in use will be surveyed, along with the options and accessories that are available. Finally, we will consider the types of batteries used in defibs and look at the testing and maintenance requirements of the devices.

1. History

The history of the defibrillator is closely tied to the history of the electrocardiograph (see Chapter 2). Scientists and physicians first needed to understand how the heart functioned, especially from the perspective of electrical signals and muscle contractions, before they could attempt to devise a means of treating the often-fatal interruptions of normal cardiac contractions.

In 1947, after six failed attempts on other patients, Claude Beck, a cardiovascular surgeon in Cleveland, successfully defibrillates the heart of a 14-year-old boy during cardiac surgery. In this case, the impulse from the defibrillation equipment was applied directly to the patient's heart.

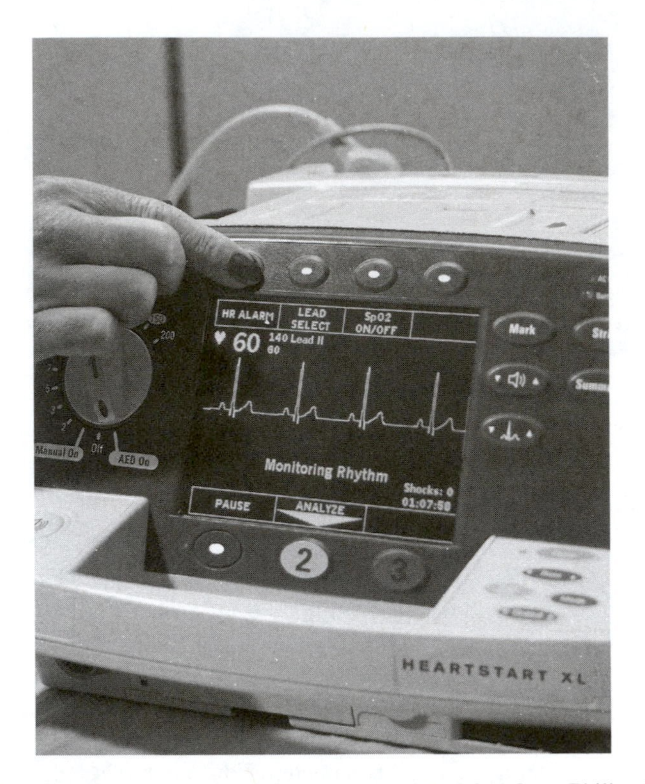

FIGURE 6.1 A typical portable defibrillator/monitor. (Modified from Philips Medical, CD provided directly, with permission. © 2006 Koninidijke Philips Electronics N.V. All rights reserved. Reproduction in whole or in part is prohibited without prior written permission of the copyright owner.)

In 1956, Paul Zoll, a cardiologist, using a more powerful defibrillator, is able to successfully defibrillate a patient by applying the defibrillator impulse externally — through the chest walls.

Research and development of defibrillators took place in Britain and the USSR, as well, including the first mobile unit built in Belfast to be used in ambulances.

2. Theory of Operation

As discussed in Chapter 1, fibrillation is the rapid, irregular, and unsynchronized contraction of the muscle fibers of the heart. Generally, fibrillation is of one of two types.

In atrial fibrillation (Figure 6.3), the atrial chambers of the heart are not contracting in an effective way, while the ventricles continue to function normally. Since the ventricles do most of the work of pumping blood, this is not usually a life-threatening condition, though it is debilitating. Correcting atrial fibrillation, a procedure sometimes called cardioversion or synchronized cardioversion, is not an emergency and is usually done in a calm, controlled clinical situation.

Ventricular fibrillation (or V fib.) results when the ventricles are contracting in a nonsynchronized manner (see Figure 6.4). Because ventricular fibrillation results

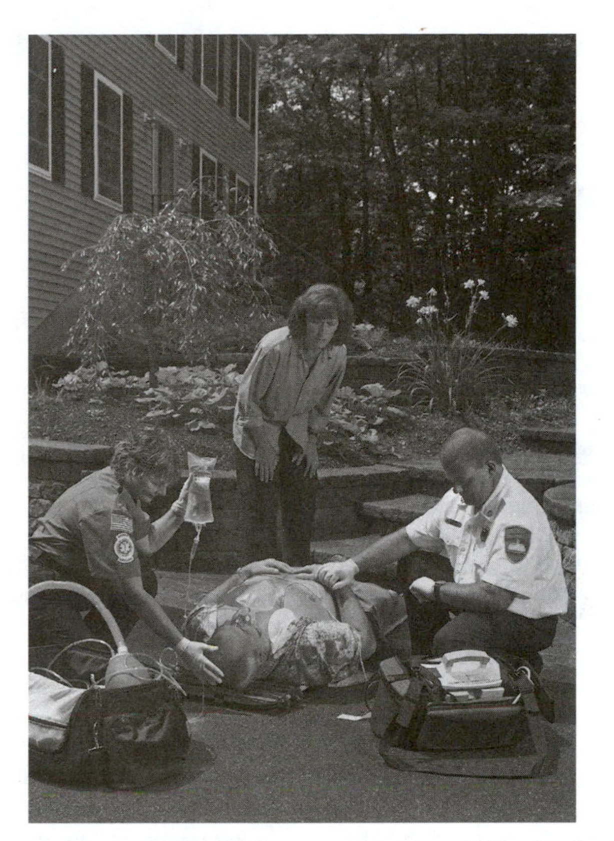

FIGURE 6.2 Paramedics using a defibrillator. (Modified from Philips Medical, CD provided directly, with permission.

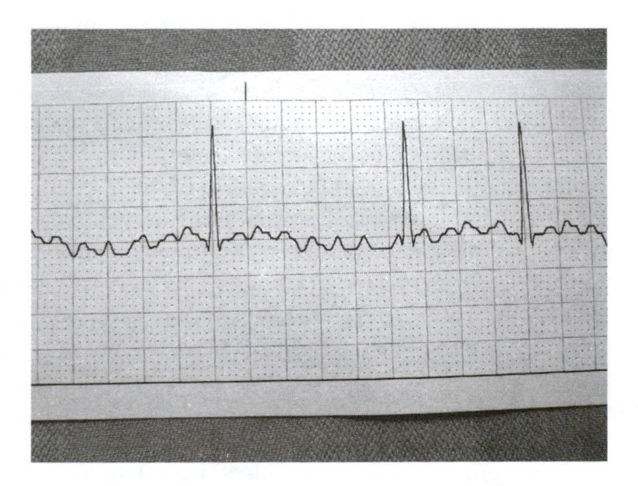

FIGURE 6.3 Atrial fibrillation waveform.

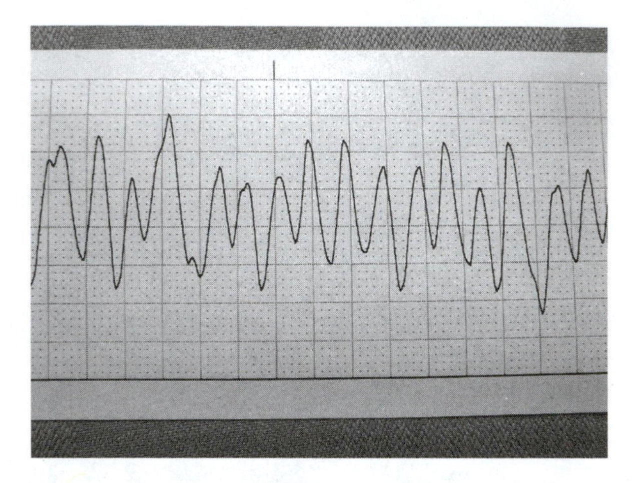

FIGURE 6.4 Ventricular fibrillation waveform.

in an almost complete cessation of blood flow from the heart, it is rapidly fatal if not reversed by defibrillation. This is an emergency procedure, and is often done after a session of cardiopulmonary resuscitation (CPR).

3. Function

Defibrillators function by delivering a short pulse of electric current to the heart. This pulse of current polarizes all of the muscle and nerve cells in the heart simultaneously and (hopefully) allows them to resume normal operation — that is, to produce coordinated contractions in the heart so that blood is pumped through the body.

A defibrillator consists of an energy source, circuitry to control the energy, and a means of delivering the energy to the heart.

a. Energy Source

The first defibrillators in clinical use derived power from AC (line) outlets and were bulky and heavy.

This meant that power was available continuously, but units were limited to operation near an outlet, and since defibrillators were often required in locations where outlets were not available, smaller, lighter battery powered units were soon developed. (Batteries are discussed in more detail in Chapter 11.)

Batteries used in defibrillators must meet a number of requirements. They must be able to supply an adequate amount of power; they must be reliable and safe; they must be able to be recharged many times; and they must be of reasonably light weight.

As battery technology evolved, different battery types were used in defibs. Early units employed nickel–cadmium (NiCad or NiCd) batteries, which had good energy density when new but were prone to developing a "memory," which prevented them from providing full power. Newer NiCd battery designs and sophisticated charging circuitry help to alleviate this problem.

Sealed lead acid batteries, which use a gelled electrolyte to prevent spills and allow operation in any orientation, have also been commonly used in defibrillator design. Their high degree of reliability made up for their relatively low energy density. Lead acid batteries generally do not do well if they are fully discharged and/or left in a discharged state for prolonged periods, and therefore should be charged immediately after use for best performance.

Lithium-ion and nickel–metal hydride batteries, having high energy density and low susceptibility to memory problems, are increasingly being used to power defibrillators; however they too must be treated carefully to ensure long and reliable operation.

b. Voltage Multiplier

The batteries powering defibrillators typically provide 12 volts DC, while the discharge to the patient is a specifically shaped wave that may have an amplitude of several thousand volts. The battery voltage must therefore be boosted to around 5000 volts. This is applied to a capacitor, which stores the electrical energy until it is delivered to the patient. Circuitry to accomplish this typically chops the DC into a square wave and passes this waveform through a high-ratio step-up transformer. The high-voltage AC waveform is then rectified and used to charge the storage capacitor.

c. Charge Storage

A capacitor with high voltage and capacitance ratings is used to hold the electrical energy until it is delivered to the patient. This capacitor must be of high quality in order to reliably and repeatedly store energy and release it at a high rate.

d. Waveforms

The first attempts to defibrillate patients used alternating (sinusoidal) current applied through paddles directly to the heart. Appropriate voltage levels had been determined in animal experiments, and further testing indicated that some type of DC waveform was more effective than AC — that is, less energy was required and success was more frequent with DC than with AC, which meant greater patient survival rates and less chance of burns.

In the early 1960s, positive-going, pulsed (monophasic) defibrillation waveforms were widely adopted by most defibrillator manufacturers. These waveforms, referred to as Edmark (the most common) or Lown waveforms after their inventors, were used until about 2000, when research showed that a biphasic waveform with both positive and negative components could provide effective results with lower power, thereby increasing patient safety while also reducing demands on batteries and other components.

Note that the period of these waveforms is a few milliseconds (biphasic longer than monophasic), while their amplitude may range from a few volts to several hundred volts depending on the application.

e. Discharge Relay

When it is time to deliver the defibrillation shock to the patient, a relay is activated to connect the charge storage capacitor to the wave-shaping circuitry and then through the paddles or electrodes to the patient. This relay must meet specific requirements. It has to be fast acting to make the charge available in a sufficiently short time. The contacts must be carefully designed to be able to withstand many high-current, high-voltage surges. Finally, the housing must be airtight to prevent open sparks in case flammable agents are being used in the vicinity.

f. Wave Shaping

Charge capacitors deliver a simple DC surge. In order to convert this into the required waveform, an array of inductors, capacitors, and resistors are used (an LRC circuit).

g. Paddles and Electrodes

In order to deliver to the patient the large amount of electrical energy required to produce effective defibrillation, a large surface area must be used so the current densities are low enough to prevent burns. External defibrillator paddles (Figure 6.5) typically have a smooth, flat, stainless steel face, and most manufacturers have smaller paddles or small slip-on attachments to accommodate pediatric patients. Conductive (saline) gel is used to help ensure even, low-impedance contact between the paddles and the patient's skin.

Defibrillation may also be performed during open-heart surgery, in which case much lower energies are needed. Being able to safely and effectively apply the paddles to a living heart requires that the paddles have relatively small, cupped faces,

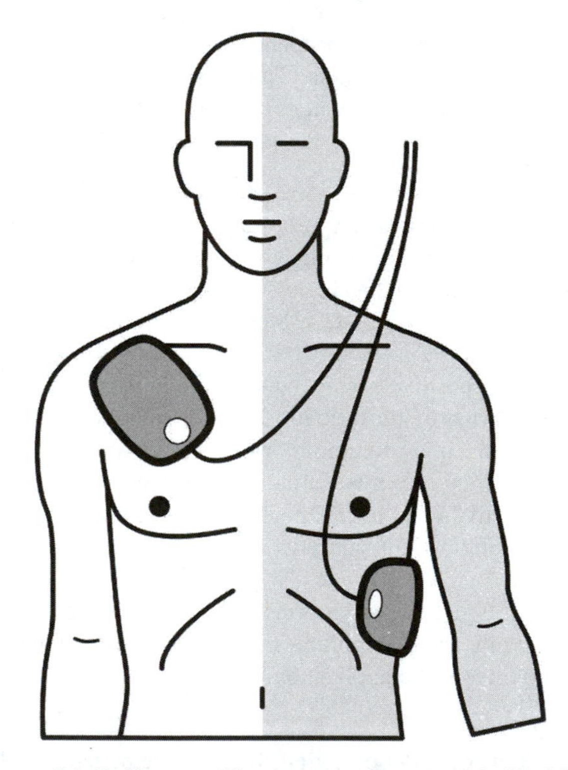

FIGURE 6.5 External defibrillator paddle placement diagram. (Modified from Philips Medical, CD provided directly, with permission. © 2006 Koninidijke Philips Electronics N.V. All rights reserved. Reproduction in whole or in part is prohibited without prior written permission of the copyright owner.)

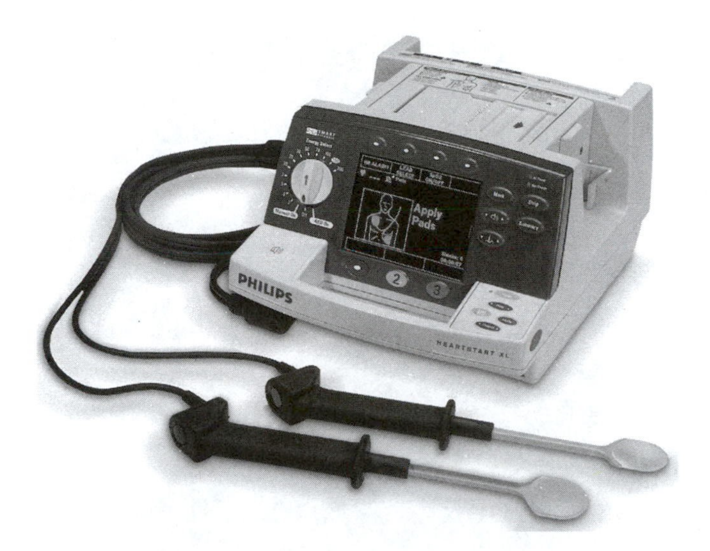

FIGURE 6.6 A defibrillator with internal paddles. (Modified from Philips Medical, CD provided directly, with permission. © 2006 Koninidijke Philips Electronics N.V. All rights reserved. Reproduction in whole or in part is prohibited without prior written permission of the copyright owner.)

with long, insulated handles (Figure 6.6). Defibrillators may have the ability to detect which type of paddle is attached and limit the maximum available energy if pediatric or internal paddles are being used.

If repeated defibrillations may be required (for example in cases of atrial fibrillation where the patient is subjected to many bouts of fibrillation), it may be more effective and convenient to apply adhesive electrodes to the patient's chest. If the patient is also undergoing external cardiac pacing, these electrodes may serve to deliver both defibrillating and pacing pulses. Automatic external defibrillators (AEDs), for use in situations where trained medical personnel may not be available, also use adhesive pads in order to simplify procedures.

"Code blue, third floor, room 315. Code blue, third floor, room 315. Code blue, third floor, room 315."

The calm but forceful voice rings through the overhead paging system throughout the hospital, and members of the code blue team react instinctively, moving quickly but carefully to the announced location.

By the time the ER physician arrives, someone has delivered a crash cart (Figure 6.7) to the patient's bedside, and there is a flurry of activity. A nurse is performing CPR, while a respiratory therapist waits to intubate the patient with an endotracheal tube, should that be necessary.

Other staff members are monitoring vital signs and preparing to provide a description of the patient, as well as the patient's condition and medications and the events leading up to the arrest, as far as they are known. Someone gets

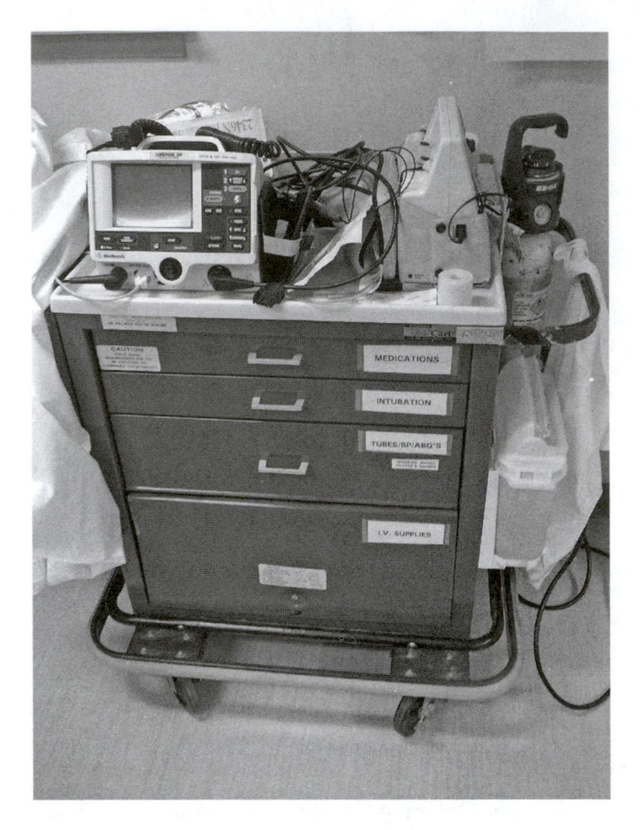

FIGURE 6.7 Crash cart.

a suction tube ready and easily accessible, another readies an oxygen supply, while syringes of epinephrine, atropine, and lidocaine are made ready for direct injection or, if there is time, administration via an intravenous line. Other medications area available in the crash cart drawers. A lab tech draws a sample of blood and rushes it to the lab for quick analysis of blood chemistry.

Most of the team members perform their tasks quickly and efficiently, with a minimum of confusion, though some of the newer members and students hang back, watching and trying not to get in the way.

The patient is a young man who had been in a car accident and who had appeared to be recovering well. His bed covers have been pulled away, and his hospital pajamas unceremoniously cut off, so that his chest is exposed. A bandage covers part of his left side where crumpled metal had pierced his skin, breaking three ribs. ECG electrodes have been applied in locations that won't interfere with defibrillation, and they are connected to the defib, where a jumbled tracing appears on the display.

The ER doctor gets a very quick rundown of the patient and current information and then asks the respiratory therapist (RT) to intubate while she selects a syringe (Figure 6.8) of epinephrine from the crash cart, noting that an intravenous line has now been started.

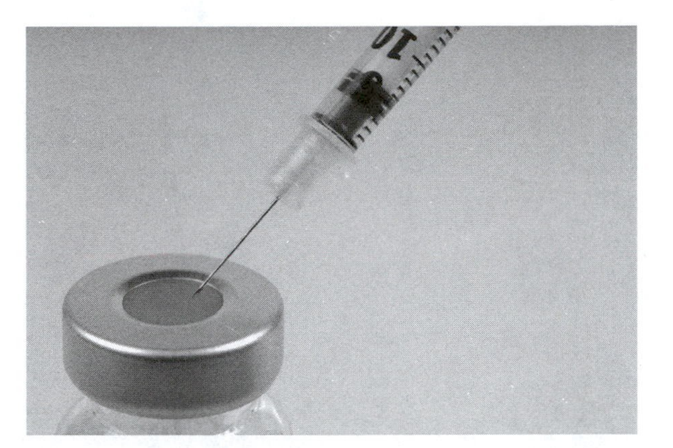

FIGURE 6.8 Syringe.

Epinephrine is injected into the IV line, and the doctor picks up the defibrillator paddles. A team member applies conductive gel to one paddle surface, and the doctor rubs the paddle faces together lightly to distribute the gel evenly, then places the paddles on the patient's chest (Figure 6.9). A small diagram on the paddle handles shows optimum placement locations, but the physician has done enough codes to know exactly where they go, only having to modify her right hand paddle position in order to avoid the bandages on the patient.

"200 joules," she says, and a nurse turns a knob on the front of the defibrillator to 200. The doctor presses a button on one handle, and a whining noise comes from the defib, increasing in pitch along with increasing numbers on the display that show how much energy is being stored in the unit. When the number reaches 200, the tone changes to a louder, steady pitch.

In a loud, clear voice tinged with tension, the doctor calls out, "I am going to shock on three; One, I am clear; Two, you are clear; Three, everybody is clear,"

A glance around shows that everyone is ready.

"One! Two! Three!"

Pressing a button on each paddle handle simultaneously causes a clunking noise to come from the defib, while at the same time the patient's body jerks spasmodically as a result of some stray defibrillation current stimulating skeletal muscles. A strip of paper starts to stream out of the defib, showing the ECG waveforms from 20 seconds prior to the discharge, with a mark indicating the exact time of the discharge along with a measure of energy delivered and patient impedance.

The display on the screen has wavered but is still indicating VFib, so the doctor asks for 300 joules, and the process is repeated, again without success. CPR continues between attempts, the third using the maximum available energy, 360 joules. The first attempt at this level fails, but the next one, after an injection of atropine, succeeds in producing a near-normal sinus rhythm.

The code team relaxes a little and goes about cleaning up the debris form the code, including gathering up the long ribbons of recording paper that will later be entered as part of the patient's record, so that the process can be analyzed.

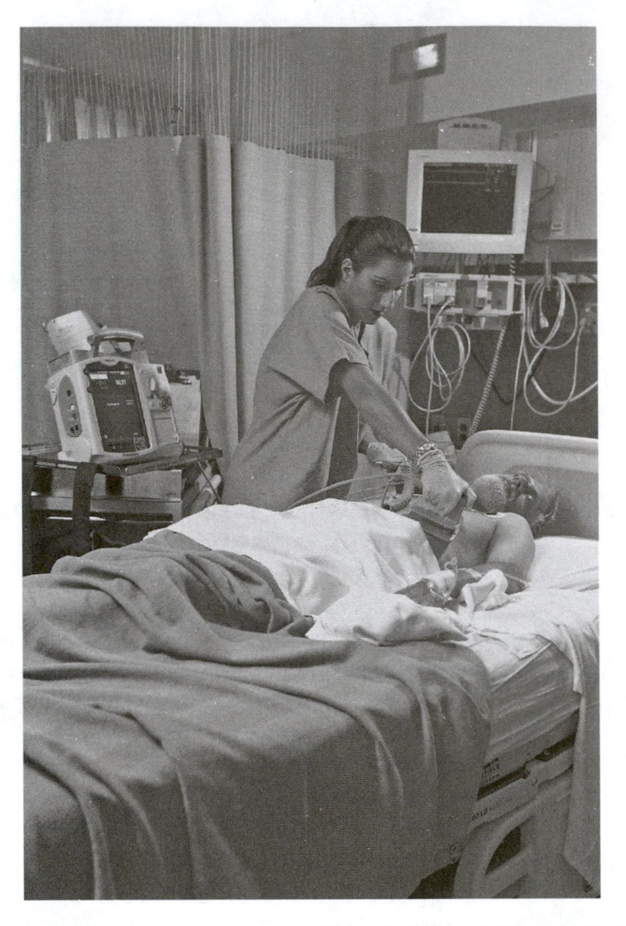

FIGURE 6.9 A defib in use in a patient room. (Modified from Philips Medical, CD provided directly, with permission. © 2006 Koninidijke Philips Electronics N.V. All rights reserved. Reproduction in whole or in part is prohibited without prior written permission of the copyright owner.)

As one of the nurses moves to the nursing station to begin the process of transferring the patient to the CCU, the ER doctor consults with a cardiologist who arrived just after all the excitement, in order to start planning a course of treatment for the patient and to try to understand why the arrest happened in the first place.

---

4. Defibrillator Types

Defibrillators can be divided into two broad categories, internal and external, while the external type can again be divided into automatic (AED) and manual groups.

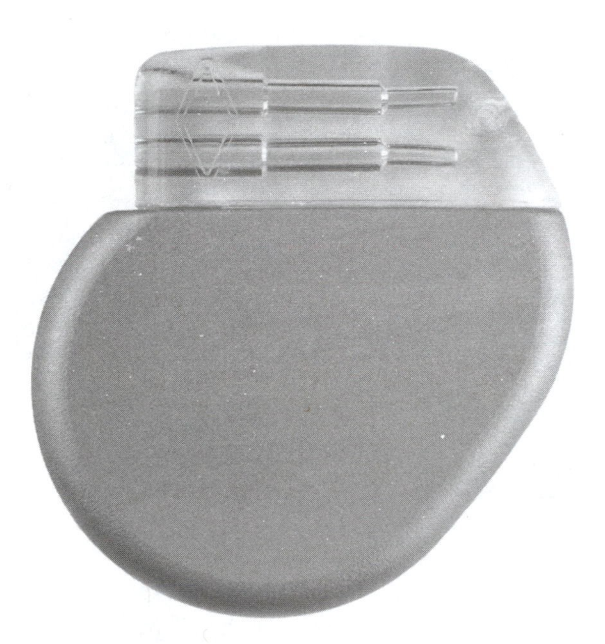

FIGURE 6.10 Implantable defibrillator. (Modified from Inmagine Corp, www.123rf.com, with permission.)

a. *Internal (Implantable) Defibrillators*

Internal defibrillators (Figure 6.10) are implanted into the patient's body, usually into a pocket made in the tissue just below the patient's clavicle, with two leads passing through a vein to the heart. Their basic function is the same as all defibrillators, but these units have a number of special requirements.

Since they are to be implanted within the body, they must be small and able to withstand fluids.

They are connected directly to the heart and thus deliver much lower levels of energy than external defibs, but since they are not directly accessible, they must have a battery that will last a very long time.

They must contain microprocessor-based circuitry that will accurately recognize ECG waveforms that indicate a need for shock delivery, as well as a radio receiver to allow for programming as well as monitoring function and battery level, and a transmitter so that stored data can be sent to an external system for analysis.

Some units have wireless connections that allow real-time monitoring of their function as well as cardiac activity.

Implantable defibrillators must be as inert biologically as possible in order to avoid rejection problems. Cases are usually made from special stainless steel alloys or titanium, and some may be coated with plastic. Leads are plastic coated, and electrode tips are usually stainless steel or some other alloy.

Some manufacturers produce units that are both defibrillators and pacemakers (see "Pacemakers," Section B of this chapter), since certain patients require both

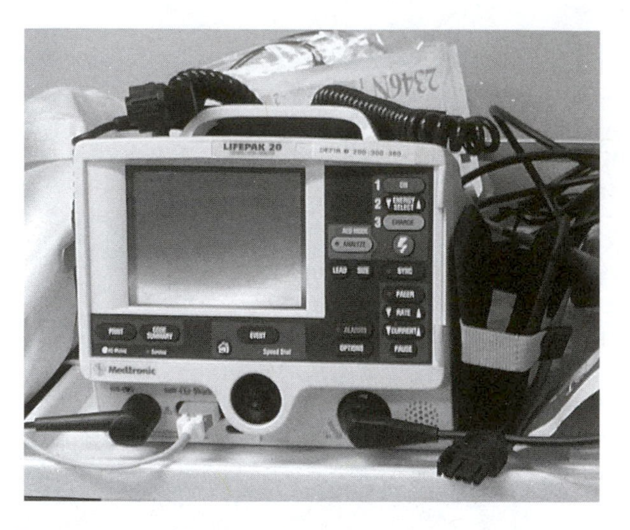

FIGURE 6.11 Defibrillator. (Modified from Inmagine Corp, www.123rf.com, with permission.)

functions. A number of components are similar in both pacemakers and defibrillators, so these components can be combined in dual-purpose units.

b. External Manual Defibrillators

These are the most common (so far) type of defibrillators (Figure 6.11), being found on crash carts and in special procedure areas of hospitals and clinics as well as in many emergency response vehicles.

Originally, external manual defibs were just defibrillators, with no other circuitry. They produced no records of the procedure, and an ECG monitor had to be used in order to see the ECG waveform. As technology evolved, features were added. First came ECG circuitry with a "bouncing ball" CRT display, then a chart recorder (which in early models had to be turned on and off manually), and more recently, extra functions such as cardiac pacing, pulse oximetry, noninvasive blood pressure, and capnography. Connectors were included to allow the ECG waveform (and later other parameters) to be transmitted to a bedside monitor or central monitoring system, or via a modem to a distant location. Alarm functions, which were nonexistent in early versions, began with basic high-low ECG settings. Paddle contact alarms and indicators helped improve patient safety and charge delivery, and low-battery warning alarms helped avoid "uh-oh" situations. Defibrillators were able to measure patient impedance and actual delivered energy.

i. ECG Measurement and Analysis

This topic is discussed in more detail in Chapter 2.

Modern defibrillators depend on the accurate automatic processing and evaluation of ECG signals in order to function effectively.

Timing discharges to cardioversion (more properly termed "synchronized cardioversion") requires that the unit be able to detect QRS complexes with a high degree of accuracy, since the relationship of the charge delivery to signal phase is critical if success is to be achieved. Harm can result if discharge timing is incorrect in atrial fibrillation, as ventricular fibrillation can be induced. Charge is ideally delivered between the R wave and the T wave of the patient's ECG.

In addition, proper evaluation of the patient's condition before and after any defibrillation effort it vital. Many new units perform some degree of automatic ECG analysis and are able to identify a variety of arrhythmias and other signal characteristics.

ii. Recorders

Clinically and, more recently, legally, it is useful and sometimes critical to have a hard-copy record of events around the time of a defibrillation attempt. Strip chart recorders have provided this function since early in the development of portable defibrillators. These units have been developed for a variety of medical and non-medical purposes and have been adapted to the specific needs of defibrillators.

The first recorders used a heated arm that moved vertically as heat-sensitive paper moved horizontally, while most new designs use a line of tiny elements that can be heated and cooled off very rapidly as the same heat-sensitive paper moves against them, thus producing a dot-matrix-like recording.

Recorders must have both a time and an amplitude scale for ECG signals, as well as the capability of printing alphanumerics for rates, time and date, energy delivered, patient impedance, alarm conditions, and various other parameters, as well as giving a graphic indication of the exact point of charge delivery. Some units print on paper that has a grid on it already, while others print the grid along with the waveforms.

The recorders may also be used to print statistical data, either graphically or in a table, as well as device information such as serial number, total number of discharges, last service date, and more. Troubleshooting codes and error logs might also be printable, which can aid greatly in servicing the units.

Most recorders can print ECG and other data from several seconds in the past. These recordings start automatically when the defib is discharged in order to provide information about the patient just before as well as after shock delivery.

Recorders may be set up to start recording when certain alarm events occur, and they may also be able to draw on stored data to print strips of past events.

iii. Additional Components

In order to help caregivers evaluate patients more thoroughly, components other than those directly associated with defibrillation and monitoring were added to defibs. All of these functions add complexity to the physical layout of machines, as well as to the internal circuitry and display requirements. Displays may be separate from the defib displays, or they may be integrated onto a multifunction graphic display.

Pulse oximetry, often using third-party circuit designs and sensors, gives an indication of cardiac pumping and respiration effectiveness, which helps in determining the best direction for treatment. It also is very useful in monitoring patients after a code, or when the unit is being used to transport a patient who has a significant risk of requiring resuscitation. A pulse ox must have a connector for the sensor as well as controls for setup and alarms, and displays of measured values and alarms settings. Pulse oximetry is discussed in more detail in Chapter 3.

Cardiac patients may need to have a pacemaker as part of their initial treatment regimen, and since much of the ECG signal processing that is needed for effective pacing is already in modern defibrillators as part of their basic design, it was relatively straightforward to add the components necessary to have pacing functions available. Pacing cables are often attached to the same port as the defib paddles, since both functions are not often used simultaneously, but the pacemaker does need its own set of controls and displays. Pacemakers are discussed later in this chapter.

In addition to pulse oximetry, a measure of exhaled carbon dioxide is useful in diagnosis. Capnography, like pulse oximetry, is usually a separate device installed in the chassis of the defibrillator, though they may share some components such as power supplies.

iv. Displays

Most modern manual defibrillators have either an LCD or plasma display. CRTs are still in use, though the CRT is bulkier and requires high voltage circuitry. More and more defibs have color displays, and the graphic displays show waveforms of various parameters as well as alphanumerics for certain measurements and alarms setting. The displays also show prompts and error codes, setup information, time and date, and a variety of other data. Color helps make increasingly cluttered screens easier to read, allowing differentiation of parameters according to hue.

Displays must be large enough to be readable, yet small enough to fit into the overall compact design of defibrillators. They must be durable, and bright enough to be visible in all lighting conditions.

v. Audio

From near the beginning of defibrillator evolution, sound has been an important design component. It is often a confusing emergency situation when the devices are used, and employing sounds to convey important information allowed code responders to better focus on the task at hand. A specialized circuit usually handles all audio signals.

High-voltage circuits such as are required to charge the storage capacitor in a defib often produced a high-pitched, rising tone as a byproduct of their design, and this characteristic was capitalized upon to allow staff to hear when the unit was charging, so they would know that a discharge was imminent. Even when newer designs no longer produced their own intrinsic sounds, engineers added audio circuitry to mimic the rising tones so this same vital information was available. A louder, steady tone was added to indicate that the set charge had been reached, and often a warbling or otherwise different tone indicates the actual discharge. Charge- and discharge-related sounds can usually be turned down but not off.

ECG beats have beeps or clicks associated with them to provide a nonvisual indication of heart function, though these sounds can often be turned right off, as defibs are often used to long periods of time for monitoring patients.

Alarm conditions obviously require staff attention, and are therefore usually indicated by both visual and audible signals, varying in intensity according to the urgency of the alarm condition. Alarm signals can generally be turned up or down, but again not off completely.

Some manufacturers use voice prompts to assist users in device operation, or to notify them of alarms or other conditions.

vi. Ergonomics

Given the kinds of situations in which they are used, ergonomics play a critical role in the design of defibrillators. Units must be as compact and lightweight as possible and still deliver adequate performance. They must be easily transportable, free of components that might hinder portability.

Units have to be tough enough to withstand the drops and bumps that are inevitable in emergencies.

Staff using defibrillators are often in an extremely stressful and busy situation, and therefore defibrillator design must allow them to use the unit effectively with minimal concentration or distractions. The operation should be as intuitive as possible, and the device should have clear, logical, and easily accessible controls and displays. Ideally, a staff member should be able to use a new defibrillator without any hesitation or unit-specific training.

vii. Testing and Maintenance

Defibrillators, being critical life support devices, require special care if they are to provide reliable, effective performance. Most units include a self-test function that checks most of their basic operations. This self-test feature is normally used by clinical staff on a regular basis, such as once a week, and the results noted in a log. Users also need to check the overall condition of the unit, that power is being delivered, and that all necessary accessories are available and in good condition.

Part of the self-test routine usually includes charging the unit to a specified level and then discharging through test terminals built into the paddle holders. This allows the unit to check for continuity of the conductive pathways, and to measure the output and compare it to what was set.

Any abnormalities, whether indicated by self-test results or otherwise, must be recorded and reported to service personnel.

Testing by trained technical staff should be done on a schedule, as recommended by the manufacturer, and results recorded. This testing includes a thorough physical examination of the unit, as well as the use of extended self-test functions. Units usually have a number of error codes that may be generated to aid in troubleshooting, and various performance logs may be accessible during testing.

Defib performance is tested using commercial test equipment, which allows precise measurement of delivered energy, waveform duration, and other parameters. Time to reach full charge will be measured and compared to manufacturer specifications. Most test devices include an oscilloscope output port so that waveforms can be examined.

Most manufacturers recommend replacing batteries regularly, perhaps every two to four years, or when testing indicates substandard characteristics.

c. Automatic External Defibrillators (AEDs)

Survival rates for victims of heart attacks are much greater when resuscitation efforts, especially defibrillation, start within a few minutes of the attack. According to the

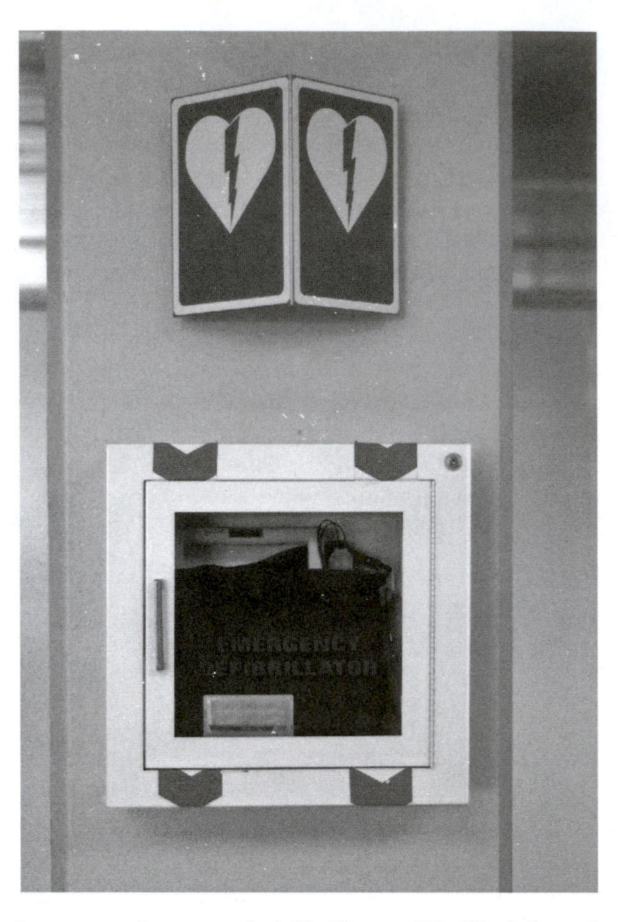

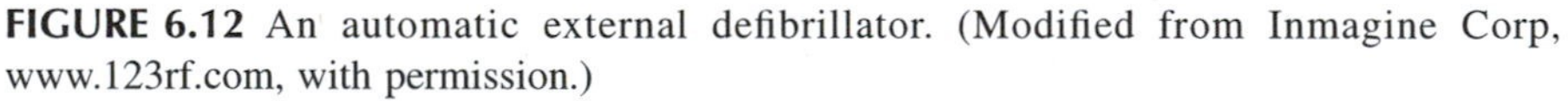

FIGURE 6.12 An automatic external defibrillator. (Modified from Inmagine Corp, www.123rf.com, with permission.)

American Heart Association, a sudden cardiac arrest victim's chances of survival fall 7 to 10% for every minute of delay until defibrillation.

Personnel trained in CPR, and especially defibrillator operation, are often unavailable when a cardiac arrest occurs, and full-featured defibrillators are generally only found in hospitals or emergency response vehicles. Because of these factors, manufacturers have developed defibrillators that are very simple to operate, performing many functions automatically, so that almost anyone can use them, and use can commence quickly.

Automatic External Defibrillators, or AEDs (Figure 6.12), contain all the basic components of a standard manual defibrillator. They have a power supply, a means of generating and storing high voltage, wave-shaping and delivery components, and ECG detection and analysis circuitry.

AEDs typically deliver lower energy levels than full-blown defibs, usually around 150 joules maximum. This amount of energy is sufficient to produce good results in most cardiac arrest situations in which a positive outcome is at all possible.

Also, higher energies are more likely to cause injury to the patient or the persons using the defibrillator.

For AEDs to be widely distributed and used, they must be relatively simple in both construction (to minimize costs) and operation (to maximize the number of individuals who can use them). Units have very clear instructions printed on their cases, with numbered pictures showing the various steps to be performed. Many units also include voice prompts to help even completely inexperienced users through the process.

Conductive adhesive pads are used instead of paddles to make application safer and more positive. These pads have pictures to show correct placement on the patient's body.

These units may sit unused for long periods of time, so their batteries must maintain a reliable charge for several years. Lithium chemistries currently provide the best performance in this regard, though some manufacturers use lead-acid batteries. All these devices require a charging circuit connected to reliable AC power.

Regular inspection and testing of AEDs is important. Someone must ensure that charging power is being delivered at all times, and most units include a self-test function that should be used regularly, for example once a week. Inspection and testing dates should be recorded.

Batteries in AEDs must be replaced at intervals specified by the manufacturer to ensure optimum performance, typically every two years.

Because defibrillator performance depends on good pad contact, the pads must be sealed in airtight packages, and still they must be replaced at regular intervals to ensure quality.

B. Pacemakers

Cardiology researchers recognized that some patients with irregular ECGs were suffering from some kind of failure in the natural pacemaking system of the heart. If an electrical signal could be injected into the heart tissue at the correct location and at the right time, more normal cardiac function might be restored.

Cardiac function is discussed in more detail in Chapter 2.

1. History

In 1950, Canadians Hopps, Bigelow, and Callaghan developed the first successful cardiac pacemaker. The large unit used vacuum tubes, and the signals it delivered through the patient's chest wall were crude and often painful to the patient.

External pacemakers were developed further in the 1950s by Zoll and others, but these external units still had the disadvantages of being bulky, requiring the use of external electrodes, and being dependent on continuous AC power.

Lillehei developed a method of inserting pacing electrodes directly into the heart, greatly reducing the power required. Lillehei's technique involved making an incision into the chest, but Furman developed a method of inserting electrode wires into a vein and threading them into the heart, where the tips could be embedded in cardiac tissue. This had the benefit of reduced trauma to the patient as well as further reducing the power required.

In 1958, Swedes Elmqvist and Senning were the first to implant a pacemaker in a human. Despite numerous problems and a large number of different models, the patient survived 43 years and died of causes unrelated to his pacemakers.

Some manufacturers have used thermoelectric generators to power pacemakers. These units contain tiny amounts of plutonium; its decay heats components and produces electrical power. Fewer than 100 patients have such nuclear pacemakers, and when the units are removed they must be transported to Los Alamos, New Mexico, for disposal.

Pacemakers now are extremely reliable and versatile and are implanted in as many as 600,000 patients every year. As well, advanced external pacemakers are used frequently, as a bridge until an internal device can be implanted or when natural pacing can be restored at a later time.

2. Theory of Operation

Pacemakers rely on much of the same design principles as defibrillators. They must be able to recognize ECG waveforms (or lack thereof) and then deliver accurately timed and shaped electrical impulses to the heart.

Internal pacing signals are several orders of magnitude lower in energy than internal defibrillation pulses, in the range of 25 microjoules as compared to up to 35 joules for implantable defibs, and therefore battery voltage can be boosted to provide these levels much more easily. Batteries must be very reliable and long lasting, typically only requiring replacement after at least four or five years of operation.

Implantable pacemakers (Figure 6.13) consume very little power, in the range of 10 to 40 microwatts, but they are often in place for seven years or more, so battery

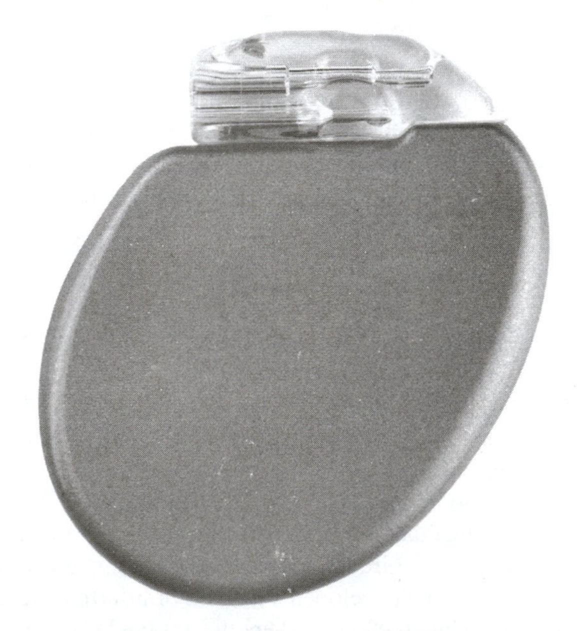

FIGURE 6.13 An implantable pacemaker. (Modified from Inmagine Corp, www.123rf.com, with permission.)

durability is critical. Newer designs can operate on only 240 nanowatts, and even further reductions in power requirements are planned.

Sensing of cardiac operation is done by picking up and amplifying ECG signals, which are analyzed by a microprocessor. The results of this analysis combined with programming parameters determines the timing and size of the pulse to be delivered, and then these parameters are fed to a wave-shaping and delivery circuit, which in turn delivers a specific pacing pulse to the heart.

Pacing may be used to "fill in the gaps" for patients with certain arrhythmias, or to increase the rate for patients with bradycardia.

Patient physical activity may be estimated by the use of an accelerometer, a microelectromechanical device within the pacemaker that detects patient motion. Increased physical activity can be taken as a signal for the pacemaker to increase the heart rate in order to increase blood flow as will be required by the activity.

Implantable pacemakers have transceivers so that their programming can be modified to suit patient requirements. Programmers (Figure 6.14) use an antenna placed over the pacemaker site to communicate with the device, and a terminal allows users to see current programming parameters and enter new ones.

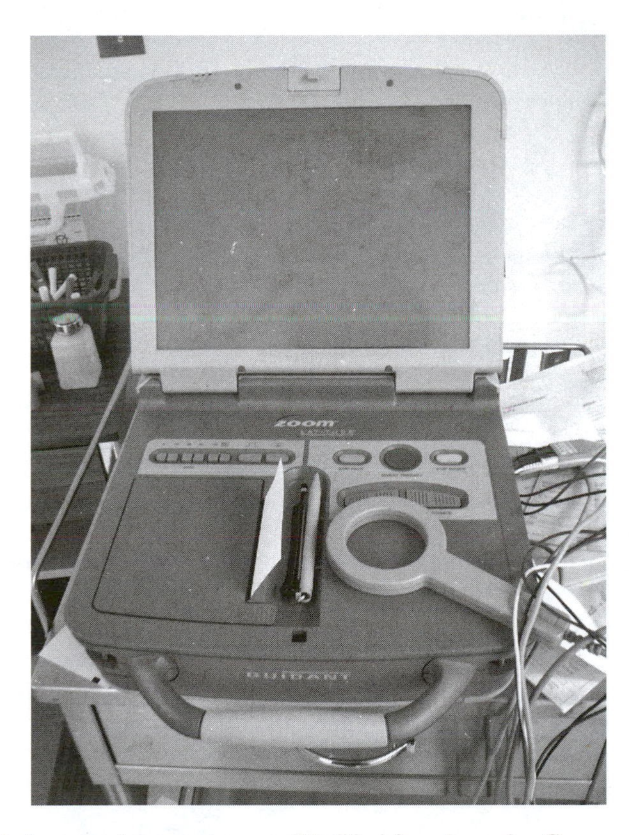

FIGURE 6.14 A pacemaker programmer. (Modified from Inmagine Corp, www.123rf.com, with permission.)

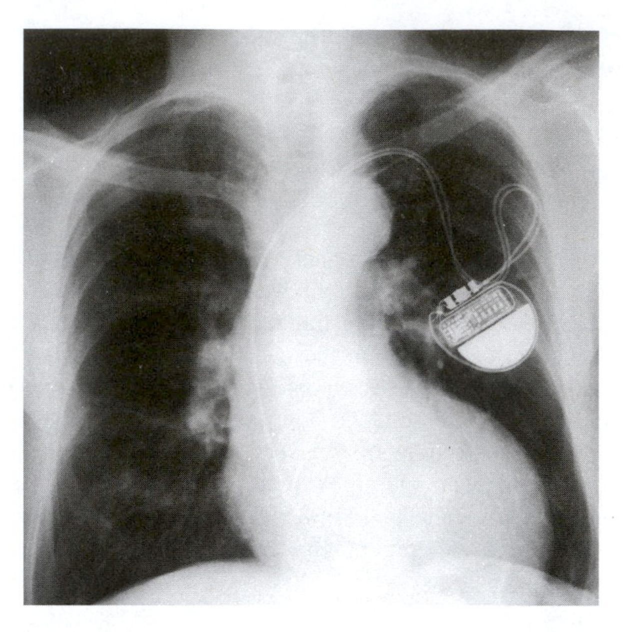

FIGURE 6.15 An x-ray showing pacemaker placement. (Modified from Inmagine Corp, www.123rf.com, with permission.)

3. Construction

The mechanical construction of implantable pacemakers is very much like that of implantable defibrillators, as described in the preceding section titled "Internal (Implantable) Defibrillators." Nuclear-powered devices require very robust cases that can withstand extreme trauma and even cremation, in order to minimize the risk of escape of nuclear material.

4. Application

Pacemakers are usually installed in a pocket made in the tissue of the patient's upper chest (see Figure 6.15). Electrodes are introduced via the left subclavian vein to the appropriate area of the heart, and the leads routed under the skin to connect to the implanted pacemaker. The axillary or cephalic veins may also be used. Electrode placement locations may include the right atrium and/or ventricle, two different areas of the right atrium and the right ventricle, or each of the right and left ventricles, as well as some other specialized locations.

Internal pacemaker signals are generally a few volts (or a few milliamps, depending on the calculation method) in amplitude and from 0.2 to 0.5 seconds in duration.

5. External Pacemakers

Some patients may need cardiac pacing urgently and/or for a relatively short duration, in which cases an external pacemaker may be used. These units utilize similar ECG pickup and analysis systems to implantable defibrillators, but physical construction and power considerations are much different. External devices can be larger, with less robust cases. Controls can be manually accessible, and power can come from AC line, or rechargeable or disposable batteries.

Some external pacers can deliver pacing signals directly to the heart via introduced (endocardial) electrodes, but most rely on external (transcutaneous) electrodes, which are less traumatic and faster and easier to apply. However, since pacing signals in the latter case are delivered through the patient's chest wall, they have to be of considerably greater amplitude than those delivered by internal devices, usually about ten times greater.

Usual electrode placement for external pacers is at the top of the sternum and near the bottom of the ribcage along the left axilla.

Since transcutaneous pacing signals travel through various surrounding muscles before they reach the heart, these muscles may contract at the set pacing rate. This may cause patient discomfort, and sensitivity reactions to the electrodes or conductive gel may also be seen.

External pacemakers may be standalone units, or they may be integrated into other devices, mainly defibrillators.

II. CIRCULATORY SYSTEM AND BLOOD

A. Artificial Hearts

As the field of cardiology developed, the replacement of diseased hearts moved from imagination to reality. The first human heart transplant was performed in South Africa in 1967. The patient survived for only18 days, mainly because rejection problems had not been successfully solved. Currently, over 100,000 patients have received heart transplants, 60,000 of these in the US. The record for survival is 28 years and counting.

The number of patients needing new hearts exceeds the number of donors, however, and artificial hearts were developed to try to meet this need. The first was implanted in 1982, with the patient surviving 112 days. So far, artificial hearts have been used with only a few patients, and many of the devices required large external components in order to function. There are trials underway of totally implantable devices, with one patient having survived 17 months. Though many hurdles remain, the day is getting nearer when hearts like that of *Star Trek*'s Captain Picard will be available to any patient in need.

B. Ventricular Assist Devices

More immediately useful than artificial hearts are ventricular assist devices (VADs), which are simple pumps that take blood from the left ventricle and pass it into the aorta. These devices are much simpler in operation than artificial hearts, and are generally used as a "bridge" while patients wait for a suitable human heart transplant.

C. Intraaortic Balloon Pumps

Another device that is used to provide temporary assistance to the patient's heart is the intraaortic balloon pump. As its name implies, it consists of a balloon that is inserted with a catheter into the descending aorta. The balloon is designed so that when it is inflated, it pushes blood along in the aorta in the normal direction of flow, thus decreasing the demands on the heart and increasing perfusion to the patient's tissues, including the myocardium.

The cycling of the balloon must be synchronized to the patient's heartbeat so that inflation occurs during diastole, otherwise it would be working in opposition to the heart. It must then deflate before systole. ECG signal detection and simple analysis allow the pump control circuitry to function in this synchronized manner.

D. Heart-Lung Machines

During some cardiac surgery, the patient's heart must be stopped so that surgeons can perform their work. Blood flow and oxygenation must be continued for this time, which may be several hours, and heart-lung machines perform this function.

The first successful use of a heart-lung machine in human surgery was in 1953 in Philadelphia, using a machine developed by John Gibbon.

Because they are used for relatively short terms in high-acuity environments, there is no need for these units to be small or portable.

The majority of total blood flow is drawn from the patient's venous system, usually the superior vena cava or the right atrium. It is then pumped into a membrane system that allows the escape of carbon dioxide from the blood and the intake of oxygen to the blood. The blood is then pumped into the aortic arch, where it continues to circulate through the patient's body. The heart and lungs are bypassed, and the heart can be made to stop to allow surgical procedures to take place.

A number of factors must be considered in the design of heart-lung machines:

- The system must have adequate and adjustable pumping capacity to maintain appropriate blood flow through the patient.
- The gas exchange system must be sufficiently effective both in removing carbon dioxide to keep blood levels below harmful levels, and in adding oxygen to simulate normal ventilation. Membranes are made of materials such as polypropylene or silicone.
- Pumping systems must cause minimal mechanical damage to blood cells. Pumps may be of the roller peristaltic type, or of a centrifugal type in which rotation of blood within the pump head produces flow. Centrifugal pumps tend to cause less damage to cells.
- An anticlotting agent, usually heparin, must be added to the blood to prevent clots forming in the system and passing to the patient. This agent must be neutralized immediately following surgery so that normal clotting can take place.
- Temperature of the blood must be controllable in order maintain, raise, or lower patient body temperature as required by specific circumstances. It may be advantageous to induce hypothermia in order to minimize tissue damage during certain procedures.

Heart-lung machines are operated by perfusionists, specially trained technologists who monitor and control system functions working in coordination with anesthetists, surgeons, and the rest of the surgical team.

E. Sequential Compression Devices

Patients who have recently had surgery on their legs or are otherwise susceptible to the formation of blood clots in the veins of their legs (usually referred to as deep vein thrombosis, or DVT) can benefit from the use of sequential compression devices (SCDs). Lymphedema, a condition resulting from the reduction of flow in the patient's lymphatic system that produces swelling of the extremities, can also be alleviated with SCDs.

Sequential compression devices consist simply of a pump that feeds a rotating valve with a number of outlet ports. The ports are connected to a multichambered sleeve, which fits snugly over the patient's limb. The chambers inflate in sequence, with higher pressures in the distal chambers and lower pressures in each of the following chambers, thus producing a peristaltic wave of compression that moves from the distal end of the limb toward the proximal end. Typical pressures range from about 45 mm Hg distally to about 30 mm Hg proximally. Inflation is maintained for several seconds, and then all chambers deflate for a minute or so before the next cycle begins. This process induces the flow of blood and/or lymphatic fluid away from the limb and toward the torso, reducing swelling and its associated problems.

It is thought that the SCD action also reduces the formation of clots in limb veins.

F. Automatic Tourniquets

When surgery is performed on limbs, blood flow to the surgical area can be problematic, both obscuring the field of view and contributing to patient blood loss.

A tourniquet placed proximally to the site can be inflated to block blood flow, but if this goes on for too long, tissue damage can occur.

Automatic tourniquets incorporate pumps and timing mechanisms that can be programmed for inflation pressure and inflation/deflation cycle timing. Many systems have two independent mechanisms to allow for placement in two different locations (see Figure 6.16).

G. Blood Warmers

Blood is stored in refrigerated cabinets in order to prolong its usefulness by slowing biological and chemical reactions that can damage blood cells and alter blood chemistry. Normally blood bags can be allowed to warm to near room temperature before infusion; however in an emergency situation, there may not be time for this. Also, when the patient is suffering from hypothermia or is otherwise sensitive to body temperature fluctuations, room-temperature infusion of blood products may not be acceptable. In such circumstances, fluids may be passed through a blood warmer before being infused into the patient.

Most blood warmers are one of two different types, dry heat or water bath.

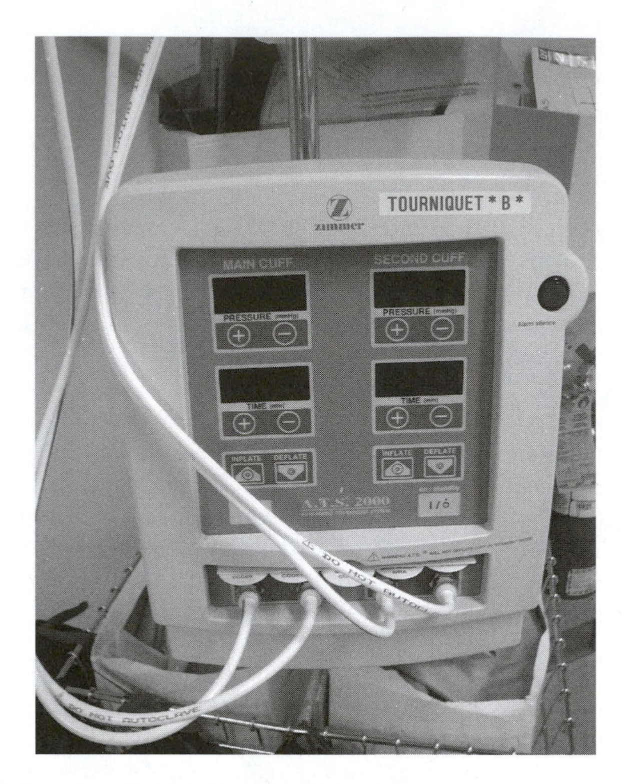

FIGURE 6.16 An automatic two-channel tourniquet.

Dry heat blood warmers use a thin plastic pad with many small channels for blood flow. This pad is placed between two metal plates that are heated to constant temperature, and the blood flows through the channels and is warmed as it goes, until it is close to body temperature at the exit. It is then carried by a short tube to the patient.

Water bath blood warmers (see Figures 6.17 and 6.18) use a double-walled tube to accomplish the same end. Blood flows through a small, inner passage while warm water is pumped in the opposite direction through a larger, outer tube. This results in a gradual but thorough warming of the blood as it passes through the tubing. The distal end of the double-walled tubing is near the infusion site, so that there is minimal cooling before the blood enters the body.

All blood warming systems must have very precise temperature control mechanisms, as overheating blood can cause very rapid degradation. Most units include a temperature display as well as an over-temperature alarm system. Some units may have a low-temperature warning indicator. Regular testing and calibration of both the control and alarm systems is important for continued patient safety.

H. Intravenous Fluid Administration Pumps

Fluids sometimes must be administered to patients when it is impractical or impossible to deliver them orally. This may be for hydration, for medication delivery, for blood transfusions, or for meeting nutritional needs.

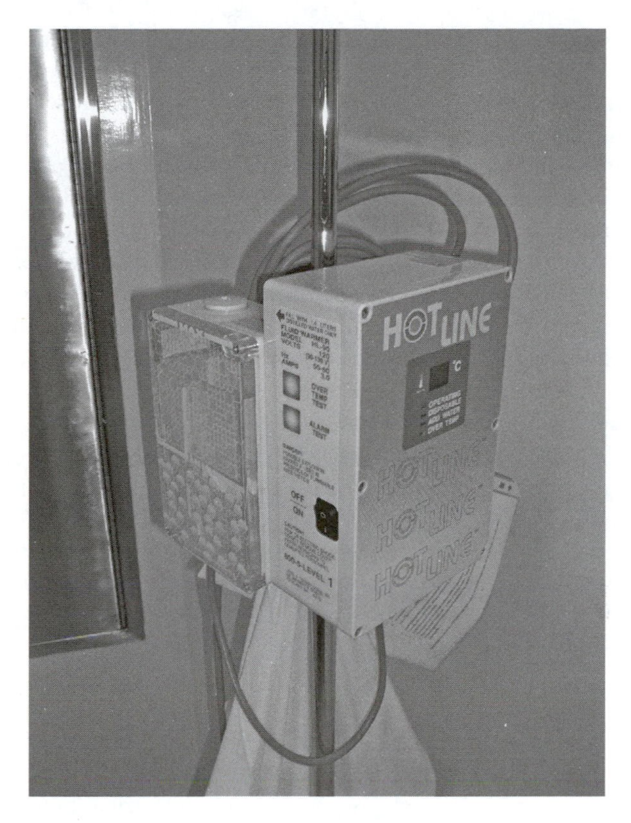

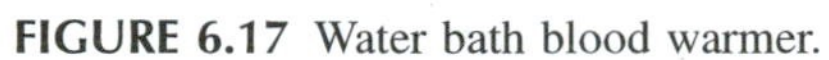
FIGURE 6.17 Water bath blood warmer.

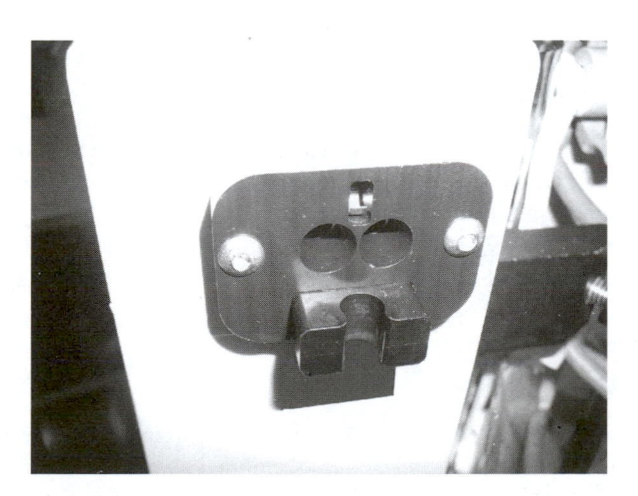

FIGURE 6.18 Female connector for the blood warmer — note two openings.

In such cases, the fluids can be delivered into the patient's blood stream using a needle or catheter connected to a reservoir of the fluid. Veins are used for this purpose rather than arteries, because blood pressure is much lower inside them, so the fluids being administered don't have to overcome a significant pressure gradient. Veins are also usually closer to the surface and so easier to locate, and they have thinner walls, which makes penetration easier.

The pressure needed to push intravenous (IV) fluids into the body can be supplied simply by gravity, but in some circumstances this can be problematic. If even somewhat accurate delivery rates are important, gravity feed lines must be carefully controlled by measuring drop rates and calculating flow rates from that. They must be closely monitored, as flow rates can vary with time. If a specific volume is to be delivered, this must be calculated and timed.

Gravity feed may not be able to deliver fluids rapidly enough in some circumstances.

For all of the above reasons, intravenous fluids are often administered using a pump.

There are a number of different types of IV pumps, depending on manufacturer preferences and delivery parameters. They can range from simple devices that can be used by patients at home, with one type of fluid only at a fixed rate, to sophisticated multichannel units that can deliver several different fluids, each at different rates.

Pumps can be grouped according to their mechanism of delivery and control.

1. Pressure Infusers

These units simply apply pressure to a flexible infusion bag, and it is assumed that constant pressure equals constant flow. The pressure may be developed using a mechanical bladder and bulb pump, or some type of electrical pump may be used. Pressure infusers are used when accurate flow rates are not critical. In some circumstances this is because large amounts of fluid need to be delivered in a short time, such as during some surgical procedures requiring quick blood pressure boosts. Other systems are found in some home-therapy applications where high accuracy is less important than ease of use and simplicity.

2. Fluid Controllers

While not strictly pumps, these devices can be used to provide controlled delivery of intravenous fluids. They operate by simply blocking or opening the fluid pathway, while at the same time detecting and counting drops of fluid as they pass through a drip chamber. Droplets are fairly consistent in volume for a given fluid, and by controlling the number of drops that are allowed through in a given time, flow rate can be controlled.

3. Syringe Pumps

As the name implies, these devices take a standard injection syringe fitted with an intravenous catheter or needle, and depress the plunger with a gear drive mechanism. Obviously these systems deal with relatively low volumes and are used in such

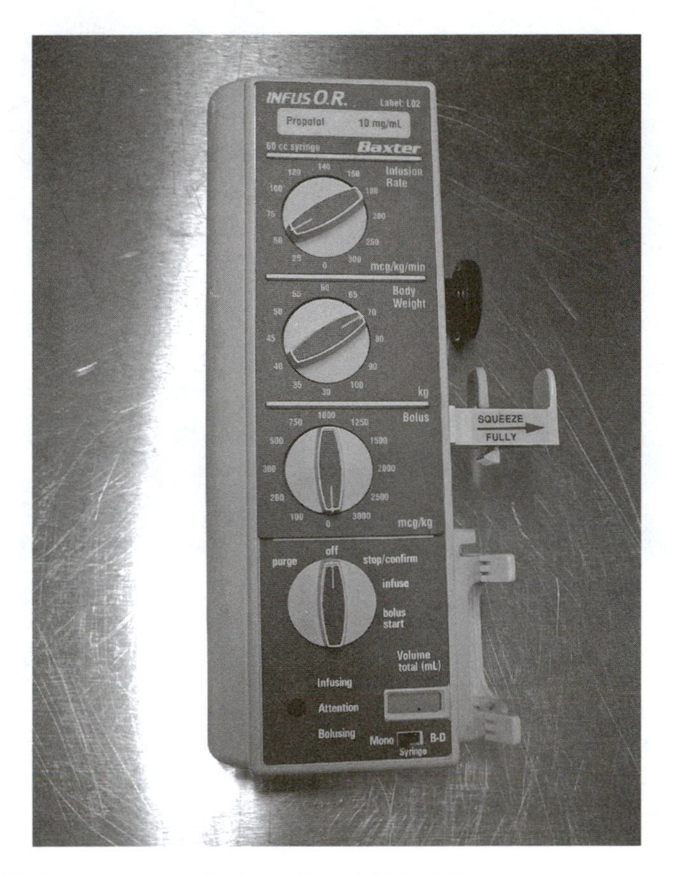

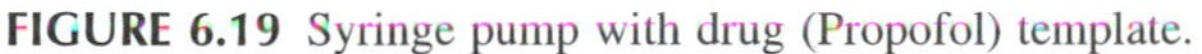
FIGURE 6.19 Syringe pump with drug (Propofol) template.

situations as delivering narcotics, spinal anesthetic agents, or certain other high-potency drugs, or for administering insulin at intervals over long periods.

Because syringes are precisely manufactured, and mechanical systems to depress the syringe plunger are relatively easy to control, syringe pumps (Figure 6.19) offer high accuracy but are limited to low flow rates and volumes.

Some pumps may have the capacity to handle various-sized syringes, while others take only one type.

Pumps have been designed so that they can be preprogrammed for specific drugs, with flow rates, volume limits, and alarms settings adjusted for each. Programming may be via selection from a list programmed into the pump, or by the fitting of a template to the face of the pump, which shows the name of the drug and interfaces with the pump to adjust settings.

General-purpose syringe pumps can be set for different flow rates, though total volume delivered is usually determined by the initial filling of the syringe.

Syringe pumps usually have a display that can show the various settings as well as volume delivered and alarm notifications.

These pumps are usually battery powered.

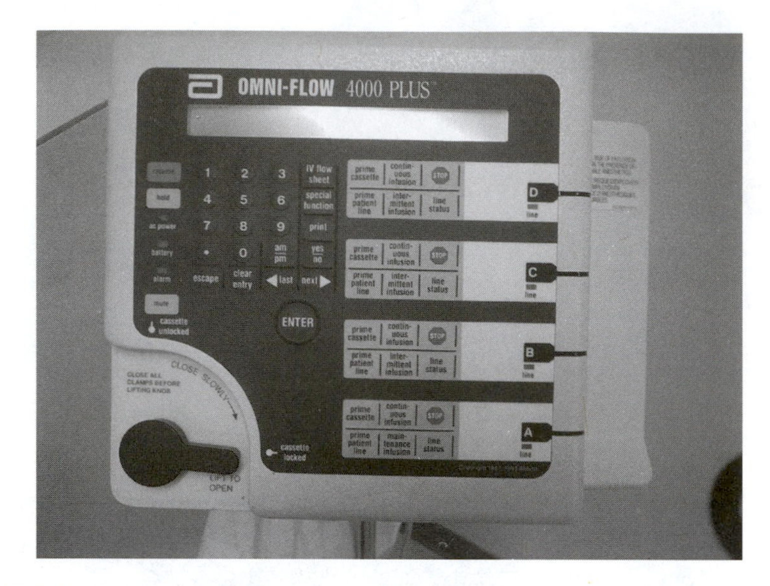

FIGURE 6.20 A multichannel piston cassette pump.

4. Piston Pumps

High accuracy can be obtained by passing the fluid to be administered through a precise chamber that can be compressed by a plunger. One-way valves control the direction of flow, and the system works like a small piston, delivering discrete pulses of a specific volume (see Figure 6.20). Flow rate can then be set by varying the frequency of the pulses.

These pumps provide high accuracy, but the complexity and precision of the piston and valve mechanism means that the costs per patient use are high. Some systems have cassettes with multiple channels, each of which can be controlled separately by the pump.

5. Peristaltic Pumps

Peristalsis is a means of moving fluids through a tube by sequentially compressing segments of the tube, pushing the fluid from one section to another in the desired direction of flow. Food is moved through the intestine by peristalsis; rings of muscle in the intestinal walls contract in a wave-like pattern to squeeze food along.

Peristaltic pumps use this method to pump IV fluids. An external mechanism compresses a section of tubing at one location, closing it off. The next section along is then compressed, pushing the fluid forward until this section is also closed off. A further section takes over, and then the first section can open up again to admit the next unit of fluid.

There are two general methods of generating peristaltic action, rotary and linear.

In rotary pumps (Figure 6.21), a flexible section of tubing is fixed tightly around a wheel that has three of four compression points around its perimeter. The compression points may have a spinning sleeve on them to reduce friction on the tubing,

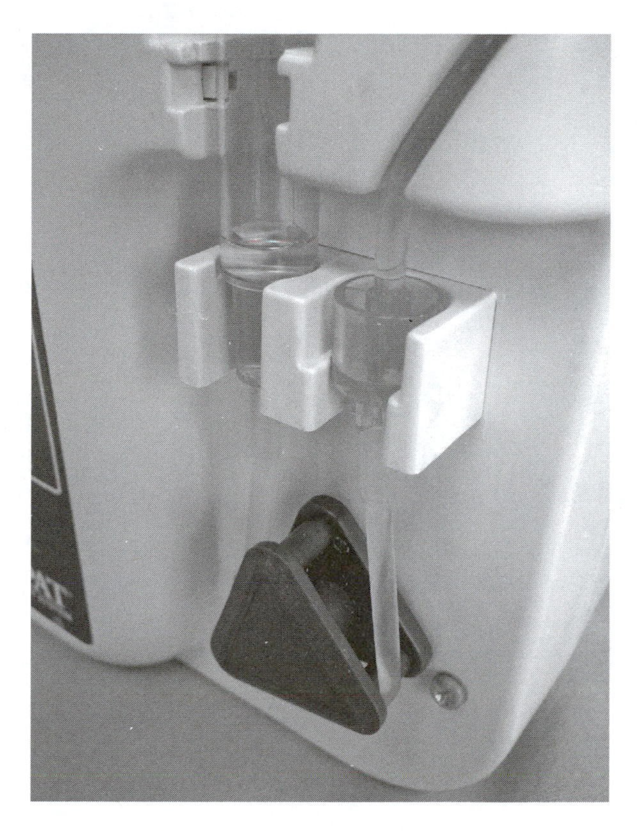

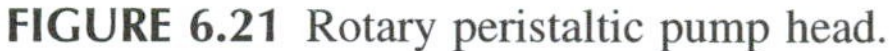

FIGURE 6.21 Rotary peristaltic pump head.

or they may simply be coated with a low-friction material such as Teflon™. As the wheel rotates, the tubing is squeezed along, and the fluid between each compression point is moved forward until it reaches the distal end where it is released to flow to the patient.

Higher pressure can be generated if there is a rim around the outside edge of the pump against which the tubing can be compressed. Without such a rim, if backpressure was great enough it could simply stretch the tubing outward until either backflow occurred or pumping became ineffective.

These pumps must use an infusion set that has a section of very flexible, durable material such as silicone rubber, with structures to hold each end of this flexible section in place on the pump. This means that set costs are relatively high.

Flow rates are determined simply by the speed of rotation of the pump head. This depends on the inside diameter of the tubing being constant; since tubing will likely stretch with time, sets must be replaced at intervals specified by the manufacturer in order to maintain volume delivery accuracy.

Linear peristaltic pumps use a set of "fingers" or bars that are moved in a wave pattern (Figure 6.22). Either a special section of rubber tubing or standard IV tubing is passed over the bars and compressed against a backing such that, when a bar is extended, it occludes the tubing, and when it is retracted, the tubing is relaxed and

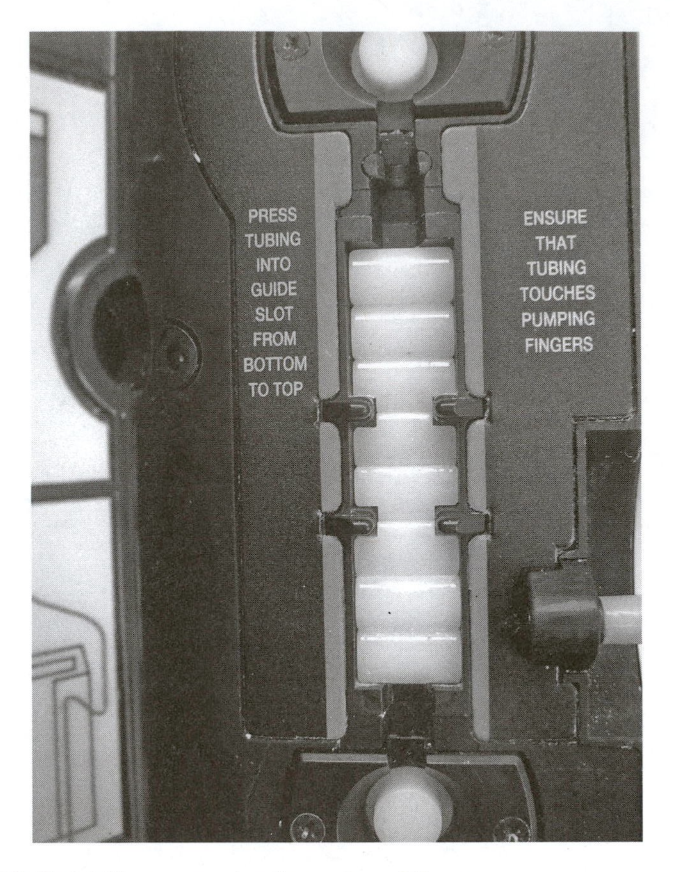

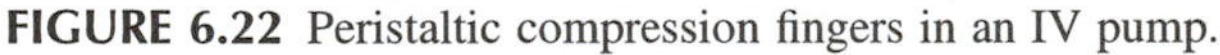

FIGURE 6.22 Peristaltic compression fingers in an IV pump.

completely open (see Figure 6.23). The wave pattern of compression and relaxation moves the fluid in the desired direction.

As with the rotary type pumps, volume accuracy depends on the inside diameter of the tubing being constant. Since regular IV tubing is not as elastic as silicone rubber tubing, it must be replaced even more frequently. If there is enough excess tubing in a line, simply moving the line along so that a new section of tubing is in the pump head will maintain accuracy.

6. Patient-Controlled Analgesia Pumps

In the administration of analgesic medications, the patient is usually the best one to determine the level of pain being felt. To this end, pumps were developed that could be controlled to some degree by the patient. By pressing a button, the patient could request an extra bolus of pain medication (see Figure 6.24).

Obviously there had to be limits to such pumps, otherwise some patients would simply keep pressing the button until an overdose was delivered.

Patient-controlled analgesia pumps, or PCA pumps, have a number of safeguards built into their design. They are programmable for rate and total volume, as with

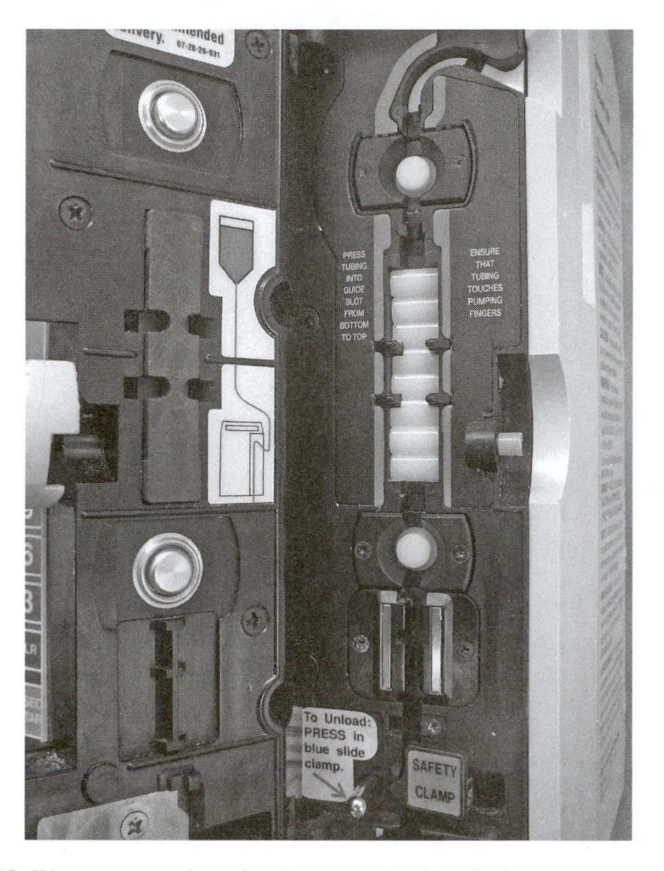

FIGURE 6.23 IV pump open door showing pump head, occlusion sensors, and air sensor.

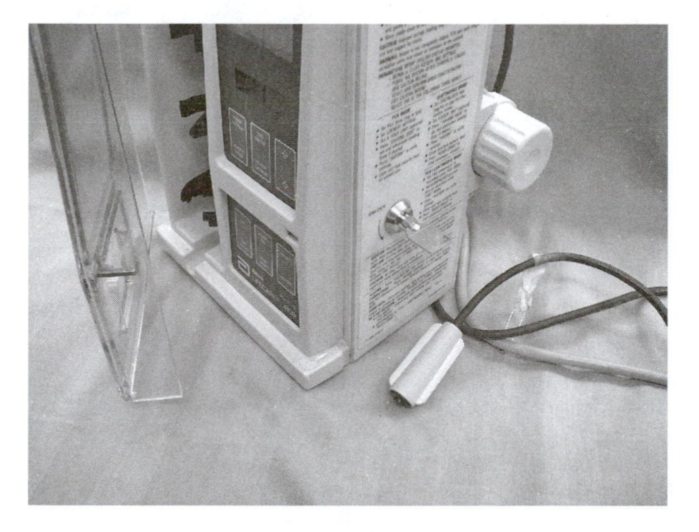

FIGURE 6.24 PCA pump showing patient control pushbutton.

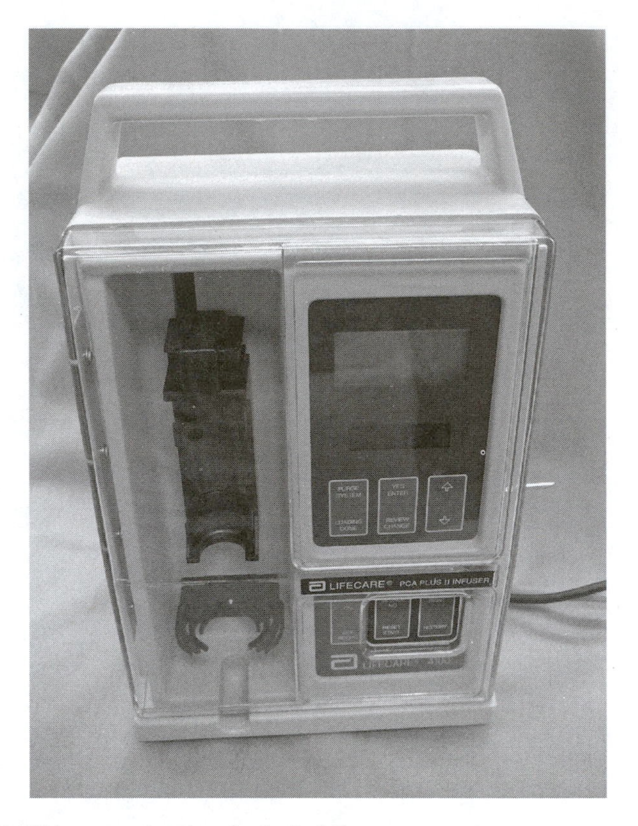

FIGURE 6.25 PCA pump showing the locked door.

most other IV pumps, but they can also be programmed to set a specific volume that will be delivered with each patient request, as well as the minimum interval between allowed requests and the maximum number of request that will be permitted within a given time.

To prevent tampering, most PCA pumps have a cover that can be locked after programming, allowing access to only the stop and start controls (Figure 6.25).

Most PCA pumps have a memory function that allows clinicians to look at how many requests have been made by the patient and how many have been allowed.

Since dosages are critical with analgesic medications, a high degree of accuracy is needed for PCA pumps, and therefore the syringe mechanism is most commonly used, often with a special syringe that has been prefilled and labeled by pharmacy (Figure 6.26).

7. Safety Features of IV Pumps

Many IV pumps have similar safety features.

Most have a mechanism that will generate an alarm if a blockage is detected downstream from the pump. This can occur if the IV line in the patient is no longer patent (no longer in the vein), if the tubing has become kinked, if the patient moves

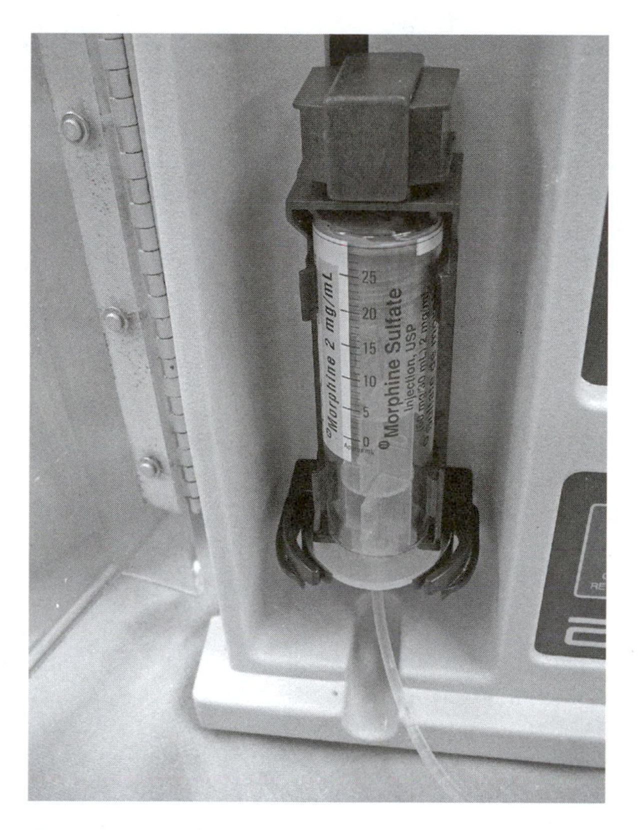

FIGURE 6.26 PCA syringe cartridge.

in such as way as to block the flow, or if clots form around the tip of the delivery needle or catheter. Alarms may be audible and/or visual, and they may also trigger a nurse call system.

Occlusion detectors often rely on the fact that tubing will become more turgid when pressure rises. This increased turgidity causes the outer wall of the tubing to bulge outward and press on a sensor such as a slug moving inside a coil, or a microswitch. Such sensors may require occasional calibration.

Most pumps signal when the set volume has been delivered, but most will keep pumping at a very low rate in order to help avoid clot formation at the end of the needle or catheter, keeping the vein open (KVO mode).

Some pumps can detect upstream occlusions as well, using the reverse mechanism of downstream occlusion detection. Tubing will tend to collapse if more fluid is being pumped out than is coming in, and a sensor can detect this reduction in diameter. Again, calibration may be required.

Since it can be harmful or fatal if air is pumped into a patient's vein, pumps often have air-in-line detectors. These typically consist of an ultrasound transmitter–receiver pair situated on opposite sides of the IV tubing. When an air bubble greater than a certain size enters the section of tubing between the emitter and sensor, the amount of ultrasound transmitted will drop, triggering an alarm. Calibration of this component is important, since small, harmless bubbles are often present in regular IV delivery, and these should not trigger an alarm, while bubbles over a certain size should always trigger an alarm. An air alarm will shut pumping off immediately.

Most IV pumps use batteries either as their sole source of power or as temporary power for when the patient is being moved from one area of the hospital to another or between facilities. Low-battery alarms are generally designed so that they give attendants time to make other arrangements for infusion before the battery fails completely.

Rechargeable IV pump batteries should be replaced at regular intervals as specified by the manufacturer in order to help avoid unexpected failures.

III. RESPIRATORY SYSTEM

A. Ventilators

Second only to cardiac function, adequate ventilation is critical to physiological survival, and therefore machines that provide artificial ventilation are of the highest importance.

When patients suffer paralysis or other trauma or disease that renders their breathing mechanisms ineffective, some form of mechanical ventilation is required if they are to live. This may be in the form of simple and direct application of air pressure to the patient's lungs by mouth-to-mouth resuscitation or by the use of a simple pressure bag, or it may be accomplished using a large, very complex and sophisticated electromechanical ventilator. Longer-term life support necessitates the use of mechanical systems.

Developments in anesthesia techniques allowed physicians to administer muscle-paralyzing agents. This made some aspects of surgery easier, especially when using electrosurgery units, but this method resulted in the paralysis of breathing muscles as well, which meant that artificial ventilation was required while patients were anesthetized.

A patient's natural breathing function may be impaired or blocked by a high-lever spinal cord injury or from brain injuries or various diseases. Poliomyelitis epidemics in the mid-twentieth century provided the impetus to develop the first widely used artificial breathing apparatus, commonly referred to as the "iron lung."

These devices enclosed all of the patient's body below the neck in a steel cylinder. Air pressure within the cylinder was then raised and lowered, causing air to be expelled or drawn into the patient's lungs. This had the advantage of being noninvasive, but was very bulky and extremely limiting to the patient, as well as making personal care of the patient difficult. Devices such as these are referred to as negative-pressure ventilators, since they rely on decreasing air pressure around the patient in order to produce inspiration.

Newer ventilator designs used compressors and tubes to supply pressurized air to the patient's trachea, either through a tight-fitting face mask, through a tube inserted in the mouth, or for longer-term situations, directly through a tracheostomy.

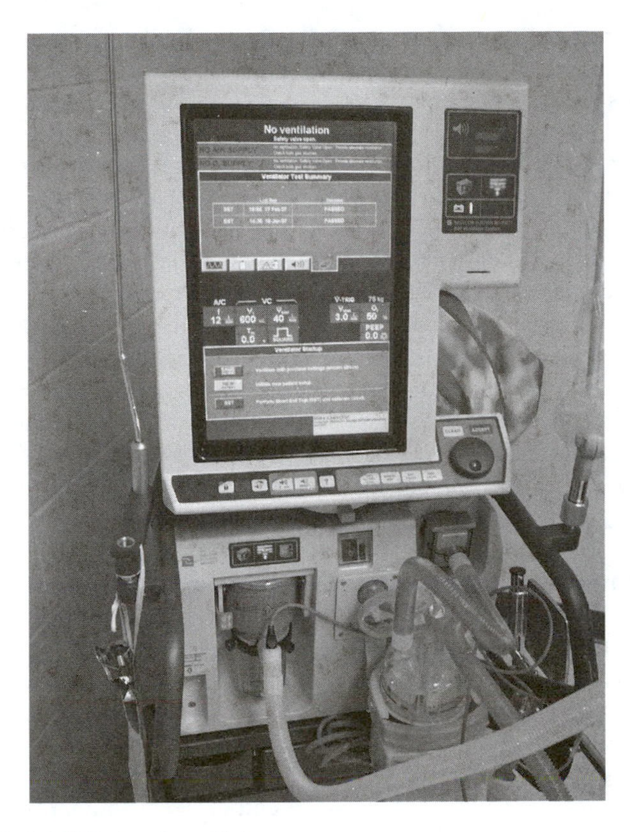

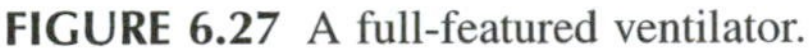
FIGURE 6.27 A full-featured ventilator.

These are the most commonly used type of ventilators today. They are referred to as positive-pressure ventilators.

Because "ventilator" can cover such a wide range of devices, from simple hand-compressed rubber bellows to large, complex machines with many controllable parameters, alarm and backup systems, monitoring circuitry, display and recording components, and various communications capabilities (Figure 6.27), it would be impossible in the scope of this text to describe all of the range in great detail. Most hospital ventilators require intensive factory training on the proper use and maintenance of the devices, and much of this information is model-specific.

In general terms, a ventilator requires a source of gas suitable for inspiration, a means of pressurizing this gas, tubing and fittings to deliver the compressed gas to the patient's lungs, and a means of removing gas from the lungs after each breath.

Gas supply may simply be room air at atmospheric pressure, but is more commonly filtered, compressed air as well as oxygen. Air and oxygen may be supplied by local tanks or piped in through a building system, or air may be compressed by a built-in compressor. The two gases can be blended in the ventilator, in proportions determined by the state of the patient.

Researchers tried using electric motors to power some of the first mechanical ventilators; however sparks produced during operation of these motors could cause fires when they came in contact with some of the very flammable anesthetic gases used at the time, such as cyclopropane and ether.

Ventilators using only compressed gas to power their operation soon came into use, bypassing the fire hazard issue and providing simple, reliable devices. Compressed gas caused a bellows to rise, and then a simple mechanism allowed the bellows to fall by gravity, thus pushing air into the patient's lungs. The natural elasticity of the lungs expelled the air at the end of the inspiratory phase. An adjustable mechanical stop controlled the volume of each breath, and varying the flow rate of the operating gas determined the breathing rate.

As medical science continued to advance, it became apparent that it would be beneficial to be able to control more aspects of the ventilatory cycle, and also to be able to monitor various parameters associated with ventilation. These features gradually became integrated into ventilator design, and the range of ventilators expanded as some applications required more complexity than others.

Following are some of the parameters that can be controlled and/or monitored on a modern ventilator:

Airway pressure — The instantaneous pressure within the patient airway of the ventilator system.

Continuous positive airway pressure (CPAP) — Pressure within the airway is always maintained at some value above atmospheric pressure.

End inspiratory pressure — Pressure in the airway at the end of the inspiratory phase.

Expiratory pause — Period of time (usually about one to three seconds) of constant pressure and no airflow at the end of the expiratory phase.

I:E ratio — The ratio of inspiratory time to expiratory time.

Inspiratory pause — As above, for the inspiratory phase.

Minute volume or minute ventilation (MV) — Total volume delivered to the patient over a one-minute time period.

Mean airway pressure (MAP) — Self-explanatory.

Tidal volume inspired — Total volume delivered to the patient in one inspiratory phase.

Tidal volume expired — As above, for expiratory phase.

Peak inspiratory pressure (PIP) — Maximum airway pressure during inspiratory phase.

Names and abbreviations of parameters may vary from one manufacturer to another, and by region.

Various modes of ventilation may be used with patients, depending on their needs. These modes may be different for different ventilators, or a single ventilator may be able to provide different modes (Figure 6.28) depending on setup:

Volume control — Tidal volume of ventilation is determined by a preset volume value. The ventilator will continue to deliver gas to the patient until this volume has been delivered, using whatever pressure is required (within limits).

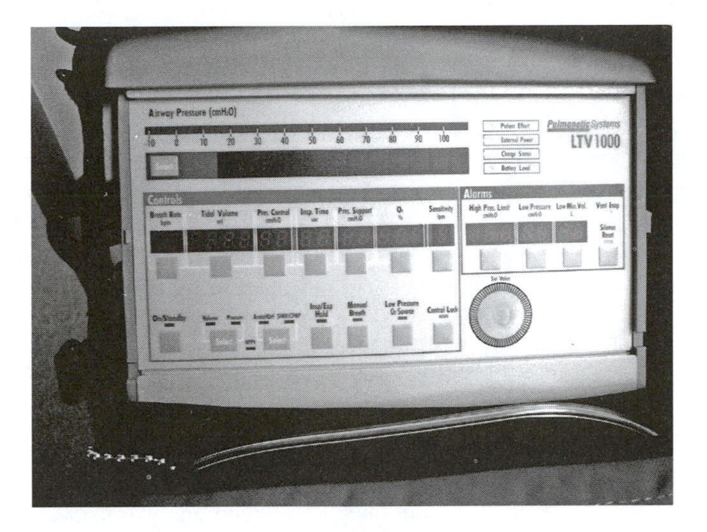

FIGURE 6.28 A compact multiparameter ventilator.

Pressure control — Tidal volume of ventilation is determined by a preset pressure value. The ventilator will continue to deliver gas to the patient until this pressure has been reached, no matter what volume has been delivered (within limits).

Positive end expiratory pressure (PEEP) — In this mode, airway pressure at the end of expiration is kept above atmospheric pressure. This has been found to prevent too-rapid movement of blood through the lungs, thus allowing better gas exchange.

Airway Pressure Release Ventilation (APRV) — The ventilator cycles between two different CPAP values, thus allowing residual gases to escape from the lungs during the lower value part of the cycle.

BiLevel — BiLevel refers to the two levels of PEEP or CPAP that are used in this mode of ventilation. The ventilator may alternate between the two levels on a set schedule, or it may switch depending on the patient's spontaneous breathing efforts. This mode is easier on patients, so they do not need to be as heavily sedated as in some other modes of ventilation.

Spontaneous intermittent mandatory ventilation (SIMV) — Ventilator operation is synchronized to the patient's breathing efforts; that is, breath cycles are initiated by the patient and assisted by the ventilator so that adequate tidal volumes are maintained.

Pressure assist (PA) — Similar to SIMV. Breathing rate is entirely set by the patient.

Pressure support (PS) — The ventilator simply provides positive pressure during inspiration, which is initiated by the patient. Pressure is supplied up to a preset limit.

Proportional assist ventilation (PAV) — Pressure assist ventilation in which the pressure supplied by the ventilator varies according to the inspiratory effort of the patient.

Inverse-ratio ventilation (IRV) — In normal ventilation, the ratio of inspiratory to expiratory times is about 8 or 9 to 1. With IRV, the ratio is reduced to about 4 to 1, and most of the inspiratory flow occurs in the first third of the inspiratory phase. This mode improves gas exchange and cardiac output.

High-frequency oscillation ventilation (HFOV) — "Normal" ventilation modes can sometimes lead to decreased cardiac output, decreased urine output, and lung tissue damage. HFOV delivers much smaller volumes per breath — in the range of 150 ml — at much higher rates — about four to five breaths per second. This method has been found to alleviate many of the problems associated with other modes of ventilation. HFOV usually is done with a completely different ventilator, specifically designed for this application.

All modern patient ventilators have monitoring and alarm systems for patient-related parameters such as pressure, flow, oxygen concentration, and expired CO_2 concentration. Ventilator systems thus include oxygen analyzers and capnographs (see Chapter 3). Additional alarms might include air leak, power failure, backup gas supply tank pressures, and backup battery capacity. A communications interface may handle such things as measured and set parameters as well as alarm conditions. This interface may connect to nurse call systems, physiological monitors, external recorders, remote monitoring systems via modem, or in-hospital computer networks or the Internet.

In order to handle all the complex functions of a ventilator, complete microprocessor systems are employed, often with hard disks and/or optical drives and flat screen monitors. These systems may be Microsoft Windows based.

The primary design parameters of a ventilator system are physiological function adequacy and reliability. Systems use multiple failsafe designs so that ventilation can continue even after one or more failures have occurred. For example, many systems can operate with an external gas supply, with self-contained tanks, with a built-in compressor, or even with manual actuation. They may be line powered but with battery backup and a gas pressure–activated mode.

Since ventilators are often used for long periods of time, they are usually designed to work as quietly and unobtrusively as possible, given their function.

Super Man

Christopher Reeve was an actor, a sportsman, and a family man. He played Superman on the big screen, but he was also a pianist and environmentalist. He participated in a wide variety of sports, including horseback riding. In 1995, at age 42, he was thrown from his horse and suffered a high-level spinal cord injury, which meant that he would be dependent on a mechanical ventilator. Through his amazing will and with the help of his loving family and friends, he was able to achieve many remarkable successes, and he inspired many people who had had similar accidents. His ventilator was usually unobtrusive when he made his many public appearances, but still it made millions of people aware of the vital role played by ventilators in many people's lives. They saw that one could live a rewarding, loving life after such severe injuries.

Christopher Reeve passed away on October 10, 2004, but his legacy lives on.

B. CPAP/BiPAP Units

Continuous positive airway pressure (CPAP) units are very simple versions of pressure support ventilators. They provide air at a pressure somewhat above atmospheric, which is delivered to the patient through a nasal mask. This helps keeps airways open during inspiration, which in turn helps prevent snoring or, more seriously, obstructive sleep apnea and other conditions. Oxygen may be added to the air before delivery to the patient.

Bilevel positive airway pressure devices are somewhat more complex, in that they sense inspiratory effort and provide slightly higher pressure at that time. After flow stops, the pressure drops to a level more like that used with CPAP units.

Because both of these types of devices are used when the patient is sleeping, they are designed to operate as quietly as possible.

C. Oxygen Concentrators

Many patients require supplementary oxygen on a long-term basis, but when living at home or in a long-term-care facility, a central oxygen supply may not be available, and relying on heavy, bulky oxygen tanks is less than ideal.

Oxygen concentrators fill this need, supplying high oxygen percentages at high enough flow rates for almost all patient requirements.

These devices rely on the properties of a material called zeolite for their function. Zeolite has the capacity to selectively absorb nitrogen while bypassing oxygen.

Oxygen concentrators (Figure 6.29) consist of two pressure tanks containing zeolite, a compressor, and a valve system. Room air is compressed and then passed through one of the zeolite tanks, where most of the nitrogen is removed, leaving oxygen at up to 95% concentration. This is delivered to the patient through a flowmeter. Once the zeolite in the first tank is mostly saturated with nitrogen, the valves switch the airflow to the second tank, so that oxygen is delivered to the patient continuously. While the second tank is being used, the first tank is pumped down to very low pressure, which draws the nitrogen out of the zeolite and passes it back into the room. Once the second tank is saturated and the first purged completely, the airflow is switched back; the first tank absorbs nitrogen and the second tank is purged. Cycles typically take about 20 seconds per tank.

Oxygen concentrators are designed to operate as quietly as possible, since they usually sit close to the patient 24 hours a day. The pumps are powerful, so there has to be effective sound insulation in the unit's cabinet.

Some units have an oxygen analyzer built in to give an alarm if oxygen concentration drops too low. All devices have power fail and airflow alarms.

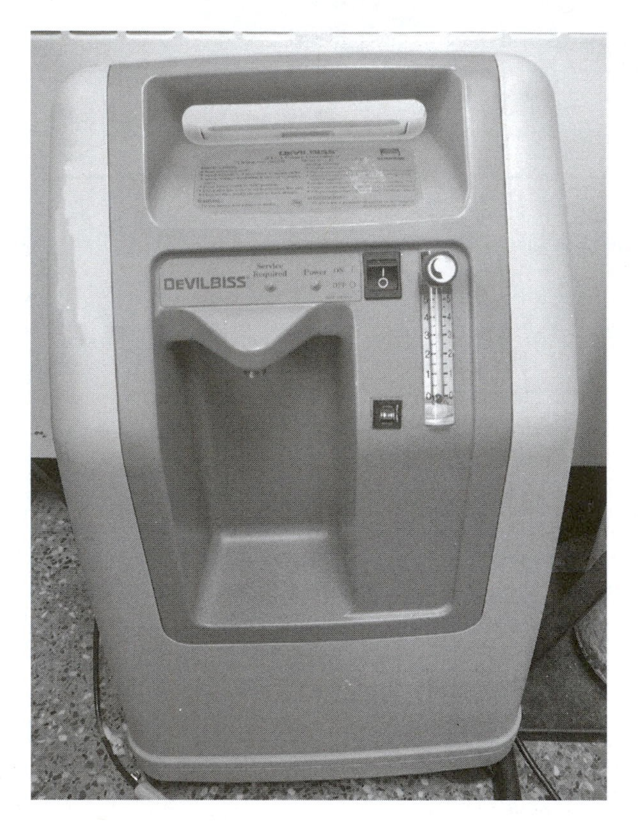

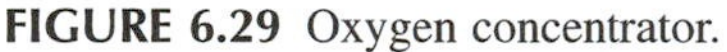

FIGURE 6.29 Oxygen concentrator.

D. Humidifiers

When gases are delivered to a patient, either via an anesthetic machine during surgery, by a ventilator, or simply as auxiliary oxygen, they are very low in water vapor content. This can cause the patient's airways to dry out, which can lead to discomfort as well as increased susceptibility to infections and tissue damage.

If the gases are to be delivered for any significant length of time, it is important that they have water vapor added by a humidifier.

There are a number of different mechanisms of humidifier function. The most basic is to simply bubble the gas through a reservoir of water. The water must be distilled to avoid contamination.

Other humidifiers use heat to vaporize water in a tank, and the gas flow passes over the surface of the water, picking up water vapor is it goes.

A third method of vaporizing water is with the use of ultrasonic crystals. High-frequency sound waves passing through water break some of it up into tiny droplets, which can then be passed into the patient breathing circuit. The droplets may pass to the patient directly, or they may, due to their small size, evaporate along the way.

Ultrasonic humidifiers, or nebulizers, have the advantage of not heating the water, which can help avoid patient hyperthermia problems.

VI. CHAPTER SUMMARY

Chapter 6 is wide ranging. The heart and its treatment is covered, including a history of defibrillators, the theory and designs of defibs, a Code Blue scenario, types of defibs, and some history and theory behind pacemakers, both implanted and exterior.

Circulation and blood are next, with topics of artificial hearts, heart-lung machines, tourniquets, and blood warmers.

IV and feeding pumps are covered, plus PCA pumps.

The respiratory system discussion includes ventilator theory and function, CPAP/BiPAP units, oxygen concentrators, and humidifiers.

7 Treatment Devices — Part Two

I. NERVOUS SYSTEM

A. Anesthesia

From the first time any kind of surgery was attempted on humans, it was obvious that it was extremely painful for the patient; the shock alone could easily be enough to cause death. In addition to this problem, the reaction of the patient to the trauma of surgery made it difficult for the surgeon to perform their tasks.

Various means were used to help alleviate the suffering of surgical patients, such as the administration of numbing drugs like laudanum (a tincture of opium) or alcohol ("Gimme a shot of that whiskey before you take the arrow out, doc!"). Patients usually had to be restrained and were often given something to bite on to help deal with the pain ("Biting the bullet").

But surgery under these conditions was still excruciating, prompting surgeons to work as quickly as possible. This, of course, often led to serious or even fatal errors, and sometimes, apocryphally, to the surgeon cutting off his own finger in his haste to complete a procedure.

Despite the claims by some that pain was natural and something that should simply be endured, most physicians and patients wished for pain-free procedures.

Dentistry, too, was advancing in both use and technique, and this helped drive the search for pain relieving agents.

1. Anesthetic Agents

In the mid-1800s, certain volatile liquids were found to produce temporary unconsciousness when administered carefully. Ether (CH_3–CH_2–O–CH_2–CH_3) and chloroform ($CHCl_3$) were used, at first simply by wetting a cloth with the liquid and having the patient breath through the material. Later designs had the cloth held on a wire framework placed over the patient's face, with a regulated amount of ether being dripped onto the cloth. Further refinements reduced the escape of vaporized gases by the use of cooling water jackets that kept the liquid below its boiling point until it was applied at the patient.

Ether had some advantages in addition to its anesthetic effect, in that it stimulated respiration and cardiac output and promoted abdominal relaxation. It didn't cause uterine relaxation, which made it useful for Caesarian sections. However it was extremely flammable, it caused bronchial irritation, which could lead to coughing fits, and the onset of its effect was slow, as was recovery from its effects.

By the mid-twentieth century, ether in anesthesia had mostly been displaced by cyclopropane (C_3H_6, arranged in a ring of carbons), trichloroethylene ($ClCH{=}CCl_2$), and halothane ($C_2HBrClF_3$), and currently the most commonly used anesthetic agents are more complex compounds such as sevoflurane (2,2,2-trifluoro-1-(trifluoro-methyl) ethyl ether), desflurane (2-(difluoromethoxy)-1,1,1,2-tetrafluoro-ethane), and isoflurane (chloro-2-(difluoromethoxy)-1,1,1-trifluoroethane), which have the advantage of both rapid onset and rapid recovery, with minimal side effects, as well as being nonflammable.

2. Anesthetic Machines

All of the anesthetic agents must be administered in a controlled manner in order to attain anesthesia that is adequate without being excessive. Anesthetic machines (Figure 7.1) were developed for this purpose, with a basic component being a vaporizer assembly to convert stored liquid anesthetic agent to a vapor form suitable for delivery to the patient.

In order to conserve anesthetic agents, they can be recirculated to the patient after exhalation, but this requires a means of absorbing the carbon dioxide exhaled. A canister containing soda lime or similar materials is included in the breathing circuit of anesthetic machines using this technique. The soda lime absorbs carbon dioxide and changes color from off-white to violet as it becomes saturated, allowing replacement before it becomes ineffective.

Surgery often involves paralyzing the patient's muscles as well as inducing anesthesia, and so a mechanism to provide artificial ventilation was required and was incorporated into anesthetic machines.

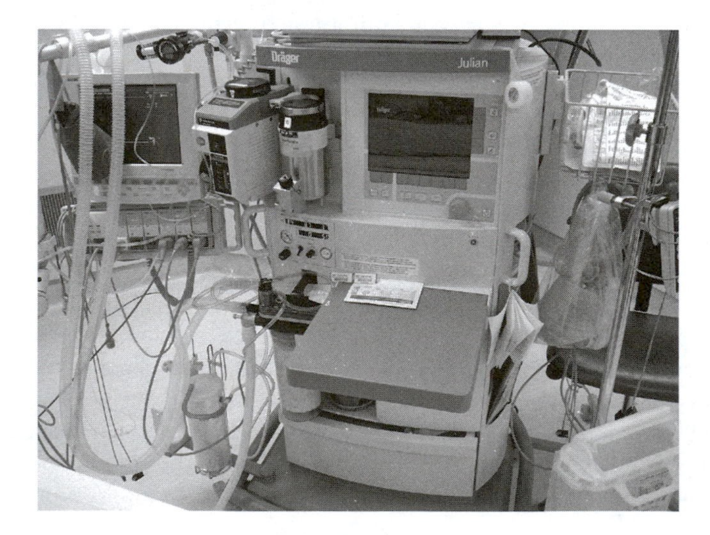

FIGURE 7.1 A modern anesthetic machine.

Oxygen, medical air, and nitrous oxide are used in the course of anesthesia, so supply and control systems for these gases are also included.

A monitor for analyzing the concentration of the anesthetic agent in use may form part of the system, either as a built-in component or as an add-on. Monitors for patient parameters such as ECG, SpO_2, temperature, and blood pressure are included in some machines, though most utilize a separate physiological monitor. There may be a means of communication between the anesthetic machine and the patient monitor, allowing anesthetic information to be included in the data being stored by the monitor.

Hypothermia is a serious side effect of surgery under general anesthesia, and it can be extremely dangerous if it advances into the malignant stage. Heated humidifiers that inject warm moisture into the breathing circuit can help prevent hypothermia, as well as alleviating the desiccation that can also be a problem.

Other components of a typical anesthetic machine include: backup gas supplies in cylinders, gauges for measuring flow and volume; backup battery power supplies to allow continued function should line power fail; alarm systems to detect leaks, pressure loss, and other malfunctions; and a scavenging system to remove excess anesthetic agents from the operating room. A suction mechanism may be present to allow removal of fluids from the patient's airways.

The details of design and operation of anesthetic machines varies from one manufacturer to another and from one model to another. Manufacturer training on these specifics and direct experience with the units are necessary for support personnel.

3. Anesthesia Vaporizers

As described above, the vaporizer used with anesthetic machines converts liquid anesthetic agents into a gaseous form suitable for delivery to the patient for inhalation. There are two main types of vaporizers found in most current hospital anesthetic machines; the characteristics of the agents determine which is used. Most machines can have two or more vaporizers installed at the same time, though interlock mechanisms must be used to prevent the delivery of two different agents simultaneously.

Vaporizers are designed to work with only one anesthetic agent and are always clearly marked to indicate which agent they take. Systems are designed to make it physically difficult to fill a vaporizer with the wrong agent.

Some agents have relatively high boiling points (isoflurane 48°C, sevoflurane 58.5°C), which allows them to be used in a specific type of vaporizer called a plenum vaporizer (Figure 7.2). Boiling points well above room temperature mean that vapor pressures of these agents in a closed chamber, or plenum, is constant (but of course different for each agent).

Medical air under pressure is applied to the vaporizer from the anesthetic machine and is split into two channels. One channel bypasses the agent chamber, while the other passes through the chamber and is then mixed back into the bypass channel. This chamber has an open space (plenum) into which some of the agent vaporizes. If the agent is kept at a constant temperature (usually room temperature — this is maintained in part by constructing the vaporizer with heavy metal walls that serve as a heat stabilizer), then the concentration of vapor (vapor pressure) in

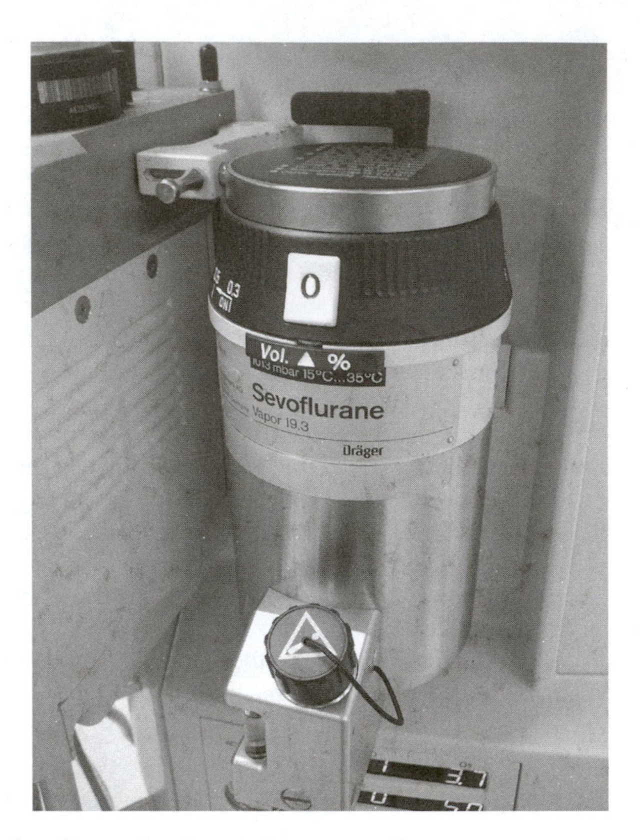

FIGURE 7.2 Sevoflurane plenum vaporizer.

the chamber is constant. By adjusting the proportion of gas passing through the chamber, the concentration of agent delivered to the patient can be controlled accurately. This mechanism works well over a wide range of flow rates.

The second type of vaporizer is designed for use with desflurane (see Figure 7.3). Desflurane has a boiling point of 23.5°C, which is close to or below normal room temperature. This means that desflurane will vaporize very readily at temperatures normally found in operating rooms, which makes the use of a plenum type vaporizer impossible; it would be extremely difficult to predict what the vapor pressure would be at any given time, and so the concentration of the agent taken by the air flowing through the plenum would vary greatly with slight temperature fluctuations, possibly even reaching lethal levels.

To overcome this problem, desflurane vaporizers are heated by an electrical element and pressurized to about 200 kPa (double atmospheric pressure). The rate of fresh gas flowing to the patient is measured by the system, and the amount of desflurane needed for a given concentration is calculated. The pressurized desflurane vapor is then injected in precise amounts into the fresh gas in order to meet the concentration requirements.

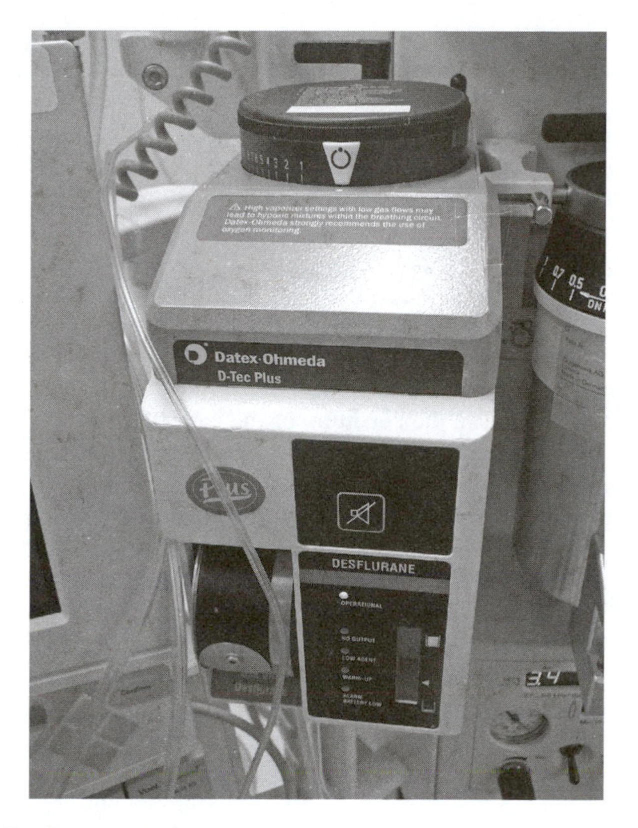

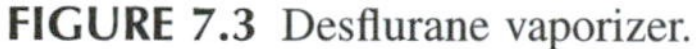
FIGURE 7.3 Desflurane vaporizer.

B. Anesthetic Gas Monitors

During surgical procedures when general anesthesia is used, it is critical to maintain anesthetic agent delivery within certain limits. Agent vaporizers are engineered to deliver specified amounts of gas, but various factors from the vaporizer through blenders and the components that deliver gas to the patient can affect the final concentration.

Additionally, some patients metabolize anesthetic agents more rapidly than others, and so might require extra amounts to be delivered to maintain adequate levels of consciousness.

Anesthetic gas monitors (AGMs) allow users to have a quantitative measure of the concentration of common agents both inspired and expired by the patient. Most systems also measure oxygen, nitrous oxide, and carbon dioxide at the same time.

Gas molecules of any substance will absorb various wavelengths of infrared light in patterns that are characteristic of that substance. By passing a broadband beam of infrared through a gas sample, measuring and analyzing the absorbance patterns, and comparing these to a table of patterns, the identity of the gas can be determined.

Further, by looking at the amplitude of the absorbance values, a measure of concentration can be taken. Accuracy of these measurements is usually best when gases are within normally used levels.

Information may be displayed on a built-in screen in both graphical and numeric forms, and/or it may be displayed on a secondary monitor. AGMs may be integrated into some anesthetic machines.

C. Electroconvulsive Therapy Machines

Mental illness has historically been difficult to treat, since there are no obvious physical causes or physiological or anatomical changes. A variety of unusual treatments have been used, some seemingly in random attempts to find something that produced an improvement in the condition of the patient.

It was discovered that some patients suffering from severe mental illness such as schizophrenia or depression responded positively to the application of electrical currents through their brains, delivered via electrodes on the head. Experimentation refined the technique to determine the optimum waveforms, amplitudes, delivery patterns, and treatment times, in order to provide the maximum benefit with minimum harmful side effects.

Electrical signals passing through any part of the body cause currents to flow throughout the rest of the body, since tissues are conductive. This means that the high-voltage signals applied to the head to treat mental illness have the potential to cause severe muscle contractions in other parts of the body, in other words, a convulsion. This gave the technique its name, electroconvulsive therapy (ECT).

When this technique was first used, patients had to be physically restrained to prevent injuries to themselves or staff when their limbs moved harshly during treatment. Despite the restraints, injuries were common. Also, if the patient was conscious during the procedure, it was often found to be a traumatic experience, although the shock usually produced immediate unconsciousness.

In current practice, the patient is first administered an agent to produce unconsciousness, and then a second agent that almost completely paralyzes their muscles. When this has taken effect, the ECT treatment proceeds. Muscle contractions, and their associated dangers, are largely avoided.

ECT machines (see Figure 7.4) may include simple ECG and EEG monitors, or separate monitors may perform these functions. Some ECT units have a motion-sensing device that can help determine if a shock has been delivered successfully; the patient's muscles still have a slight ability to contract, and a twitch of one of the patient's toes is a good indicator that the shock was delivered.

Originally, ECT machines used AC almost directly from the mains supply, but modern units deliver pulsed stimuli at a constant current of up to 750 mA (set by the operator) for a period of one to six seconds (again, set by the operator). Since current is constant, the voltage is determined, via Ohm's Law, by the impedance of the patient, although maximum voltage is limited by circuitry, to perhaps 200 or 225 volts.

ECT was originally developed because it was thought that epilepsy and schizophrenia were opposite maladies, and that if convulsions similar to that or epilepsy could be induced in schizophrenic patients, the effects of their disorder might be

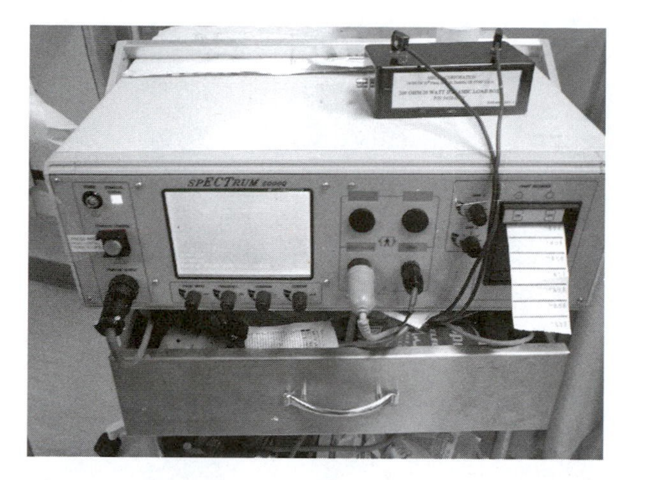

FIGURE 7.4 Electroconvulsive therapy machine.

reduced. This theory has long been abandoned, but controversy remains as to the exact mechanism of ECT. Generally, it is thought that the process acts on either the electrical function and blood flow in the brain, or on neurotransmitters in the brain, or on hormonal systems. In any case, it does seem to help certain patients who do not respond to other forms of treatment.

Side effects of ECT may include those commonly seen in response to the anaesthetizing and paralyzing agents, mental confusion, memory loss, and muscle aches. Some of these effects, particularly confusion and memory loss, may persist for long periods.

II. DIGESTIVE SYSTEM

The human machine needs both fuel and building materials in order to grow and function and also a means of getting rid of the waste products of living. The digestive system (see Figure 7.5) provides these services.

Human digestive systems are made up of the mouth and throat, the stomach, the small and large intestines, the rectum and anus, and associated organs such as salivary glands, the pancreas, and the liver.

Other than those involved in surgery, there are few devices used to support the digestive system.

A. Feeding Pumps

Patients are often unable to take food by mouth. They may be suffering from surgical or accidental trauma to their mouth or throat, they may be unconsciousness or otherwise unable to swallow, or they may be on a ventilator, whose mechanism blocks swallowing.

In such cases there are two means of providing the needed nutrition: intravenously, with a total parenteral nutrition program; or through the use of a tube that is passed into the stomach.

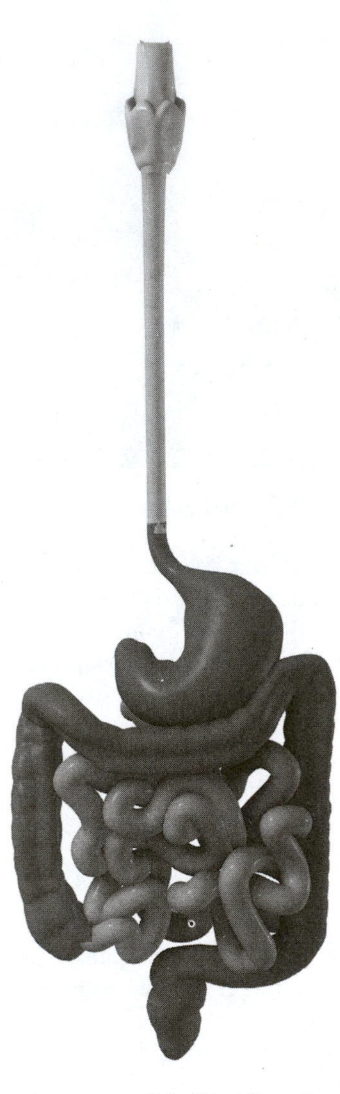

FIGURE 7.5 The human digestive system. (Modified from Inmagine Corp, www.123rf.com, with permission.)

Liquids delivered to the patient through a feeding tube may be simply gravity driven, but this does not have accurate controls and may be blocked by stomach structures. A feeding pump provides control and sufficient pressure to ensure delivery.

As with intravenous pumps, enteral feeding pumps (Figure 7.6) have controls for setting flow rates and total volume to be delivered. Flow rates typically range from 1 to 300 ml/hour, and volume limits from 1 to 9999 ml.

Because feeding solutions have different characteristics than intravenous fluids, pump details are different in some aspects:

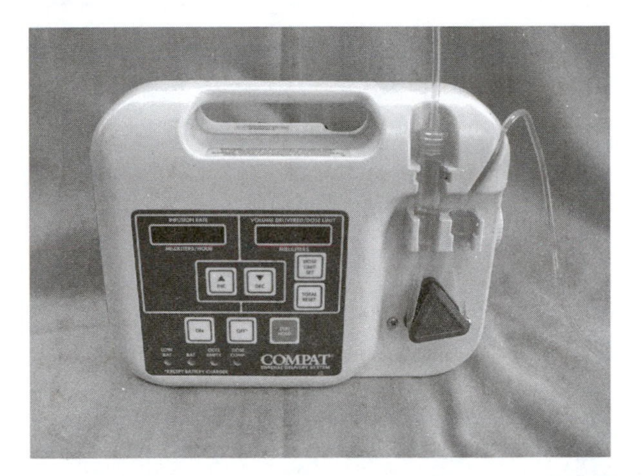

FIGURE 7.6 An enteral feeding pump.

- Feeding solutions are more viscous than IV fluids, so pump mechanisms must be robust, and channels must be relatively large. Most feeding pumps use a rotary peristaltic mechanism, with a rubber section of tubing to fit into the pump head (Figure 7.7).
- A few air bubbles entering the stomach will not cause any problems, so air-in-line detectors are not needed.
- Blockages are not as critical as with IV pumps, but alarms are needed to alert staff that flow has been interrupted. Typically, the delivery tubing set has a drip chamber that fits into a drip-sensing receptacle in the pump. Drips are counted and correlated to the set flow rate. If a discrepancy is found, an alarm sounds. Drops may have stopped because the fluid reservoir is empty, the line is kinked at some point, or the exit of the tubing in the stomach is occluded by tissue.

Enteral feeding pumps normally have batteries to allow them to function when the patient is being transported from one area to another.

III. RENAL SYSTEM

The renal system in humans consists of a pair of kidneys with associated blood supplies, ureters to drain urine from the kidneys, the bladder to store urine, and the urethra to empty the bladder.

The kidneys perform a number of important functions in the body, with one of the most important being the removal of certain waste products by filtering them from the blood. Urea, a breakdown product of proteins, is the main waste to be removed; others include uric acid, creatinine, and other metabolic breakdown substances. The kidneys can also remove excess water and glucose as well as sodium, potassium, and other electrolytes.

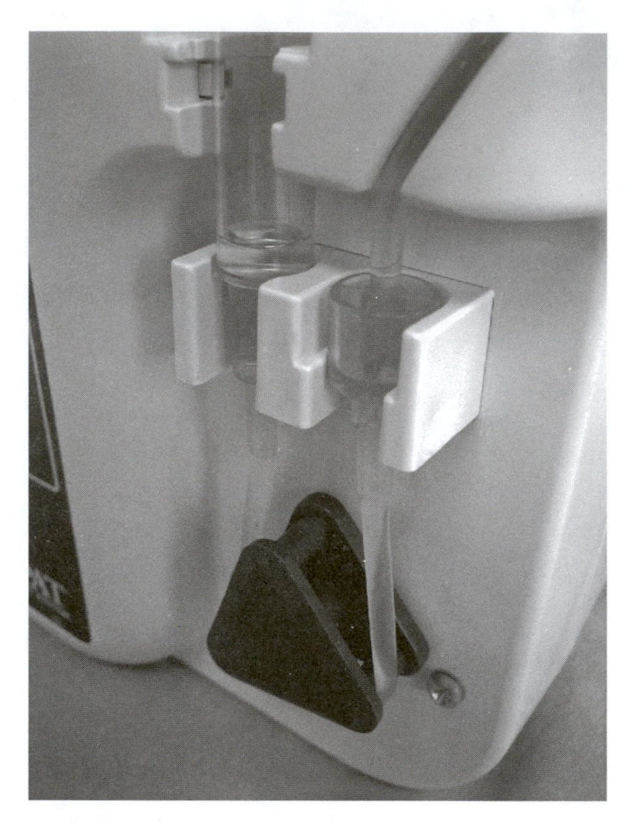

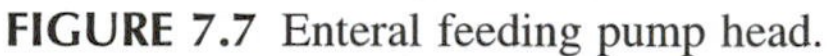

FIGURE 7.7 Enteral feeding pump head.

If the kidneys are not functioning adequately, waste products can build up in the body, and a variety of symptoms appear, including high blood pressure, weight loss, nausea, fatigue, muscle cramps, a yellowish-brown discoloration of the skin, and loss of mental acuity. If not treated, death can eventually result.

A. Hemodialysis

Various means have been used throughout history to try to treat the symptoms of kidney failure, including hot baths, sweat lodges or steam baths, enemas, and bloodletting. There was some basis to these treatments, as some toxins can be excreted in sweat, they can diffuse into an enema solution through the walls of the colon, and if some "bad" blood is removed, new "good" blood is generated to replace what was lost. There are limits to the amounts of toxins that can be removed by these methods, however, so more effective means were sought.

As scientists learned more about such matters as diffusion and osmosis, and about blood chemistry, it became apparent that there might be ways of temporarily removing blood from the body of a kidney failure patient, removing much of the impurities, and returning the cleansed blood to the patient. This process would have to be repeated regularly. In some circumstances, the kidneys may regain their function, but most of the time, the only two alternatives to continued hemodialysis are kidney transplants and death.

In 1945, Willem Koff performed the first successful human hemodialysis treatment, in the Netherlands.

The term hemodialysis comes from the roots "hemo," referring to blood, "dia" meaning through, and "lysis," meaning a loosening. Impurities are *loosened* from the *blood* by passing them *through* a membrane.

A modern hemodialysis system consists of a water purification system, an access point to the patient's blood stream, a number of different monitoring components for both patient and hardware, and the dialyzer itself.

1. Water Purification System

Since dialysis involves the use of large quantities of water, any impurities such as minerals or bacterial toxins can enter a patient's blood. Normally, the kidneys would remove much of these impurities, but of course for dialysis patients, this isn't an option. Therefore, the water used must be extremely pure. A very high-quality reverse osmosis system is generally used, with monitoring for specific contaminants such as chlorine and conductivity monitoring to detect the smallest amounts of any other ions.

2. Access Point

Hemodialysis is a long-term treatment method, and access to the patient's blood stream must be safe and reliable. Repeated insertions of large-bore needles would soon exhaust the available sites, which would be the end of the road for the patient.

Semipermanent catheters provide a simple, reliable access point (Figure 7.8), but are only suitable for relatively short-term applications, such as when recovery of kidney function is expected or a transplant is pending. Catheters, inserted into veins, may be "nontunneled" or "tunneled." Nontunneled catheters are simply passed through the skin above the vein insertion site; this is only suitable for very short term use because veins accessible for this purpose are too small to allow high flow rates. Tunneled catheters are passed through the skin at a somewhat convenient location, such as the chest wall, and are "tunneled" under the skin to a larger artery such as the internal jugular and then to the vena cava.

Both catheter type access points are susceptible to infection and so are not suitable for long-term (more than about 10 days) use.

The ideal method of accessing the blood system is through an arteriovenous (AV) fistula. A surgeon constructs this by joining a vein and an artery together, which allows a high rate of blood flow through the joint, since the capillary system is bypassed. Once this structure is healed, needles can be inserted in opposite directions, one to withdraw blood and the other to return it to the patient. AV fistulas are usually placed on the patient's arm. Infections are much less common with fistulas than with catheters as the needles are only present for relatively short times, during all of which the sites are closely monitored. AV fistulas may reduce blood supply to the lower part of the limb in which they are used.

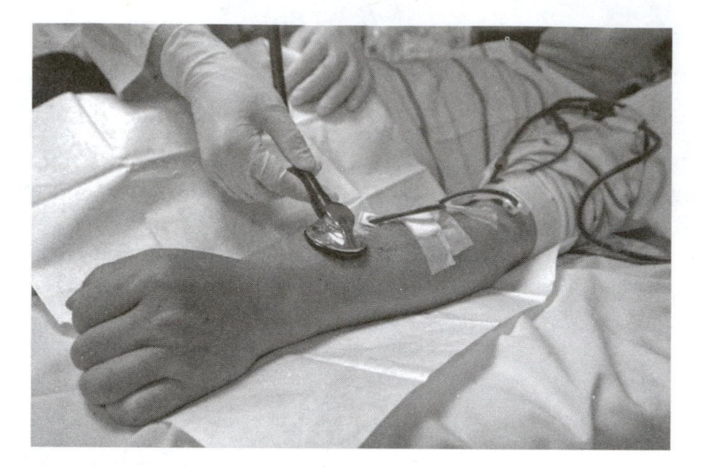

FIGURE 7.8 Hemodialysis access point. (Modified from Inmagine Corp, www.123rf.com, with permission.)

A variation on the AV fistula uses an artificial material to connect (or graft) the artery and vein, which results in faster healing; they can also be installed in more locations than a fistula. However, such grafts are more prone to infection, and the joint can become narrowed, restricting blood flow.

3. Monitoring Components

As mentioned previously, water purity must be continuously monitored, and access points must be visually monitored for signs of infection or other tissue damage.

Additionally, the patient must be carefully monitored.

Since large amounts of fluids are being removed from and replaced in the patient's body, balance is very important, so the patient is weighed precisely and continuously during treatment. Since fluids are retained in patients with kidney failure, staff must accurately estimate what patient's weight should be with normal fluid levels, which is the target weight. Blood pressure can fluctuate considerably with dialysis, and so this is monitored as well using a noninvasive blood pressure machine. Temperature and ECG are also monitored.

4. Dialyzer

Once blood is removed from the patient, it is pumped through the system using a peristaltic pump mechanism. This uses much larger tubing than either intravenous or feeding pumps. The peristaltic method allows pumping without having the pump mechanism come in contact with the blood, and also, especially with a large-diameter, relatively slowly rotating pump head, mechanical disturbance of blood cells is minimized.

Blood passes from the pump into a large number of fine parallel tubes made of semipermeable material. The tubes are immersed in a bath of body-temperature fluid (the dialysate), which contains isotonic levels of the chemicals that should stay in the blood, but hypotonic levels of the components that are to be removed. The dialysate is pumped in the opposite direction to the blood flowing in the tubules, and impurities diffuse from the blood into the dialysate. Since fluids have been retained by the patient as a result of their kidney failure, this excess must also be removed. This is accomplished by applying higher pressure to the blood than to the dialysate, causing water to move through the membrane from the blood into the dialysate.

When treatment is concluded, the access connections are removed and the patient transferred to a recovery area, where vital signs, especially blood pressure and temperature, continue to be monitored until the patient is able to leave.

B. Peritoneal Dialysis

For patients who cannot tolerate hemodialysis for any reason, or if their kidney failure is not complete, peritoneal dialysis offers an alternative.

It is a much simpler process than hemodialysis, and the equipment is portable and simple enough to be used in patient's homes or even while traveling.

Peritoneal dialysis takes advantage of the fact that the abdominal cavity, or peritoneum, has a very large total surface area of well-vascularized membranes. By filling the peritoneum with a carefully formulated dialysate solution, urea and other waste products in the blood will diffuse across the peritoneal membranes and into the dialysate. The composition of the dialysate can also cause excess water to diffuse out of the blood stream if this is required. After a set period of time, the dialysate and waste products are drained from the abdomen; the process maybe repeated, depending on circumstances.

Because large volumes of fluid are entering the body, they must be heated to near body temperature before infusion, or hypothermia can result. Only low pressures are required to move the fluid into the abdomen, so gravity feed is adequate; dialysate bags are simply hung a short distance above the patient.

A catheter, which can be opened or closed, must be installed into the abdomen and left in place more or less permanently. This requires that the patient be diligent in keeping the site clean in order to avoid infection. A passage to the peritoneum means that infections can move beyond the surface, where they might be relatively minor, into the abdomen, where peritonitis can result. Peritonitis is much more difficult to treat and can be fatal.

Peritoneal dialysis may be done in three somewhat different ways:

1. Continuous cyclic peritoneal dialysis (CCPD) uses a relatively large volume of fluid per cycle and longer cycles, one cycle following the other immediately. The process is repeated perhaps once every 24 hours and may be done at night while the patient is sleeping. A machine with a timer and valves controls the filling and draining cycles.
2. Intermittent peritoneal dialysis (IPD) can use the same cycling device as CCPD, but set so that there is a time gap between one drain phase and the next fill phase.
3. Continuous ambulatory peritoneal dialysis (CAPD) involves slower fluid exchanges with smaller volumes. Warmed fluid is instilled into the abdo-

men and then left there for four or five hours. During this time, the patient can go about daily activities. After the preset time (signaled by a timer, or simply when the patient sees that the time is up; no machines are required), the old dialysate is drained from the abdomen, and a fresh batch is instilled again. Cycling goes on continuously. The timing of cycles is somewhat flexible and can be adapted to the patient's lifestyle. Because of its simplicity and ease, CAPD is the most commonly used form of peritoneal dialysis.

C. Lithotriptors

The renal system is in the business of filtering waste products from the blood and concentrating them for removal from the body. Under some circumstances, related to diet, body chemistry, altered kidney function, or certain disease conditions, some of the waste products can become so concentrated that they precipitate out of the urine. If this happens over a prolonged period of time, the precipitated material can bond together to form kidney stones, also called renal calculi.

Kidney stones can form from a variety of chemicals:

- About 80% of stones are formed from calcium oxalate.
- Some stones are formed by the action of bacteria in relation to ammonia, which forms crystalline stones called struvites. These stones can become very large, filling the renal pelvis and taking on a "stag horn" shape. These stones can be very difficult to remove and very harmful to the kidneys. They are most often seen in women who have frequent urinary tract infections.
- Uric acid stones form due to an excess of, you guessed it, uric acid. Uric acid can also precipitate in joints, causing the painful condition known as gout.
- A rare genetic condition can cause high levels of the amino acid cystine in the urine, which can result in stone formation.

Kidney stones can be removed from the body in three different ways: by passing them through the urinary system, which can be extremely painful, and if the stone is too large, impossible; by surgery, which has its own set of dangers, especially involving the kidneys; or by breaking them into small pieces so they can pass with a minimum of discomfort. The process of breaking the stones into pieces is called lithotripsy, literally "stone crushing."

Some systems use a probe that is threaded up through the urinary tract until the tip comes in contact with the stone. The tip has an electrical terminal that produces a spark when triggered with a high-voltage pulse. The spark vaporizes a small amount of water, which in turn creates a sonic shock wave. Repeated over and over again, the sonic pulses can eventually break the stone apart. Fluoroscopic or ultrasonic imaging is used to locate the stone and guide the probe tip. It can be difficult to maintain contact with the stone, especially after it starts to break apart.

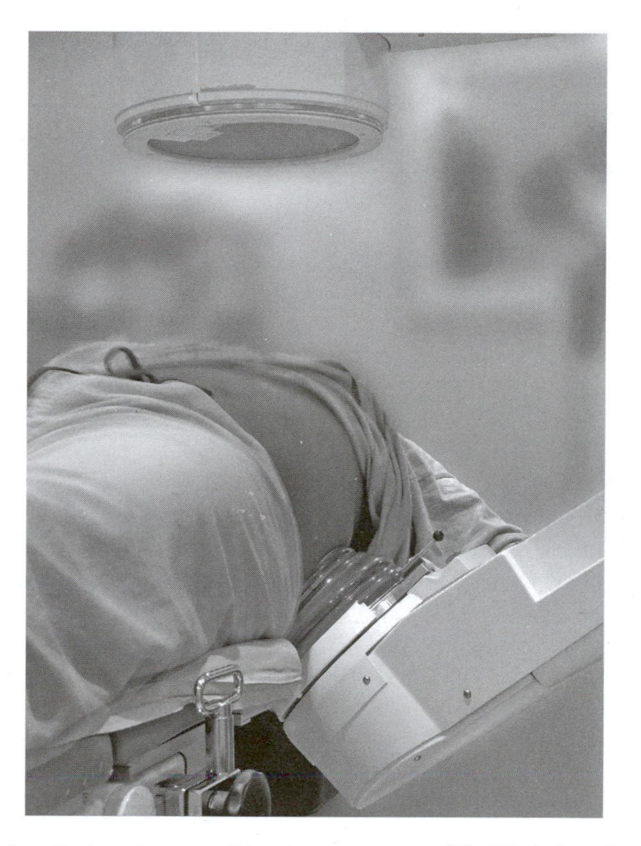

FIGURE 7.9 A patient undergoing lithotripsy treatment. (Modified from Inmagine Corp, www.123rf.com, with permission.)

Extracorporeal shock wave lithotripsy (ESWL) takes advantage of the fact that sound waves can be made to focus in a very small volume. The sonic intensity at the focal point can be extremely high, and if it is located in the same space as the kidney stone, it can, with repeated applications, cause the stone to break apart.

ESWL is performed by placing the patient in a water bath, or alternately by having bags of fluid contact the body at certain specific locations (Figure 7.9). In the latter case, coupling gel helps to ensure optimal transfer of sonic energy from the generator to the patient. This method is both more convenient and more common.

Patients are sedated, or sometimes anaesthetized, and usually connected to an ECG monitor.

An imaging system is used to locate the stone, and targeting mechanisms adjust the focal point of the sound generator so that it coincides with the position of the stone.

Sonic pulses are initiated, and power levels increased to a set level. Eventually the stone begins to break up, and treatment is continued until only small particles remain, usually in about an hour.

The sound waves break up the stone by a combination of shear forces, where adjacent parts of the stone are trying to move in opposite directions due to the crest and trough of the sound wave being very close together, or from cavitation, where the low pressure in the trough of the sound wave is sufficient to produce a vacuum "bubble"; collapse of the bubble creates a mechanical shock.

Sonic waves are generated by two methods.

- Immersed in water, a spark gap, somewhat like the spark plug of a car's engine, carries a high-voltage pulse across its gap. This produces an explosive vaporization in the immediate area, which in turn produces a high-intensity sound wave in the fluid.
- More recently, ESWL systems use a large array of piezoelectric crystals. Again, a high-energy electrical pulse stimulates the crystals and causes them to produce a sound wave directly.

With either method, the maximum intensity of the sound waves is at one focus of an ellipse. The spark gap method uses a metal reflector to focus the waves on the stone. The piezoelectric crystals are arranged in an elliptical pattern that has its focal point at the stone.

IV. SENSORY ORGANS

A. PHACOEMULSIFIERS

Cataracts are a common cause of vision loss, especially in older patients. They form when the proteins that make up the lens of the eye (Figures 7.10 and 7.11) change shape and orientation, reducing the clarity of the lens. Eventually, complete loss of vision can occur.

Surgical techniques were developed in the eighteenth century that simply removed the clouded lens, which restored limited vision. Extremely thick eyeglasses provided some further improvement.

During World War II, pilots sometimes suffered eye injuries when the plastic canopy of their plane was shattered. Doctors found that the shards of plastic were biologically inert, and not rejected by the eye.

In 1949, one of these surgeons, Howard Ridley in Britain, had a lens fabricated from the same material as the airplane canopies and inserted it in a cataract patient's eye after removing the clouded natural lens.

Techniques and material evolved, and now only very small incisions are required to perform lens removal and replacement surgery.

One of the main developments that allowed surgeons to use such small incisions was the phacoemulsifier (Figure 7.12).

Removal of the old lens was always a limiting factor for the size of incision, since the lens is quite hard and inflexible.

Phacoemulsifiers use ultrasound produced at the tip of a small probe to break up (emulsify) the lens, sometimes within its outer capsule, which usually remains clear in cataract patients. A plastic lens is then folded and inserted through the same

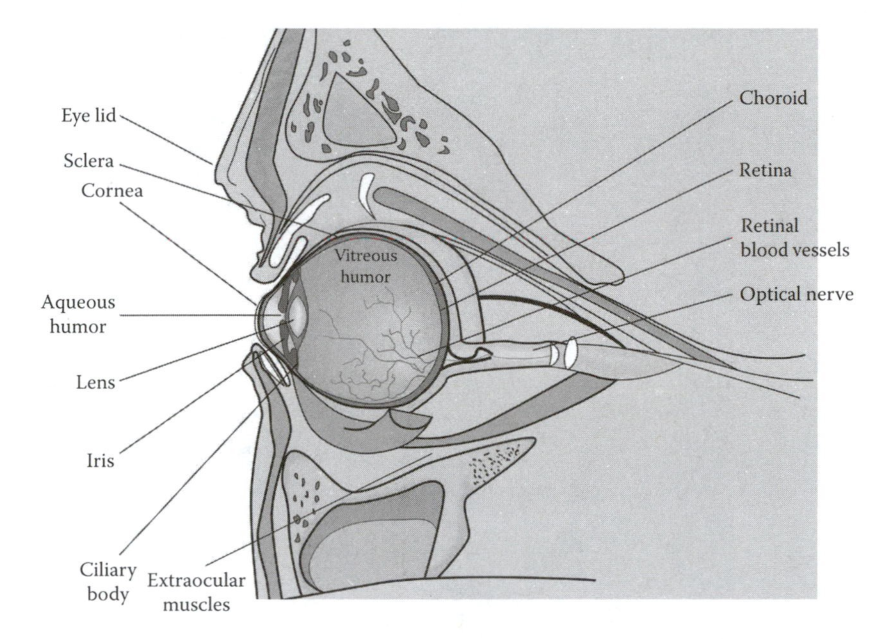

FIGURE 7.10 Anatomy of the eye. (Modified from Inmagine Corp, www.123rf.com, with permission.)

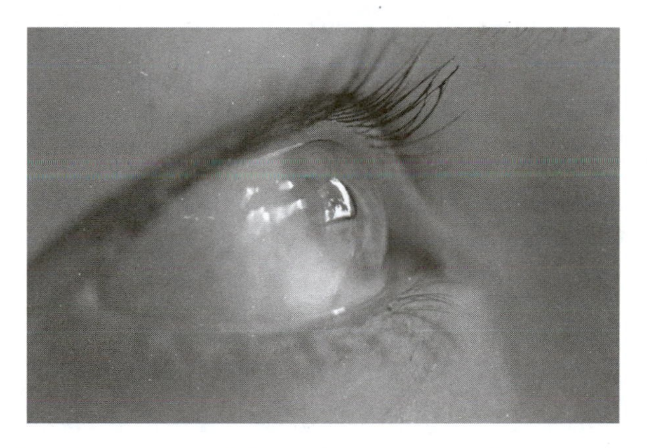

FIGURE 7.11 Eye looking up. (Modified from Inmagine Corp, www.123rf.com, with permission.)

incision as used for the probe. It is unfolded within the lens capsule, and small tabs on its rim help hold it in position.

The incision in modern cataract/lens replacement surgery is so small that sutures are not required; this, combined with the small size, makes the healing process quite short. Patients are usually discharged within a few hours of the procedure.

Surgery is performed with the aid of an operating microscope (see Chapter 8).

The phacoemulsifier system includes the components required to generate and control the ultrasound signal, as well as a means of removing the broken-up pieces

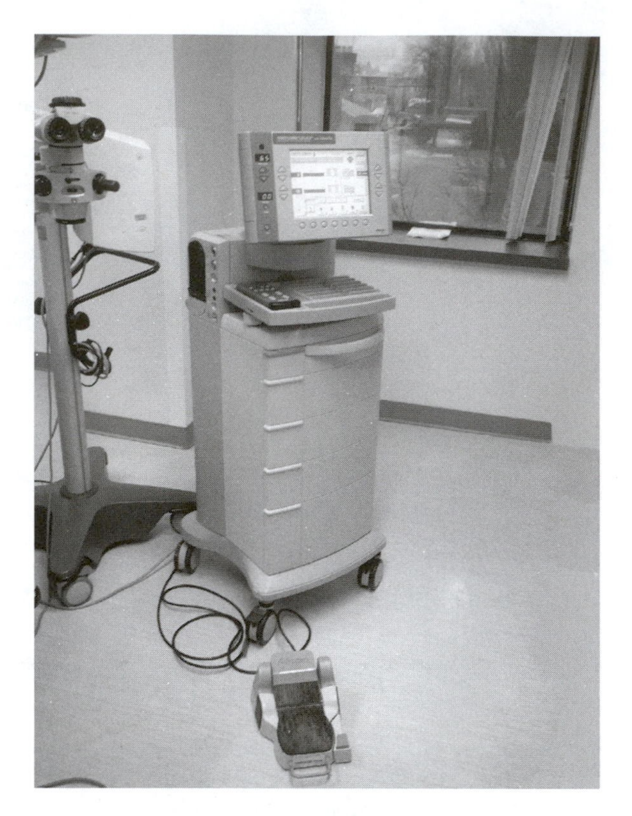

FIGURE 7.12 Phacoemulsifier system.

of lens. Intraocular pressure must be monitored and maintained throughout the procedure. A footswitch allows the surgeon to control most functions of the system, such as ultrasound power, suction and irrigation (Figure 7.13), while keeping hands free for doing the actual surgery.

B. Ophthalmic Lasers

Ophthalmic lasers are much like the surgical lasers described in Chapter 8, but they have special design features that make them more suitable for ophthalmic procedures.

The most common eye surgery using lasers is for vision correction. The cornea is part of the focusing system of the eye (Figure 7.14), and its shape helps determine where an image is focused. If this focal point is not at the retina, vision is blurred and corrective lenses are needed to move the focal point to the retina, producing clear vision. Laser surgery can reshape the cornea sufficiently to correct focusing on its own, so that patients will no longer need glasses or contact lenses for clear vision.

The patient's vision is first measured carefully, and then the cornea is scanned to produce a three-dimensional model. This data can be analyzed to determine what adjustments must be made to the cornea to correct vision. The parameters are fed into a laser control system, which applies the laser beam in such a way as to produce the desired results.

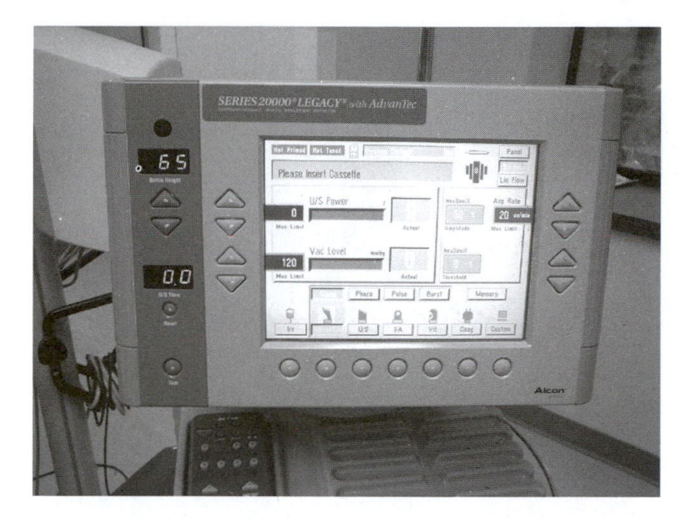

FIGURE 7.13 Close-up of phaco screen.

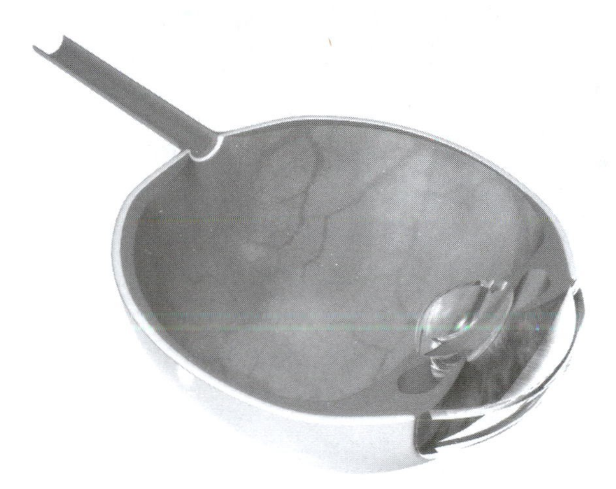

FIGURE 7.14 Eye diagram. (Modified from Inmagine Corp, www.123rf.com, with permission.)

The most common methods of corneal vision correction are PKR and LASIK.

PKR stand for Photo-Refractive Keractectomy, in which the surgeon removes the outer layer of the cornea before the laser comes into play, vaporizing tiny parts of the cornea to adjust focusing.

LASIK is Laser Assisted in situ Keratomileusis, and is more invasive than PKR. The surgeon cuts a very small flap into the cornea, and then the laser is directed through the flap onto the underside of the cornea, where it burns away enough tissue to produce corrected vision.

A typical LASIK laser wavelength is 193 nm.

Lasers (Figure 7.15) are used in other ophthalmic procedures as well, such as retinal repair and to remove protein films on implanted lenses.

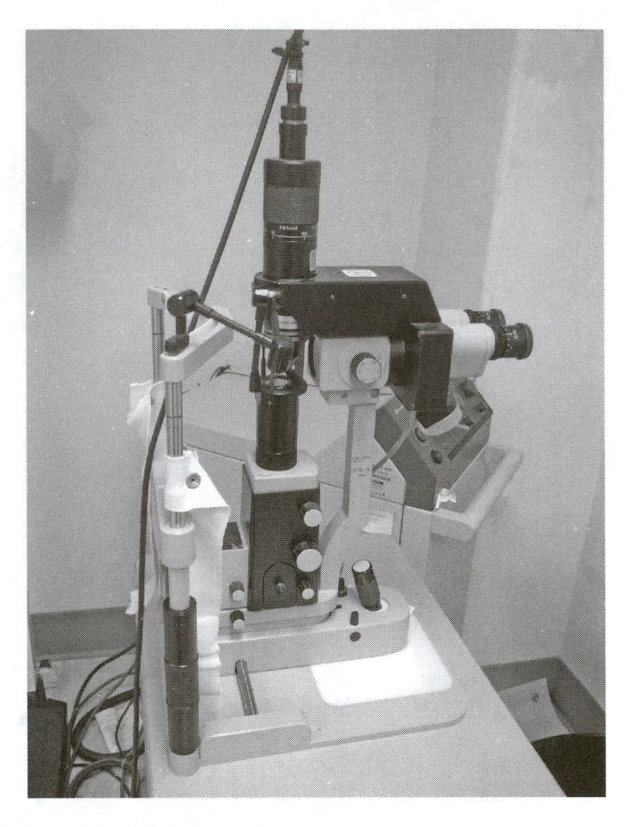

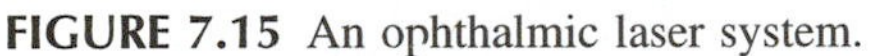

FIGURE 7.15 An ophthalmic laser system.

V. CHAPTER SUMMARY

Chapter 7 covers equipment relating to the nervous system. Anesthetic machine history and technology, types of anesthetic agents, and anesthetic machine features are described. Electroconvulsive therapy units are discussed.

Enteral feeding pumps are covered.

Relating to the renal system, kidney function is outlined, as well as hemodialysis system features and theory, and methods of treatment. Peritoneal dialysis is described, plus the physics of lithotripter and a section about the treatment process.

The sensory system focuses on the eyes, with a discussion of cataracts and lens replacement using phacoemulsifiers, and the theory and applications of ophthalmic lasers.

8 Treatment Devices — Part Three

I. REPRODUCTIVE SYSTEM

A. Bilirubin Therapy Systems

Newborn babies often have an excess of bilirubin in their bodies. Bilirubin is a breakdown product of red blood cells that is normally excreted via the liver. If liver function is not up to normal capacity, the bilirubin can build up in tissues including the skin, giving it a yellowish color, a condition called jaundice.

If bilirubin levels are too high, they can cause brain damage, so it is important to remove excess amounts as quickly as possible.

Bilirubin in the skin can be broken down when exposed to certain wavelengths of light, with the greatest effect occurring at about 510 nM. The breakdown products can then be safely excreted in urine.

Since light sources usually have a somewhat broad bandwidth, and since some photochemical breakdown of bilirubin occurs at wavelengths above and below 510 nM, lights with a bandwidth in the range of 360 to 520 nM are often used to treat hyperbilirubinemia in neonates. Light of the 510 nM optimal wavelength is green, but 360 nM is in the near-ultraviolet range, with violet and blue in between. The overall effect is that most treatment lights appear to be blue.

This light may be delivered by an overhead bank of special fluorescent tubes (Figure 8.1), either through the Plexiglas™ canopy of an infant incubator or directly through the air above a bassinette. In this case, as much of the infant's skin must be exposed to the light as possible in order to maximize the therapeutic effect, but then environmental and body temperatures must be controlled and monitored carefully.

Since incident radiation varies with the square of the distance from the source, and since Plexiglas™ absorbs some light, and further since light output at the relevant wavelengths can vary with bulb age, light levels should be measured with an accurate, calibrated photometer (Figure 8.2) that is sensitive to the relevant wavelengths.

Some systems reduce both the issue of light distance and the amount of exposed skin for the baby by using a blanket with embedded fiberoptic channels that are fed by a light source of the appropriate wavelength. This system is also less bulky than the overhead lighting system.

In all cases, as mentioned, measurement of light output using a calibrated photometer is very important.

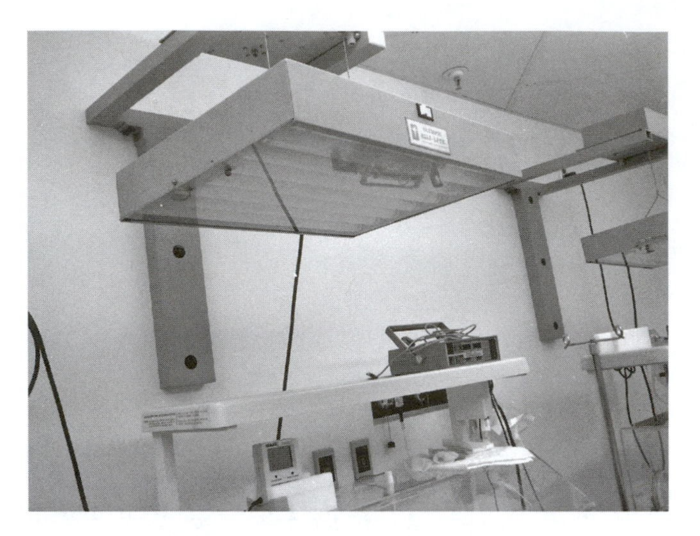

FIGURE 8.1 An overhead bilirubin therapy light.

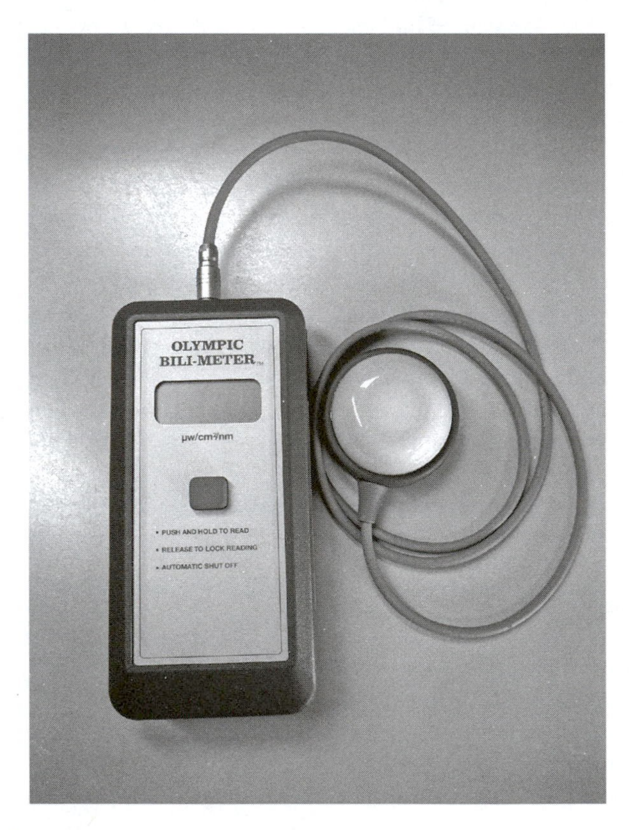

FIGURE 8.2 Bililight photometer.

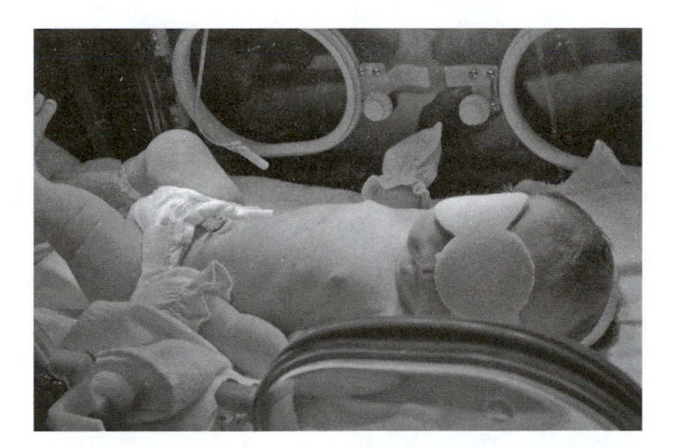

FIGURE 8.3 A baby undergoing UV therapy — note eye covering. (Modified from Inmagine Corp, www.123rf.com, with permission.)

Since prolonged exposure of the eyes to light of these wavelengths can cause damage, infants must have a mask fitted to cover their eyes while undergoing light therapy (Figure 8.3).

B. Infant Incubators

Neonates, especially if of low birth weight and/or born prematurely, or if there are other medical conditions, may not have adequately developed thermoregulatory systems. In these cases, the infant is best kept in an environment with closely controlled temperature and humidity.

Such infants may also have breathing difficulties, so an oxygen-enriched atmosphere may be beneficial.

Infant incubators are designed to meet these needs. A number of design criteria must be met:

- Temperature control must be precise and responsive. The temperature must be able to be set to an appropriate range of values, with alarms for over- and under-temperature. Since the incubator may have to be opened frequently for care purposes, exposing the interior to room temperature, the system must be able to return to the set temperature quickly. A heater element of adequate capacity is needed, along with an effective air circulation system. Most systems use double-walled construction to help insulate the interior. Air flow between inner and outer walls helps to maintain temperature and even out heat distribution. Temperature control may be done according to air temperature or infant skin temperature; control must be maintained should a sensor in use fail or become disconnected, which requires an independent, permanent temperature sensor located somewhere else in the system.
- Access for routine care procedures must be easy, but still restrict heat and oxygen loss. Systems use multiple access hatches with gasket-sealed

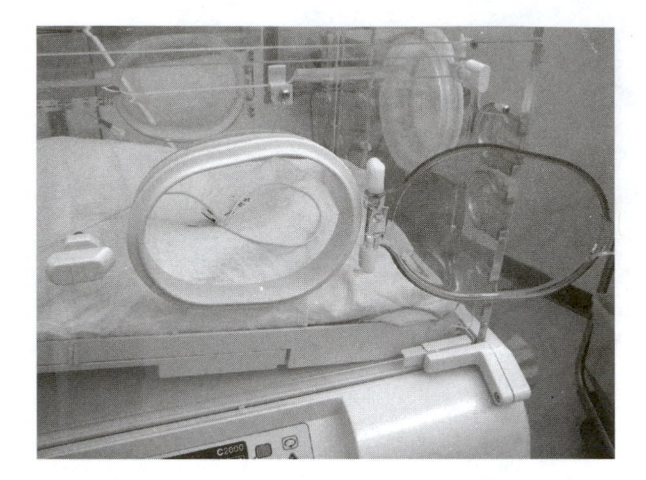

FIGURE 8.4 Incubator — doors open.

doors, along with elasticized collars to fit around the arms of caregivers. There is usually a large side door to allow the infant to be moved in and out of the incubator as necessary (Figure 8.4).

- Oxygen systems must provide sufficient flow to maintain maximum set levels when the incubator is closed, and return to set levels in a short time after hatches or doors have been opened. Oxygen should be monitored continuously, with alarms for over- and under-measurements (Figure 8.5). Excess oxygen can cause problems with eye development in neonates, while too little oxygen may not be therapeutically adequate. Incubators are generally used in hospitals where line oxygen is available.
- Humidity systems should be easy to use and effective, ideally with a humidity monitoring capability.

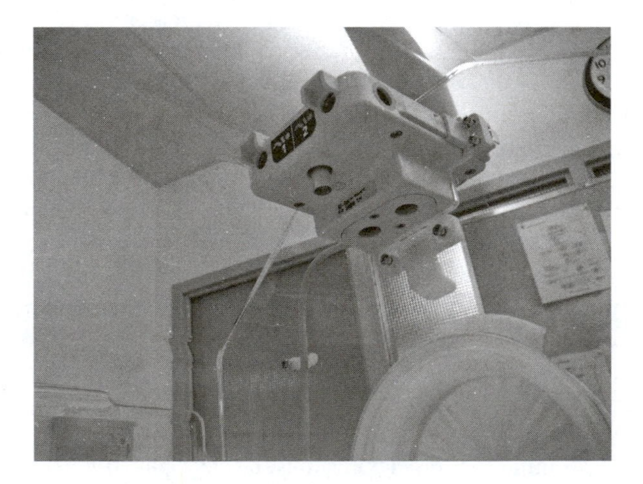

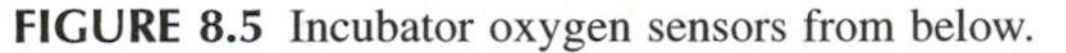

FIGURE 8.5 Incubator oxygen sensors from below.

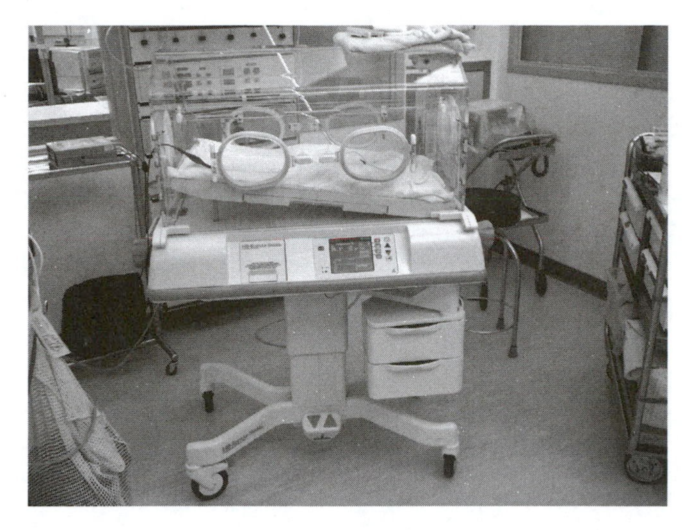

FIGURE 8.6 Full view of incubator.

- The infant must be easily visible at all times (Figure 8.6). Incubators use Plexiglas™ canopies for this purpose, with minimal obstructing hardware.
- Since the interior of the incubator has many hard, flat, sound-reflecting surfaces and newborn ears are very sensitive, sounds inside the incubator should be kept to a minimum. This mainly relates to the air circulation system, which must use high-quality, quiet motors and well-designed fans that move air effectively but quietly.
- Ideally, the body of the incubator should be able to be raised or lowered to accommodate different staff as they work with the infant.
- Certain medical situations may require that the infant be placed in a head-up or head-down position. This should be possible using external controls.
- Air-tight access points should be available for SpO_2 or ECG cables, ventilator hoses, or IV or feeding tubes.
- Since infant weight is an important parameter for monitoring growth as well as fluid balance, an integrated weigh scale is a valuable feature.
- X-rays may need to be taken of the infant, so a tray for x-ray film cassettes under the bed means that the infant does not have to be removed from the incubator.
- A display system that shows values for current temperature (skin and/or air), set temperature, current and set humidity, and current and set oxygen levels is very useful. Such displays may also show graphs of the various parameters, as well as infant weights and other data, and alarm information (Figure 8.7).
- An audible alarm to indicate loss of AC power is vital.
- Built-in compartments for accessories and supplies are important.

Transport incubators are specialized versions of infant incubators that are designed to fit into emergency vehicles (with smaller dimensions and collapsible

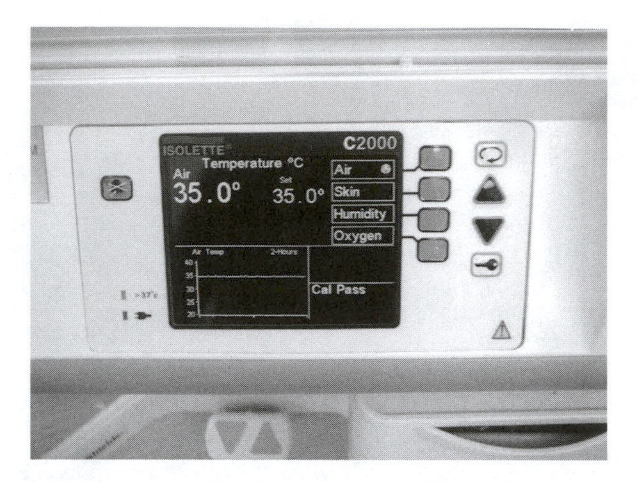

FIGURE 8.7 Incubator display panel.

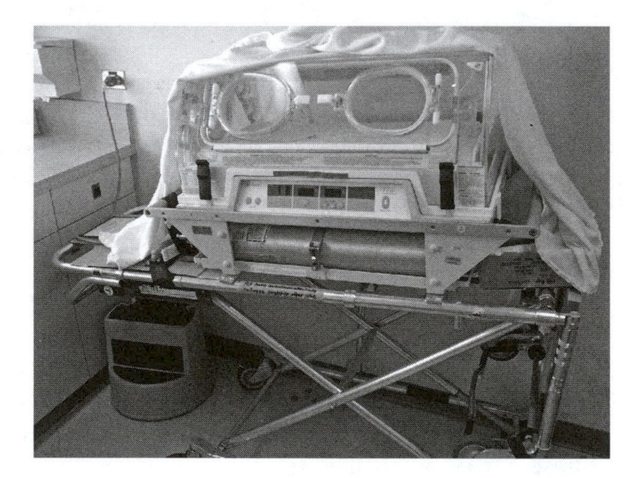

FIGURE 8.8 Transport incubator.

undercarriages), and include oxygen tanks and powerful batteries to maintain functions while away from line power (Figure 8.8).

C. Infant Resuscitators

Immediately following birth, babies may need intensive treatment. Airways may need to be aspirated, oxygen administered, tests performed, and breathing augmented, in an environment that provides quick heat and bright light.

Infant resuscitators (Figure 8.9) are devices that fulfill these requirements.

Since they may need to be moved to other areas of the hospital (babies do not always chose to be born in convenient locations), they usually have oxygen tanks onboard, though they can run on line oxygen if it is available. Oxygen flowing through a venturi can produce suitable suction if wall suction is not available.

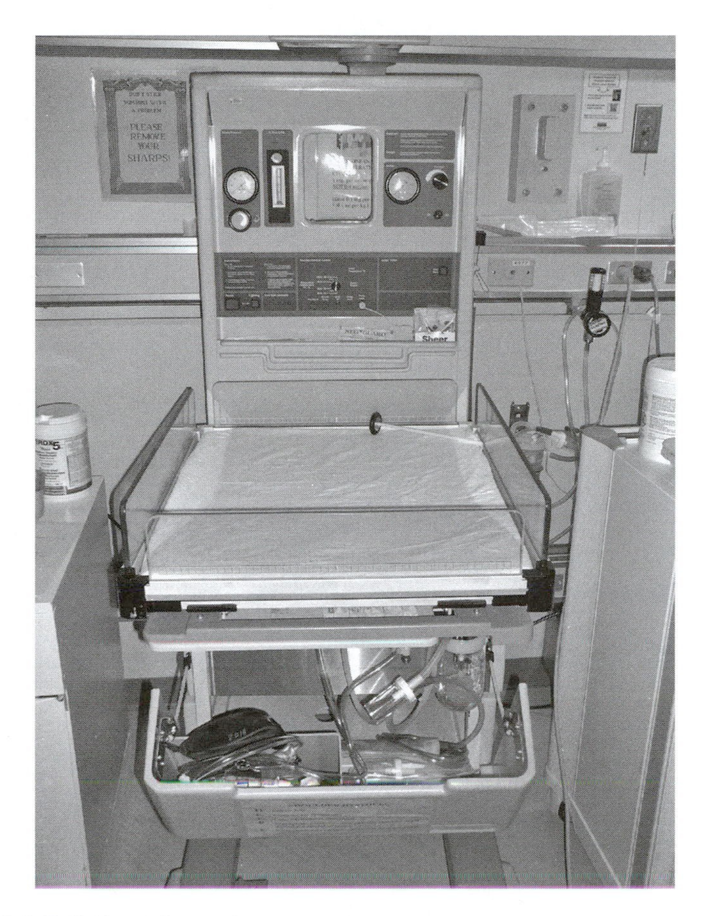

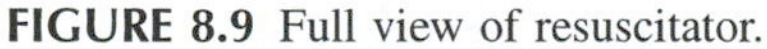

FIGURE 8.9 Full view of resuscitator.

Suction and oxygen must be readily available, and their controls easy to access. Because several people may be involved in the care of the neonate, access from three sides must be clear, with controls and support for heaters and lights on the fourth side (Figure 8.10).

Since the working area is open, radiant heat is the best option, with overhead heating elements controlled by a skin sensor. This overhead heat and light fixture (Figure 8.11) should be able to move aside to allow access for a C-Arm x-ray machine, which also needs a film cassette chamber under the working surface of the resuscitator.

D. Nitrous Oxide Units

Nitrous oxide (N_2O) has been found to be a safe, effective means of alleviating some of the pain of labor when delivered at the correct concentration. It is mixed about half and half with oxygen. The gases may be available from wall outlets or from portable tanks. The mechanism for delivering the mixture to the patient is usually

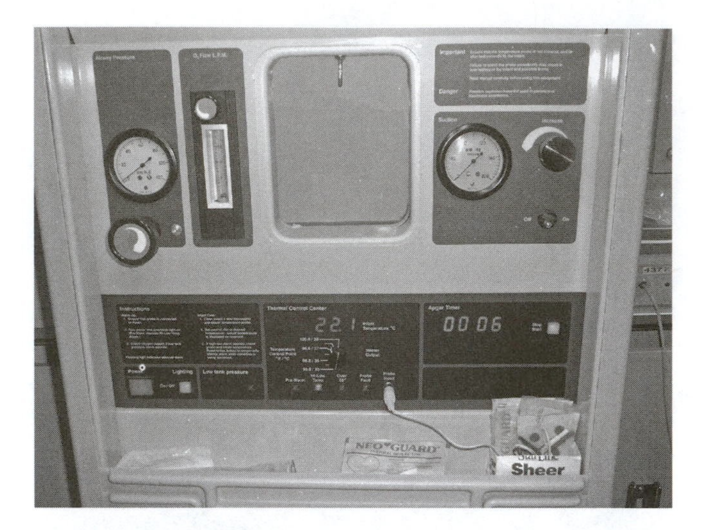

FIGURE 8.10 Resuscitator controls + Apgar timer.

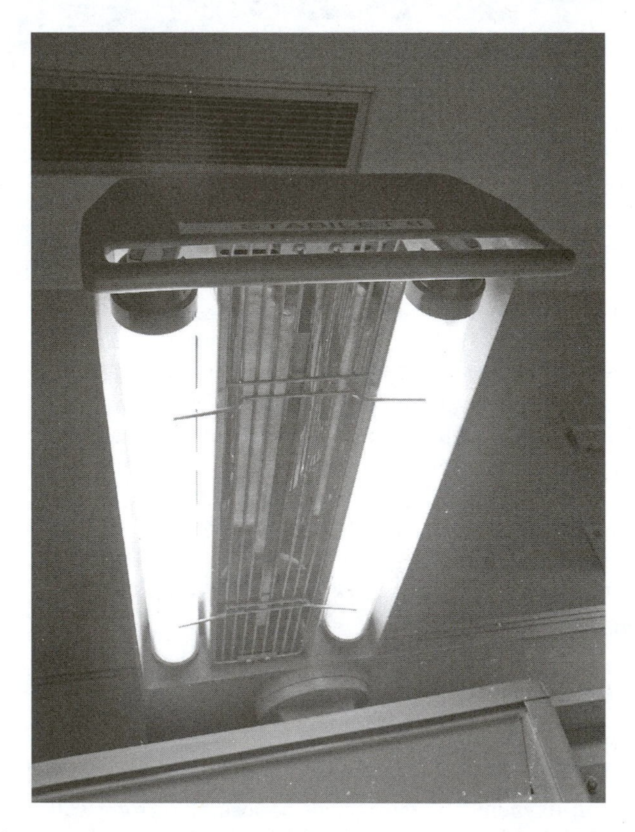

FIGURE 8.11 Resuscitator overhead arm with lights and heater elements.

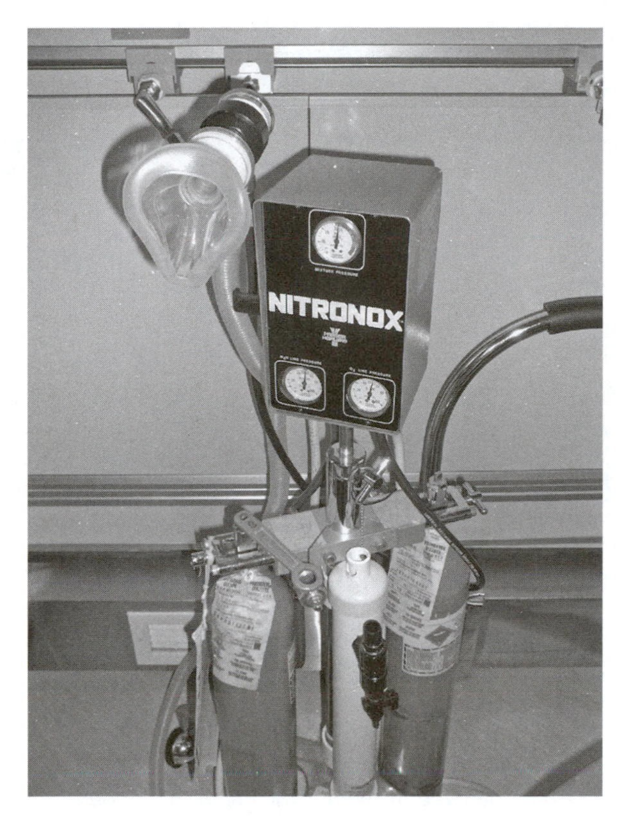

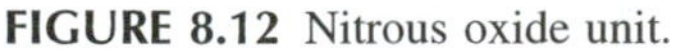
FIGURE 8.12 Nitrous oxide unit.

nonelectrical, consisting of the necessary supply hoses and connectors, and a box containing regulators, a blender, overpressure alarms, possibly pressure gauges, and fittings to connect a patient line (see Figure 8.12). The patient line carries the blended, pressure-reduced gas mixture to a demand valve, which only opens when the patient inhales. The demand valve fits on to a soft, snug-fitting mask that covers the patient's nose and mouth. To prevent buildup of nitrous oxide in the area, a scavenging system may be in place that collects exhaled gases and draws them into the building air handling ducts where it dissipates to harmless levels.

II. SKIN, BONE, MUSCLE, AND MISCELLANEOUS

A. Electrosurgery Machines

The art of surgery has been practiced for thousands of years, but bleeding was always a problem. Cutting into flesh in order to remove a body part or foreign object (including demons), or to repair some kind of damage, resulted in many small and large blood vessels being severed. Larger vessels could sometimes be tied off, but the smaller ones were impossible, and the surgeon and patient just had to wait until the body's natural clotting mechanism stemmed the flow, hopefully before the patient

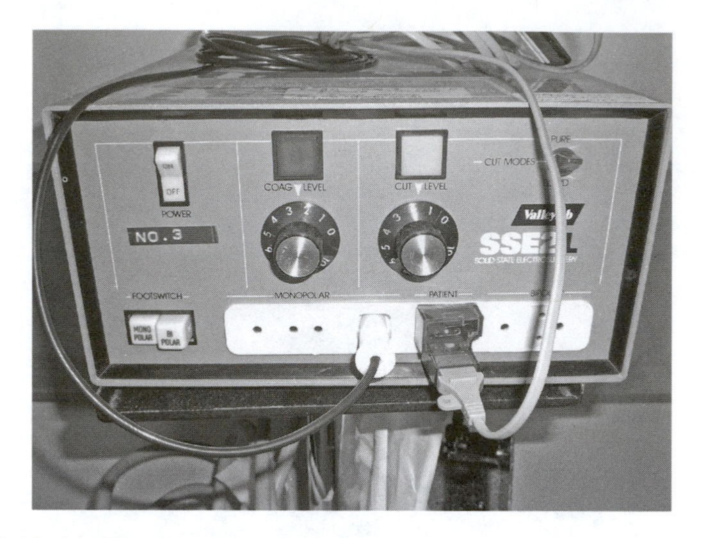

FIGURE 8.13 An older electrosurgery unit.

bled to death. Besides this rather inconvenient side effect, bleeding obscured the surgical site, making it hard for the surgeon to see what he was doing.

Whether discovered accidentally or by experimentation, it was found, also long in the past, that high heat would sear, or cauterize, tissue and stop much of the bleeding from a wound or incision. A red-hot iron did the job, but was inconvenient and potentially extremely painful, as it was used long before the advent of anesthesia.

A side benefit of cauterization by any means is that it kills most bacteria and viruses in the tissue being cauterized.

When experimenters began working with electricity, one characteristic they noted was that electric current passing through an object generated heat. Eventually it was found that this characteristic could be used to cauterize tissue, and if applied carefully, electricity could cut tissue as well. In 1920, William Bovie built the first practical electrosurgery generator. More models improved on his original (see Figure 8.13), and his name was associated with the field for decades afterward — in fact, it is not unusual to hear OR staff referring to electrosurgery units (ESUs) as "Bovies," in the same way that photocopy machines are often called "Xeroxes."

With experimentation, it was found that certain frequencies of electricity caused more nerve and muscle stimulation than others, and ESUs were designed to avoid these frequencies. Most units operate in the range from 100 KHz to 10 MHz.

Applying electrical current to tissue results in the tissue being heated, but the specific features of the signal determine what happens to the tissue. As with any electrical circuit, there must be a complete pathway. In electrosurgery, the source of the current is called the active electrode (Figure 8.14), while the sink is called the return or grounding electrode.

When a high-intensity, continuous sine wave signal is applied, the cells in the tissue rupture and any water rapidly boils away. This has the effect of cutting the tissue. However, the rapid drying of the material makes it less conductive, and so the current doesn't spread very far from the point of application. The cut is thin,

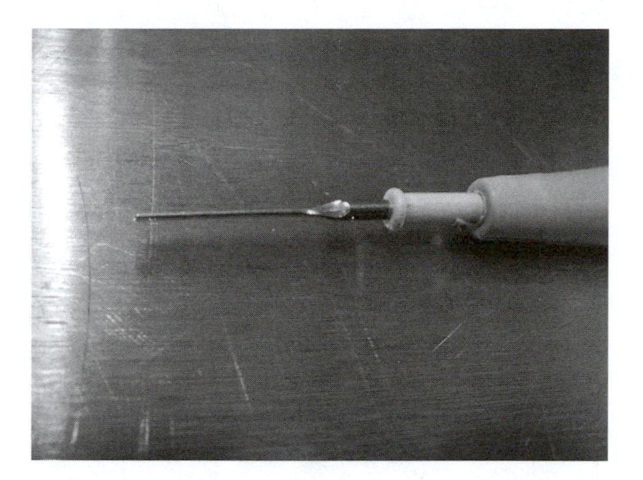

FIGURE 8.14 ESU pencil tip.

and heating is minimal away from the cut point. Current is high enough in the cutting process that the active electrode does not directly contact tissue; instead, sparks jump from the metal electrode to the tissue to carry out the action.

If the same signal is cycled rapidly on and off, the cutting effect is reduced, and heating occurs in a larger area. This has the effect of coagulating the tissue, that is, drying a wider path and stopping any bleeding.

In some situations, it is useful to be able to dry out, or desiccate, larger areas. In this case, the duty cycle of the sine wave is further reduced, allowing greater current penetration to produce the desired result.

Increased application of such signals will burn away the desiccated tissue, a process called fulguration. It is used to remove such structures as cancer tumors when simple excision is not possible, or to destroy sections of the vas deferens or fallopian tubes in sterilization procedures.

Most ESUs have a "Blend" setting, which is intermediate between "Cut" and "Coagulate." The settings used are often determined by individual surgeon preferences, though experience has shown that specific settings work best for some particular procedures. Staff members often attach notes to the ESUs with a list of settings and procedures.

There are two general modes of operation for ESUs: monopolar and bipolar.

1. Monopolar Electrosurgery

In monopolar operation, surgical current is applied through an active electrode at the site. Active electrodes may be turned on and off using a foot switch, or they may have switches on the hand-piece (Figure 8.15). Both types can select CUT or COAG.

Once past the immediate area of application, current spreads out through the body, reducing current density enough that no significant heating occurs. The monopolar return electrode (Figure 8.16) has a large surface area to keep current densities low. It is usually applied to an area of the body with a large, relatively smooth surface, such as the thigh or buttock.

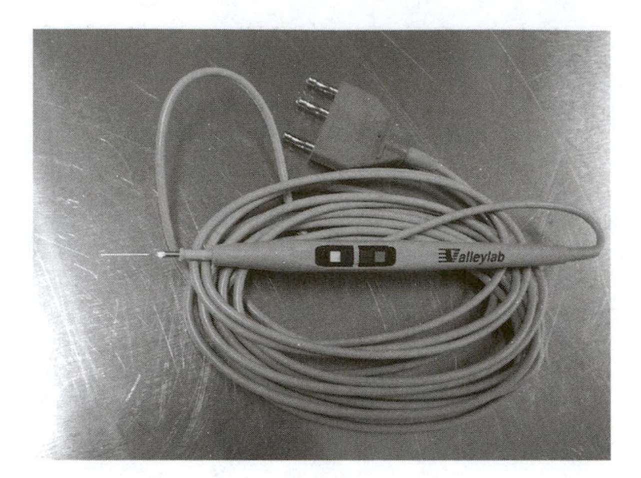

FIGURE 8.15 ESU pencil with hand switches.

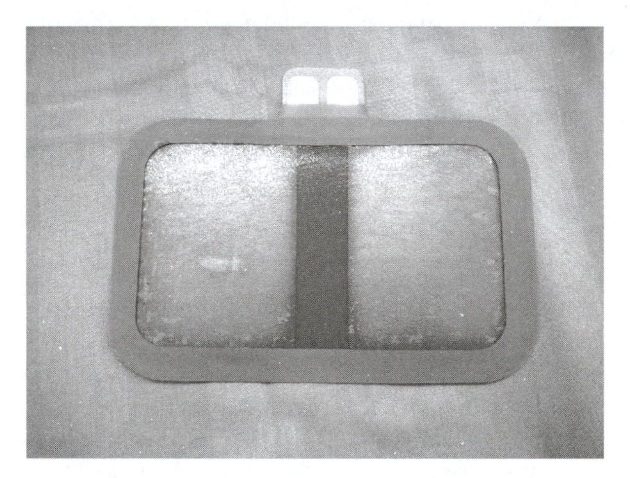

FIGURE 8.16 Return electrode monitor pad.

It is critical for the return electrode to maintain a large contact area to keep current density low enough that burns do not develop at the electrode site. To this end, most ESU manufacturers have developed a system to measure contact quality. Valleylab uses an electrode with two sections, which applies a small voltage across the two sections and measures the current flow. If it is too low, indicating inadequate contact, an alarm will sound, and operation of the ESU will be blocked. On the other hand, if the test current is too high, for example if the two sections of the electrode have come away from the skin and contacted each other, or if some conductive material like blood has run between the sections, an alarm is also triggered, preventing machine operation. As in the story of Goldilocks, contact has to be "just right" in order for electrosurgery to proceed.

2. Bipolar Electrosurgery

In some procedures, especially those performed laparoscopically (see Chapter 8), a return electrode arrangement as described earlier is not practical. In such circumstances, a bipolar arrangement is used, in which the source and sink of current are close to each other.

This is usually in the form of forceps or pincers in which one jaw is source and the other sink (Figures 8.17 and 8.18).

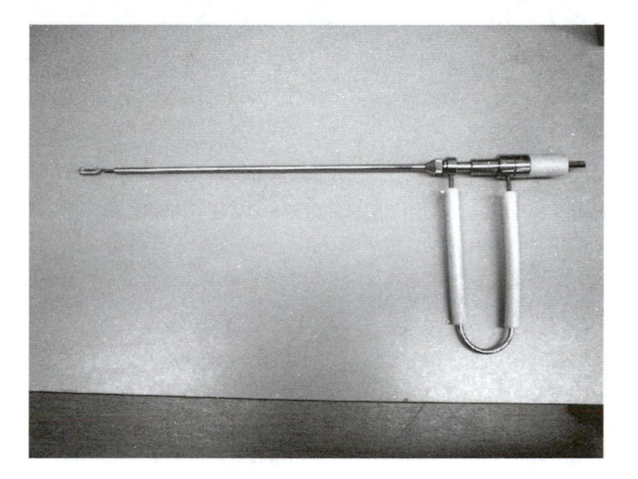

FIGURE 8.17 ESU bipolar forceps.

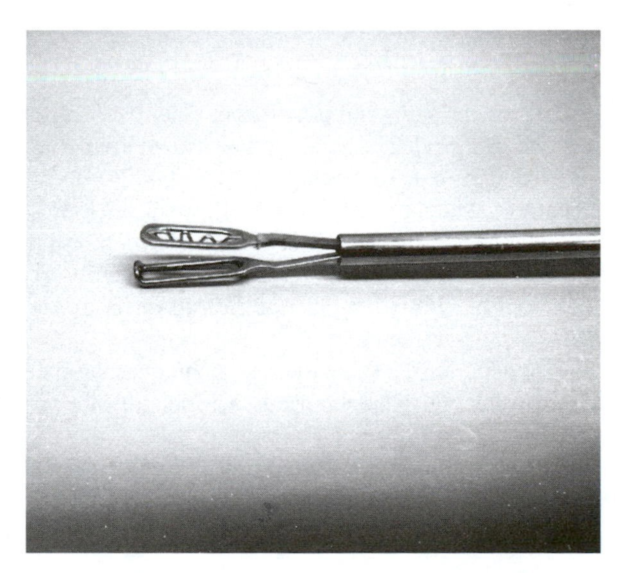

FIGURE 8.18 Bipolar forceps tip.

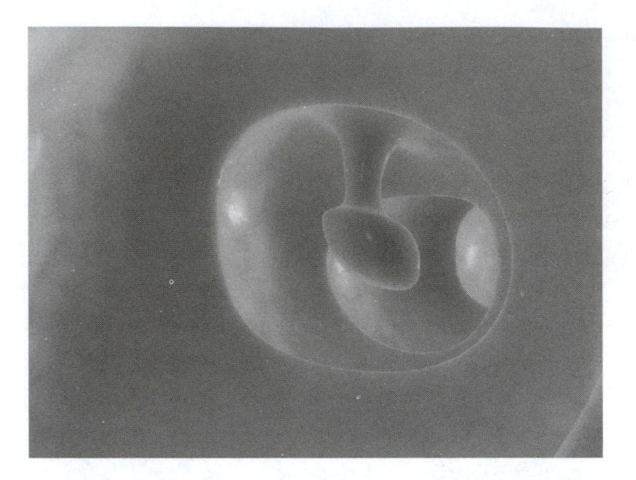

FIGURE 8.19 Endoscopic view of an intestinal polyp. (Modified from Inmagine Corp, www.123rf.com, with permission.)

This makes a separate return electrode and associated wiring unnecessary, but is only useful for small structures such as fallopian tubes or intestinal polyps (Figure 8.19).

When cutting tissue, ESUs can produce smoke, which rises in a plume above the surgery site. This smoke can contain both toxic chemicals produced by the burning tissue, and also possibly virus particles, should the patient be infected. The use of a smoke evacuator system is highly recommended in order to remove such smoke plumes from the area.

B. Surgical Lasers

Surgical lasers operate on the same end principal as electrosurgery machines, in that rapid heating of tissue can produce cutting and/or coagulation.

Surgical lasers use their coherent beams of laser light to do the heating rather than an electrical current, which has advantages in certain situations. The laser beam can be very precisely focused to allow it to act on small structures without damaging adjacent tissues; it can be directed around corners and into very confined spaces; and it can be controlled in such a way that almost all of its power is focused at a specific, precise distance from the emitter.

By using different materials and construction techniques, lasers can be produced that have different wavelengths. These various wavelengths are absorbed differentially by different tissues.

Lasers are named according to the material used in the lasing tube.

1. Carbon Dioxide Lasers

Carbon dioxide lasers have a wavelength of 10.6 μm (10,600 nm), which means that the light is strongly absorbed by water. Since soft tissue in the body is composed mostly of water, the CO_2 laser will cut them very effectively, but will only penetrate slightly. Cutting action extends only about 0.1 mm into the tissue, while coagulation is only about 0.5 mm deep. With such characteristics, very precise procedures can be carried out.

Because bone and teeth have much lower water contents than soft tissue, CO_2 lasers are not used on them.

Light at this wavelength does not travel well through fiberoptic channels, and therefore CO_2 lasers are mostly used on structures that are directly accessible, especially the skin.

2. Neodymium-Doped Yttrium Aluminium Garnet Lasers

Nd:YAG lasers operate at a wavelength of 1064 nm, and beams are not absorbed preferentially by water. This means that cutting depth is up to 4 mm, much greater than with CO_2 lasers. Coagulation effects are also deeper.

Nd:YAG laser light will pass through fiber optics, so it can be used in endoscopic procedures.

3. Argon Lasers

Argon lasers produce various wavelengths of light, with most of the power being concentrated at 488 nm and 514 nm.

4. Excimer Lasers

Excimer lasers use an inert gas such as argon or krypton combined with chlorine or fluorine to produce an ultraviolet laser beam. This beam can be very tightly focused and controlled, and its energy level means that tissue on which it is used vaporizes rather than burning. Excimer lasers are used to reshape the cornea of patients to correct their vision; by vaporizing specific areas, the cornea is deformed in such a way as to change the focus of the eye, reducing or eliminating the need for corrective lenses.

5. Laser Safety

Since surgical lasers emit high-powered beams of light energy, extreme care must be taken not to allow it to contact the wrong materials. Unlike ESU currents, laser light maintains its power over considerable distances through open air.

Patients and staff must wear eye protection when lasers are in use, and doors must be closed and windows covered. A prominent sign must be posted outside the room warning others that lasers are in use. The retina can be seriously and almost instantaneously damaged by high-powered laser light.

Flammable materials must be avoided in the area. Items such as surgical drapes must be dampened with water to prevent ignition should the laser beam come in contact with them. Any other flammable objects that can't be removed should be covered with a damp cloth.

Reflective surfaces should avoided in the procedure room, since a stray beam could bounce off such a surface and enter the eye of a staff member who thought they were safely looking away from the procedure.

When cutting tissue, lasers can produce smoke that rises in a plume above the surgery site. This smoke can contain both toxic chemicals produced by the burning tissue, and also possibly virus particles should the patient be infected. The use of a smoke evacuator system is highly recommended in order to remove such smoke plumes from the area.

C. Surgical Ultrasound

High-intensity, high-frequency ultrasound waves can be focused in such a way as to heat tissue very rapidly, in much the same way as electrosurgery or surgical lasers, but without the need for return paths as in electrosurgery or the dangers of laser beams. Beams can be focused in tissues below the surface without damaging the overlying tissue, which has made the process especially suited for prostate treatment.

D. Cryosurgery Units

As long as humans have been venturing outside in winter, it has been known that exposure to extreme cold can kill tissue. By using carefully controlled applications of super-cold objects to surface tissues such as warts, skin keratoses, and certain skin cancers, the tissue in question can be frozen and killed, with very little effect on the surrounding structures. After a few days, the "frostbitten" area will dry up and slough off, leaving almost no sign of it having been there. As caution is important in such applications, the first treatment may not get all of the offending tissue, so a follow-up may be required.

The simplest cryosurgery technique uses a small piece of absorbent material on the end of a rod made of low-heat-conductivity material such as wood. The rod and material are dipped into a vacuum flask containing liquid nitrogen. The liquid nitrogen is absorbed by the material and stays in liquid form long enough for the rod to be removed from the flask. The soaked material is then applied to the target area. A few seconds of contact is usually sufficient to produce the desired result.

Liquid nitrogen may not always be available or convenient, or may not last long enough for some procedures. Cryosurgery machines take advantage of the fact that gases cool rapidly when they expand. If a highly compressed gas is released from a cylinder and passed over or through a metal surface, the metal itself will cool rapidly. By repeating the gas release as necessary, the metal can be kept cold (Figure 8.20).

Cryosurgery units (Figure 8.21) use either carbon dioxide or nitrous oxide to effect cooling of the metal probes used. Compressed carbon dioxide is readily available and inexpensive, and is harmless when released into room air (unless it reaches very high concentrations), but it doesn't reduce probe temperatures as effectively as nitrous oxide. Nitrous oxide can be harmful at relatively low concentrations, especially with prolonged exposure, so a scavenging system must be used with nitrous oxide cryosurgery units in order to remove most of the exhaust gas from the area.

Probes come in various shapes and sizes for different applications. Most systems have two controls, one to pass the expanding nitrous oxide through the probe to cool

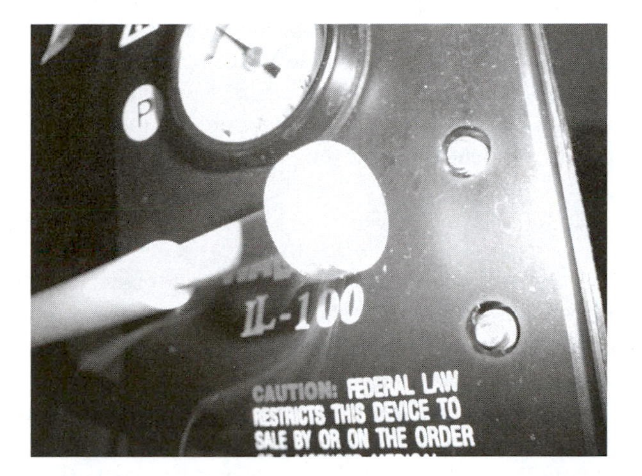

FIGURE 8.20 Frosty cryosurgery probe.

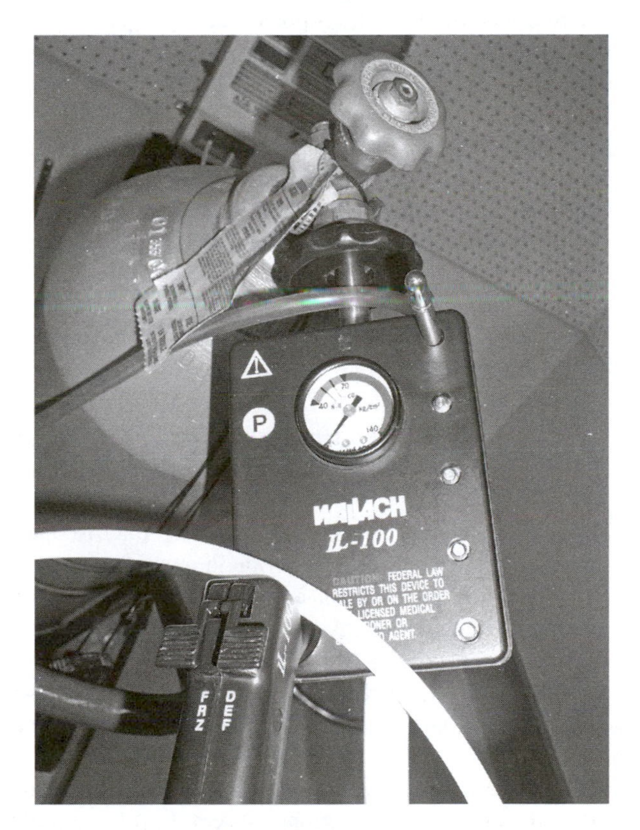

FIGURE 8.21 A cryosurgery unit.

it off, and the other to draw room air through the probe in order to warm it rapidly, as super-cold probes can be dangerous if left out in the open after a cryosurgery procedure; they may inadvertently come in contract with the flesh of the patient or staff, causing damage, or they may freeze to other objects they come in contact with, which may cause an accident when moved.

E. Microscopes

Human eyesight is limited in its ability to see very small objects. With the invention of lenses in about the eleventh century, these limitations were overcome, and by the sixteenth century, scientists were using simple microscopes to examine the previously invisible world of the very small.

Single lens microscopes gave way to compound, or multilens devices that offered much greater magnification with larger fields of view (Figure 8.22).

These eventually led to the modern laboratory microscope (Figure 8.23), with its high power and binocular eyepieces.

Lab scopes are outside the "scope" of this book; however specialized microscopes are used in both direct diagnosis and in treatment situations.

Operating microscopes mount a high-powered, high-quality binocular microscope on an articulating arm that can be maneuvered in order to look at various structures during microsurgery (Figure 8.24). The arm may be placed on a mobile stand or fixed to a wall, floor, or ceiling mount.

Controls for adjusting position, focus, and magnification are located on the head of the device, but usually they have servomotors attached that allow the controls to be operated using a special foot switch (Figure 8.25). Surgeons become adept at using the footswitch without looking at it, thus freeing their hands to perform surgical procedures.

Operating microscopes (sometimes called OPMIs, though this is actually a model name for a specific device) are designed to provide the levels of magnification, field of view, and depth of focus that are required in microsurgery. Compared to a lab microscope, the magnification levels are considerably less, since it would be impossible to physically work on extremely small structures. Lab microscopes may magnify up to 1000× or more, while operating microscopes are usually limited to about 20×.

Also, depth of focus is much greater for operating microscopes than for lab units, because the objective lens must be far enough away from the observing area to allow access for surgical instruments and the surgeon's hands, and because structures being viewed are three dimensional.

Some operating microscopes have two sets of binocular eyepieces (Figure 8.26), for instructional use, and they may also have a video camera integrated into the optics to allow viewing on a large video monitor, and also so that procedures can be recorded for later review.

Illumination of the surgical field is critical, so high-intensity, color-correct light sources form part of the operating microscope system. Light is usually delivered to the site by fiberoptic cables. Systems may include various colored filters to help in imaging certain tissues or structures.

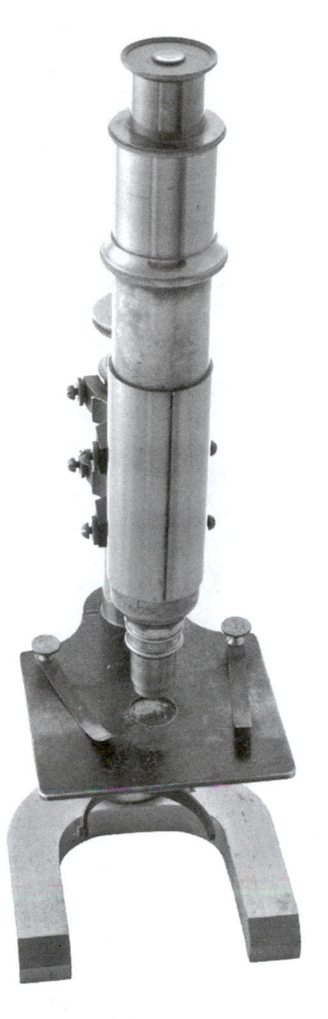

FIGURE 8.22 An old microscope. (Modified from Inmagine Corp, www.123rf.com, with permission.)

F. Sterilizers

Although biomedical staff does not usually support hospital sterilizers (Figure 8.27), they will be discussed here briefly.

Many types of medical equipment may come in contact with contaminated material, which means that they must be cleaned and sterilized before they can be used again. There are three general types of sterilizers: gas, heat, and liquid.

1. Gas Sterilizers

Gas sterilizers use a poisonous gas such as ethylene oxide or chlorine dioxide. Instruments to be sterilized are placed in a chamber which is sealed and pumped full of gas. The interior is heated moderately (for example, to about 55°C), to promote

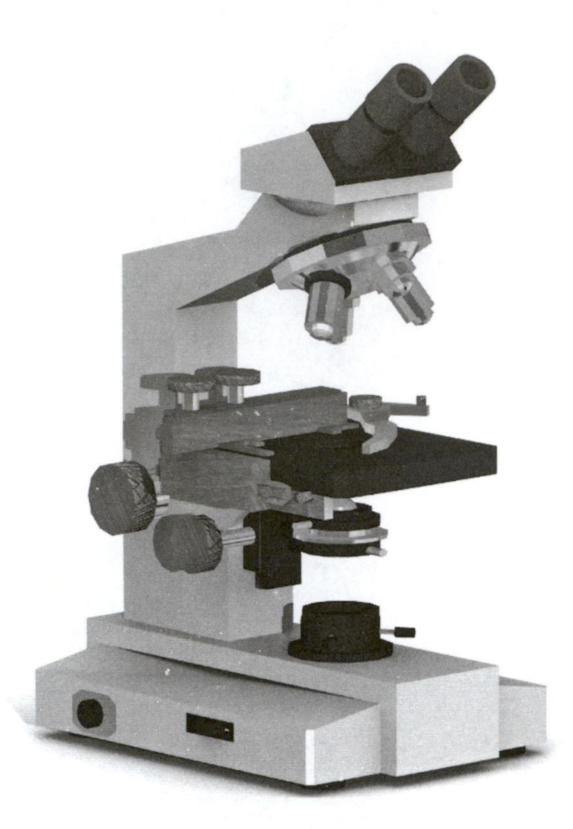

FIGURE 8.23 Modern microscope. (Modified from Inmagine Corp, www.123rf.com, with permission.)

more rapid chemical action. Systems may have controls for temperature, humidity, gas concentration, and process time; certain parameters may have preset values for specific sterilization procedures.

The gases in use must be safely evacuated from the chamber before opening to remove the instruments.

Gas sterilizers are typically used for equipment that cannot tolerate high heat levels and/or liquid immersion.

2. Heat Sterilizers

For devices and parts that can tolerate high levels of heat, this method of sterilization offers faster processing than low-temperature gas sterilizers.

Toxic gases and steam may be added to the chamber, though some systems may use dry heat only, especially for instruments such as scalpels whose edges may be degraded by contact with steam or corrosive chemicals.

Steam sterilizers, or autoclaves, are pressurized so that they can be heated to about 120°C to increase sterilization effectiveness and reduce cycle times.

Controls are otherwise similar to those of gas sterilizers.

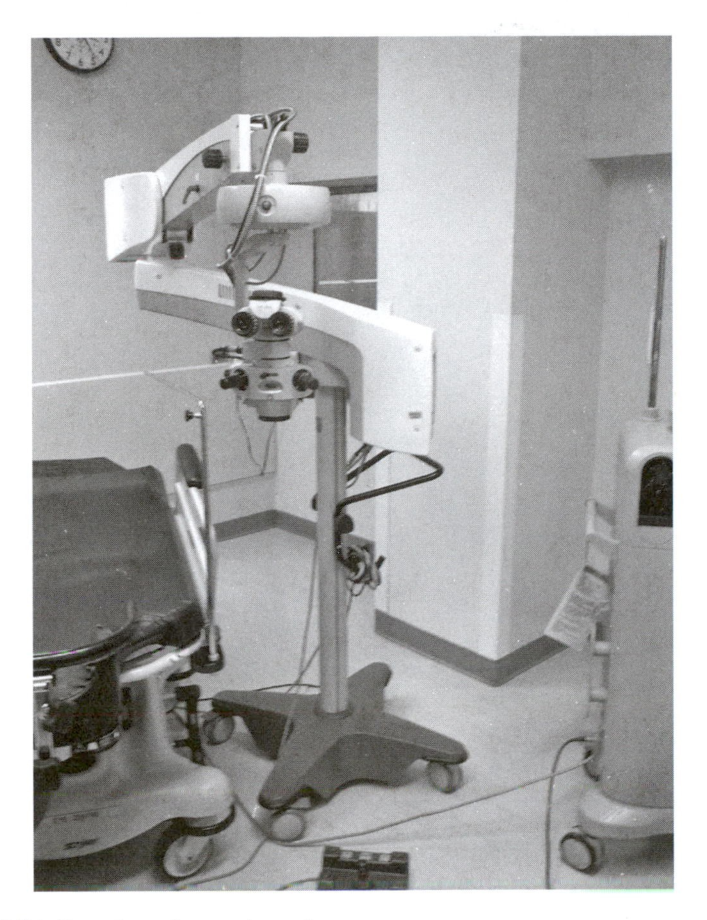

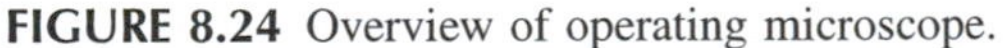

FIGURE 8.24 Overview of operating microscope.

3. Liquid Sterilizers

As their name implies, these units utilize toxic liquids to carry out sterilization. This is especially useful for instruments with small crevices or internal passageways that gas and heat may not reach effectively.

These instruments must first be thoroughly cleaned physically before attempting sterilization.

A specialized type of liquid sterilizer is used to clean endoscopes, since they have long internal passageways that can become contaminated with body fluids and possibly solids (Figure 8.28).

Scopes are placed in the washer and connected to a fitting. The washer goes through a cycle, either preprogrammed or user set. The scope is first flushed with water and then with a water–detergent combination, followed by another water flush. Then a sterilizing liquid such a glutaraldehyde is introduced into the scope and is left for a set time. Flushing with water and/or alcohol follows, and finally air is blown through the scope to prepare it for its next use.

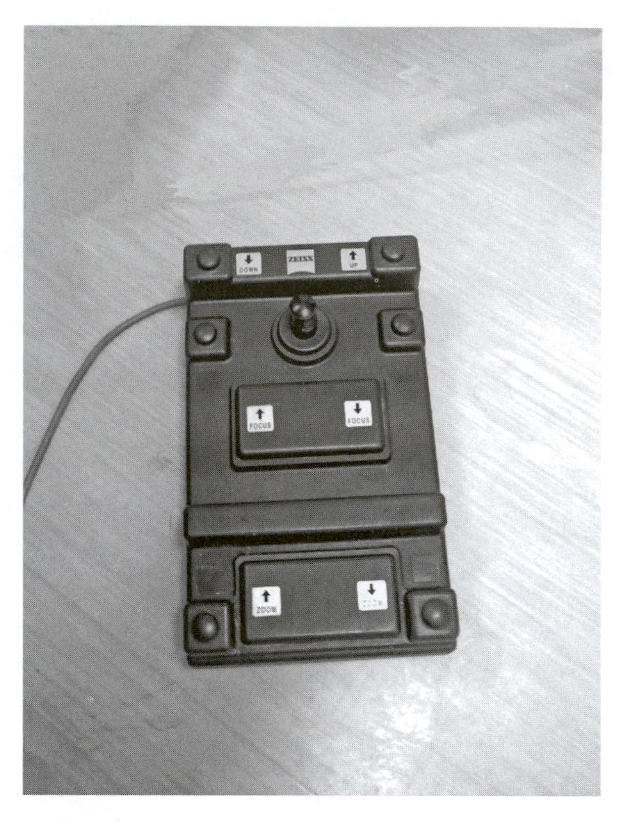

FIGURE 8.25 OPMI footswitch.

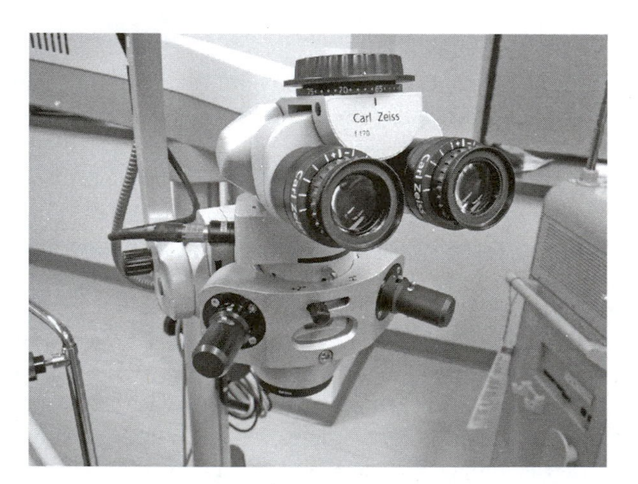

FIGURE 8.26 OPMI binocular head.

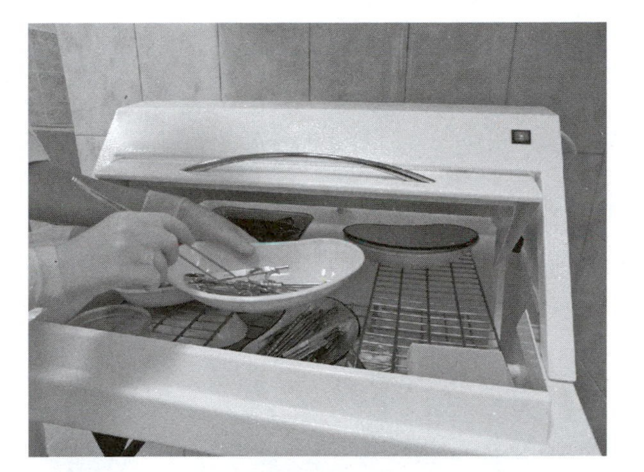

FIGURE 8.27 Small steam sterilizer. (Modified from Inmagine Corp, www.123rf.com, with permission.)

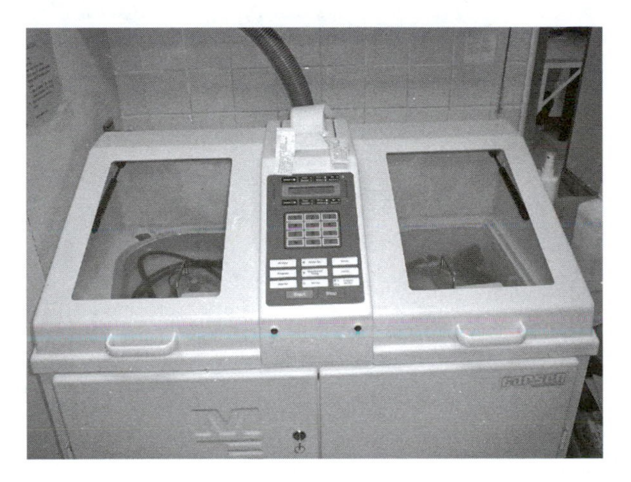

FIGURE 8.28 Endoscope washer.

G. Physiotherapy Equipment

Devices used in physiotherapy or rehabilitation departments may or may not be supported by biomed; some devices are strictly mechanical, while others include varying levels of electronics.

Generally, physiotherapy equipment is designed to maintain or improve range of motion, to relieve pain, or to promote healing; sometimes two or more of these goals may be attained through the use of one mode of therapy.

1. Continuous Passive Motion

Much range-of-motion work with patients is done by direct physical manipulation by the therapist, but machines can do some repetitive, simple actions.

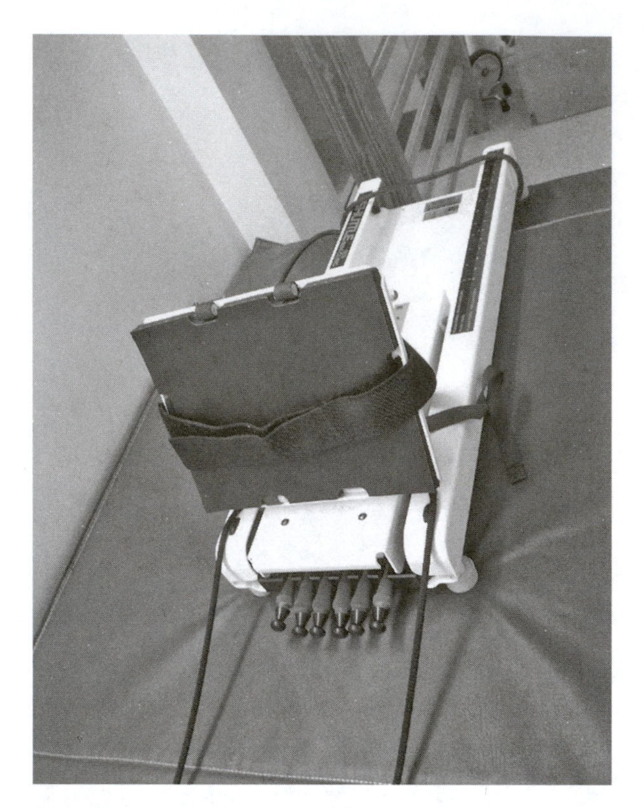

FIGURE 8.29 CPM device.

These continuous passive motion (CPM) devices (Figure 8.29) simply flex and extend joints, especially knees, by gripping an extremity such as a foot and moving it back and forth. The rate and degree of motion can be set for each patient, and a timer may be used to set treatment duration.

2. Pain Relief

A number of different techniques may be used for pain relief, many of which involve the use of heat.

a. *Direct Heat*

Heat may be applied to a muscle group or joint by simple transfer, using a wax bath, moist hot packs, or whirlpool baths (Figure 8.30). Generally, controls on this type of equipment are limited to temperature adjustments and over-temperature alarms and treatment timers.

b. *Induced Heat*

In the past, radio waves were used to deep-heat tissue, with technology much like that found in a microwave oven. Possible negative effects were common with these short-wave diathermy machines, and they are rarely used today.

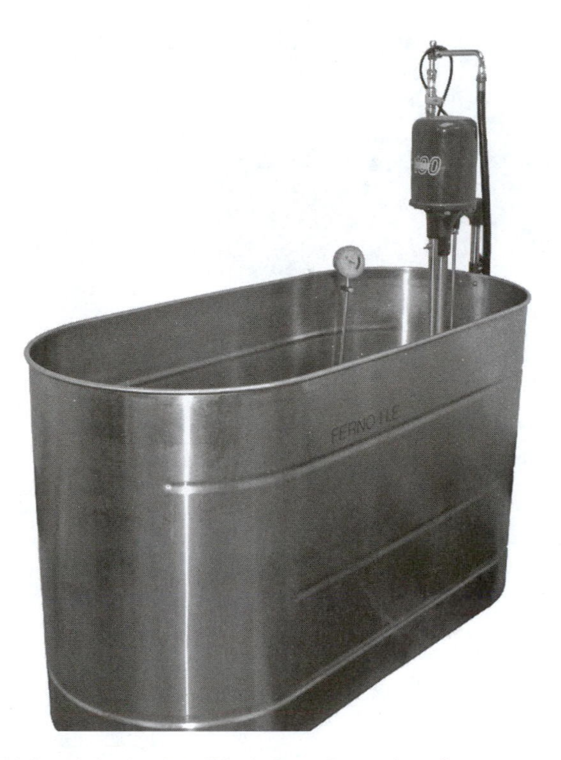

FIGURE 8.30 Whirlpool bath. (Modified from Inmagine Corp, www.123rf.com, with permission.)

Ultrasound can produce similar deep tissue heating much more safely. These units consist of ultrasound generators, various power heads to provide heating at different depths, and controls for power output and length of treatment. Ultrasound is produced in the power head with piezoelectric crystals.

Some ultrasound therapy machines are combined with interferential therapy units (Figure 8.31; see below).

c. *Interferential Therapy*

These devices apply stimulating electrical currents to two pairs of electrodes, placed on the skin so that the currents cross each other diagonally. This sets up an interference pattern of muscle stimulation that has been found to be helpful in relieving some types of pain.

These units may also use a suction cup system in conjunction with electrical stimulation. Large cups (with electrodes built in) are placed over muscle groups and suction is applied alternately to the cups, producing a massaging action.

d. *Laser Therapy*

Certain wavelengths of laser light can penetrate surface tissues and produce deep heating. As with ultrasound therapy units, power levels and treatment times are controlled, and different applicators can determine the depth of heating.

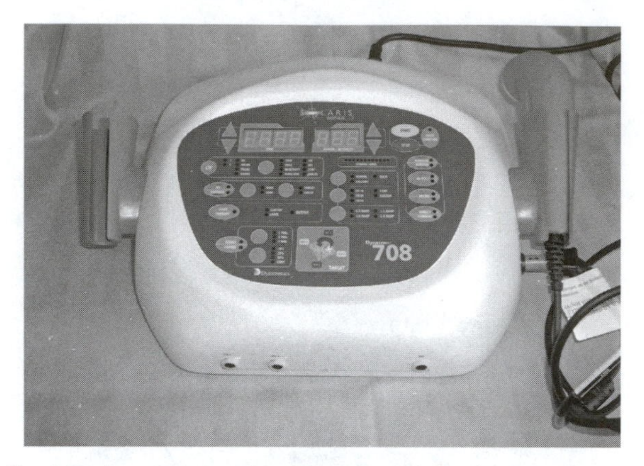

FIGURE 8.31 Combination ultrasound and interferential unit.

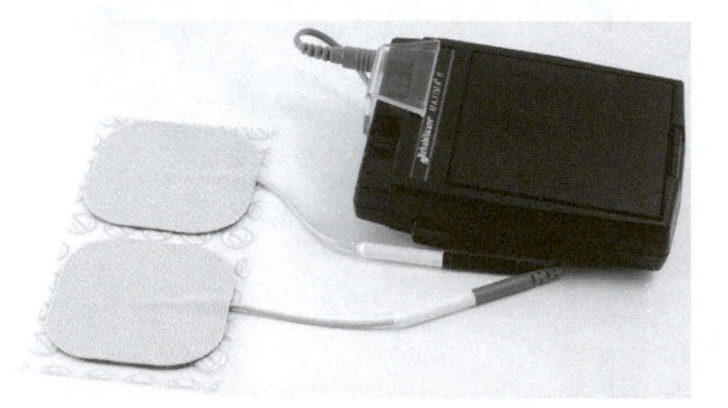

FIGURE 8.32 TENS device. (Modified from Inmagine Corp, www.123rf.com, with permission.)

e. Transcutaneous Electrical Nerve Stimulators

It has been found that applying electrical signals of a specific amplitude, wave shape, and duration to particular locations on the body can result in reduction of pain sensations in other areas, almost like the needles used in acupuncture. Transcutaneous electrical nerve stimulator (TENS) units are small, battery-powered devices with controls for the parameters mentioned above (see Figure 8.32). Stimulation signals are delivered by small electrodes, often made of conductive rubber, which are placed on the designated skin locations.

3. Promotion of Healing

a. Ultraviolet Light Therapy

Ultraviolet light has been found to help certain skin conditions such as psoriasis. By exposing as much skin as possible to UV rays, maximal benefit is achieved (see Figure 8.33).

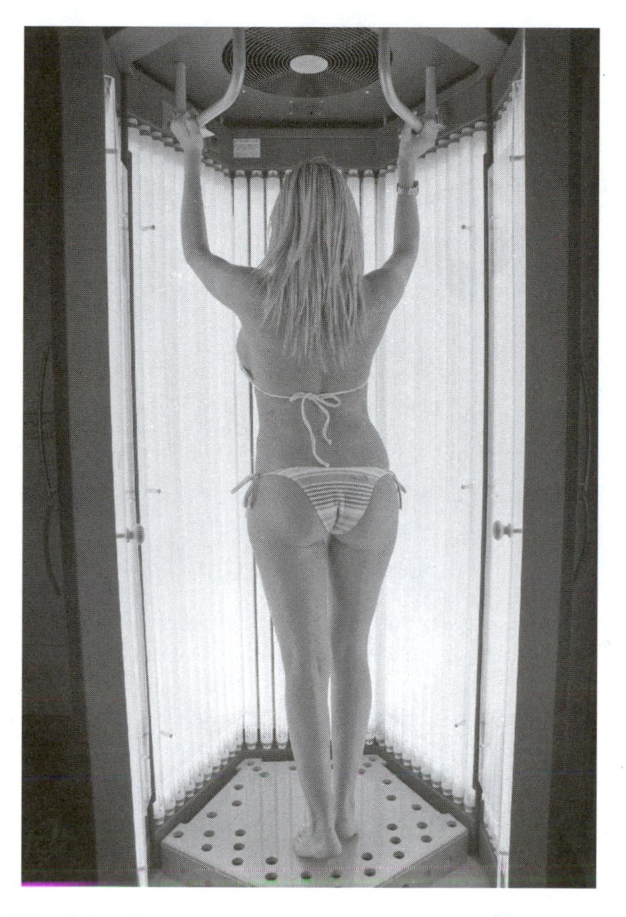

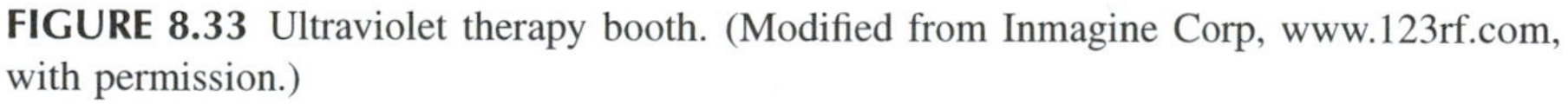

FIGURE 8.33 Ultraviolet therapy booth. (Modified from Inmagine Corp, www.123rf.com, with permission.)

Since UV rays can be harmful to the eyes, patients must wear a properly fitted, effective mask during treatment.

A timing circuit turns lights off after the specified treatment is completed.

b. Sequential Compression Devices

After certain surgical procedures or with some medical conditions, lymphatic fluid does not return to the central venous system as quickly as it should. To aid in this process, devices were developed that use a large, compartmentalized cuff that is placed around the patient's arm or leg. By inflating the compartments sequentially, the limb is compressed in a peristaltic fashion, with the wave moving from the area furthest from the body to the area closest to the body (see Figure 8.34). In this manner, lymphatic fluid is pushed up through the lymph ducts toward the heart.

The control unit contains a pump, a valve system, and a distribution header, as well as a timing circuit.

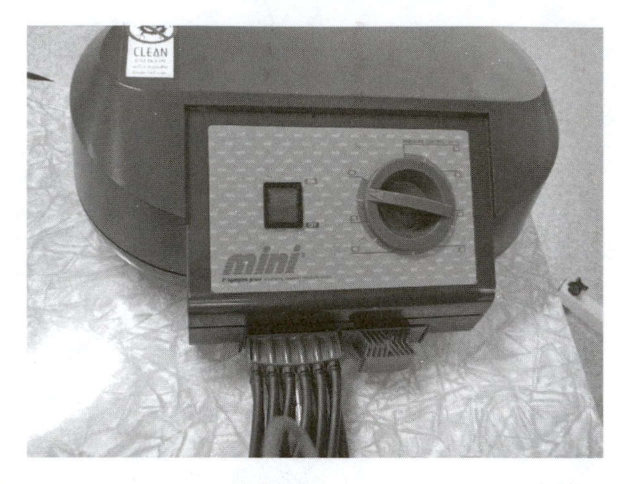

FIGURE 8.34 Sequential compression device.

III. CHAPTER SUMMARY

Chapter 8 deals with equipment for the care of neonates including bilirubin therapy systems, incubators, and resuscitators, plus a section on nitrous oxide delivery units.

The section titled "Skin, Bone, Muscle, and Miscellaneous" covers the rest of the chapter, including electrosurgery unit history, theory, and applications, surgical laser types, and cryosurgery.

Microscopes and especially operating microscopes are discussed, with sterilizers and physiotherapy equipment rounding out the section.

9 BMET Work

I. OVERVIEW

Biomedical engineering technologists can work in a wide variety of jobs. Many will be part of an in-hospital biomed department, large or small, but others will work for outside companies providing support to hospital equipment, or doing repairs and calibrations off-site. Equipment vendors and manufacturers need skilled people to do bench repairs of equipment under warranty, to install new technology in hospitals, or to provide technical expertise to sales teams. Being part of the team researching, designing, and building new devices is an exciting and challenging option. The Armed Forces have hospital equipment that needs support and may provide their own training programs for biomed techs. Finally, there is a need for people with a talent for education, to teach biomeds in model-specific factory training courses, or in the many educational institutions that have BMET programs.

This chapter will focus mainly on the work of biomeds in hospitals; the other areas of employment are almost too broad and varied to describe in any useful detail.

II. ELECTRICAL SAFETY

One of the original, primary functions of BMETs in hospitals was to ensure that electrical devices that might come in contact with patients were not going to kill them. Electrical safety was big, partly because equipment design was not as closely regulated as it is now, and partly simply because it was an easy target. Almost anyone could design, build, and sell equipment to hospitals, and these devices might not have adequate grounding, they could be designed with very "leaky" components, or they could have potentially lethal output settings.

The whole issue was exacerbated by a coincidental convergence of engineering and physiology. Power plant and grid designers throughout the world found that alternating current with a frequency of 50 to 60 Hertz was effective for distributing electricity to customers. Medical researchers discovered that many functions of the human body, such as the vital beating of the heart, were mediated electrically. Experiments showed that outside electrical stimulation could disrupt the electrical signals in the heart, causing it to enter into a state of uncoordinated contractions. In this state, called ventricular fibrillation, the heart no longer pumped blood, and death soon followed. Different frequencies of electricity were found to have differing effects, and testing showed that the most dangerous frequencies, those that were most likely to cause fibrillation, were from 50 to 60 Hertz. Fate had conspired to make the most common form of electricity also the most dangerous.

Hospital administrators were terrified of having patients electrocuted while in their facilities, and since testing for electrical safety was fairly simple, programs were put in place to rigorously check every electrical device as it entered the hospital and on a regular schedule thereafter. Hospital wiring, too, was subject to scheduled tests to ensure safety.

Modern building codes and precise, well-designed manufacturing standards for medical equipment have made it so that it is very rare to find a new device that has inadequate grounding or excessive electrical leakage.

Electrical safety is still a concern, however, since failures can occur in equipment, especially as it ages, and especially if it is subjected to harsh conditions. These failures can include those that can reduce grounding effectiveness or increase electrical leakage. When repairs or modifications have been made to equipment, testing should be performed to ensure that safety systems have not been compromised.

A. Rationale

As described above, the common 50- or 60-Hz line power found in most areas of the world is the most dangerous in terms of causing fatal disruptions in cardiac rhythms.

When line-powered electrical equipment is used with patients, there are two factors that must be present for harm to occur:

- There must be a source of electrical current that can come in contact with the patient through an exposed surface.
- There must be a pathway, or sink, for that current to flow through the patient to complete a circuit.

Current sources can result from a number of reasons:

- Equipment may be built with components that have high intrinsic leakage, such as some transformers and capacitors. This leakage can find its way to patient contact surfaces.
- Circuit design may bring current pathways or components together in such a way as to produce capacitive or inductive coupling to patient contact surfaces.
- Components or conductors may connect with patient contact surfaces through improper design or through warping or breakage of structures.

Current pathways are mostly to various ground points, such as through the grounded chassis of another electrical device, through the grounded frame of a hospital bed, or through plumbing fixtures.

If only one fault is present, no harm will result, but testing should catch single faults before there is a chance of the second fault occurring.

B. Testing Methods

Electrical safety testing of medical equipment must include measurement of grounding resistance and of electrical leakage under various conditions, including power to the device being on or off, ground wiring being open or closed, and the hot and neutral supply wiring of the device being normal or reversed.

If the device includes conductive components that normally come in contact with patients, such as ECG leads or defibrillator paddles, the leakage from these must be tested as well. Leakage between ECG leads can be dangerous and so should be included in the testing process.

Grounding and leakage testing can be done using appropriate bench test devices such as digital multimeters, but testing is made much more convenient using a specially designed electrical safety testing unit.

Ground continuity is a simple measurement, though the test equipment must be able to measure low values of resistance. Typically, ground resistance is required to be less than 100 milliohms, so testing equipment must be accurate at these levels. Note: the actual ground resistance limit may vary depending on national, local, or institutional standards.

Electrical leakage measurement is somewhat more complex. A sensitive meter could measure the total leakage current produced by a device by simply connecting it between the device and ground. Human beings have a characteristic impedance, however, and for measurements to be relevant, they must be made though a load that has an impedance approximately equivalent to that of the human body. Typical "patient loads" are resistor-capacitor networks that have been designed to simulate body impedance.

Electrical safety testers, or analyzers (Figure 9.1), have been designed to streamline the testing process. They include circuitry to measure ground resistance both through the ground wire of the device being tested (sometimes referred to as the device under test, or DUT) and through its chassis with the ground wire disconnected. A switch or an internal relay can open or close the ground connection. Ground resistance is usually measured using a double-wire circuit that is designed to eliminate the resistance of test leads and contact points from the measurement.

Safety analyzers also have a built in patient load, which is used in conjunction with a microammeter circuit to measure electrical leakage. Switches or relays can open or close ground, open or close the neutral supply line, or switch the hot and neutral supply lines.

In order to facilitate measurements from ECG leads, testers have a set of contact posts that can accept a variety of common lead connectors, usually color coded and labeled.

The power cord of the device being tested is plugged into an outlet in the tester.

Analyzers have a common display for the various parameters being measured and for set-up and self-test information.

Some extra features that analyzers may have include:

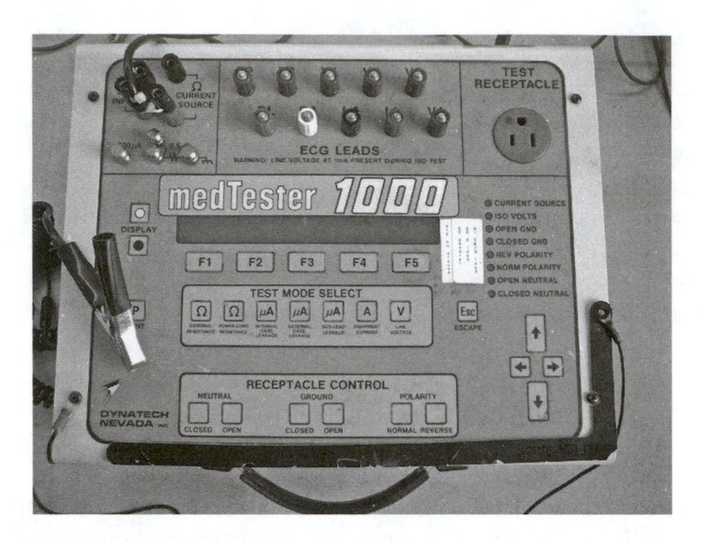

FIGURE 9.1 Electrical safety analyzer.

- Circuitry to measure the current being drawn by the test device.
- Measurement of line voltage. Some units can monitor line voltage over time to help detect line fluctuations, voltage spike, or other anomalies in supply that may affect instruments.
- An internal clock, which is used in conjunction with test result printing.
- A printer port, for test results.
- A data communications port to connect to a computer, to allow test result transfer and computer control of test functions.
- Automated routines for common testing situations. User-developed routines may be accommodated.
- A bar code scanner or other input device to identify the individual device being tested. This information would then form part of the test results and may be used to determine what type of tests are to be performed.

Some systems work in conjunction with an equipment management software package to collect and organize test results and to schedule preventive maintenance testing.

III. OTHER SAFETY CONSIDERATIONS

Electrical safety is only one aspect of overall safety in a hospital setting.

A. Fire Safety

As in any building, fire safety is important. Staff members need to know fire alarm sounds and codes, fire extinguisher (Figure 9.2) locations, fire response protocols, and fire escape routes.

Hospital staff members may be assigned specific duties for patient evacuation in case of fire or other disaster.

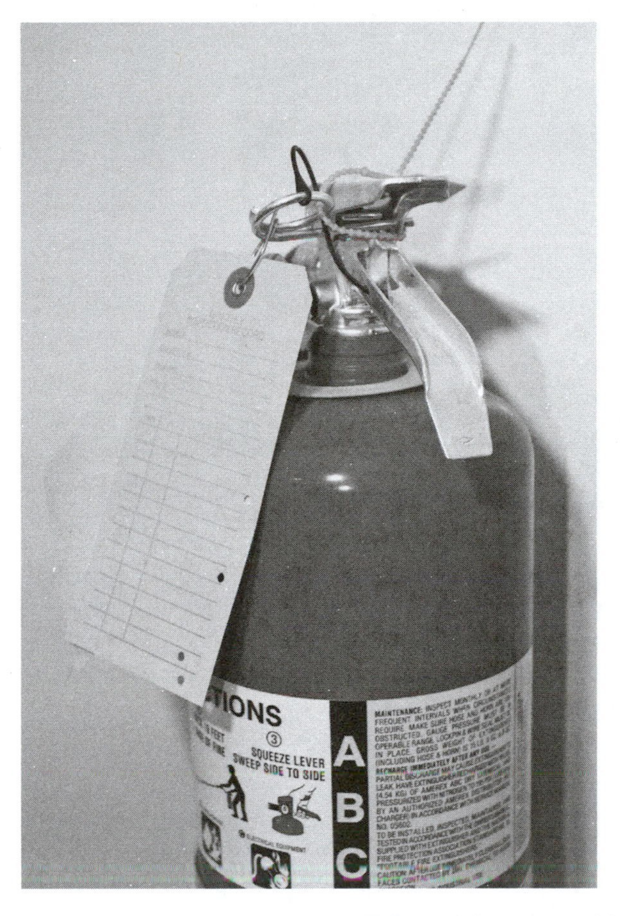

FIGURE 9.2 Fire extinguisher. (Modified from Inmagine Corp, www.123rf.com, with permission.)

Typically, new employees are given fire safety training; this may be repeated on a scheduled basis.

B. Chemical Safety

Biomed staff may come in contact with hazardous chemicals during the course of their work. They should be familiar with the variety of chemicals in their workplace and with the hazards associated with each.

Material safety data sheets (MSDS) should be available in every area for each hazardous chemical found in that area; staff should know where the MSDS information is located, and be familiar with the characteristics of the chemicals.

MSDS provides information about flammability, melting and boiling points, toxicity, health effects, first aid measures, chemical reactivity, requirements for protective gear, safe storage methods, spill or leak handling procedures, and proper disposal methods.

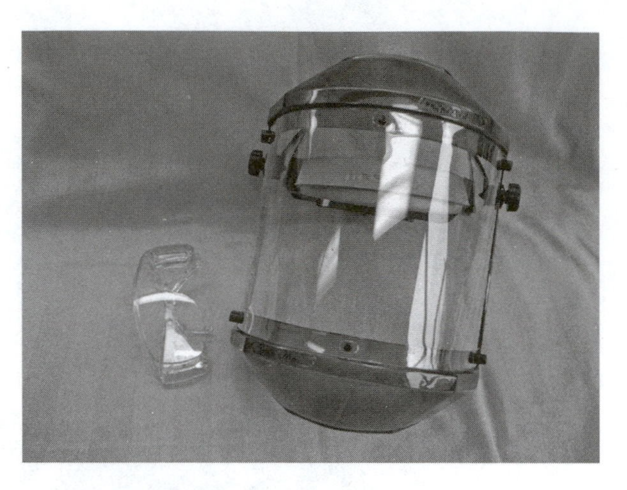

FIGURE 9.3 Goggles and face shield.

C. Mechanical Safety

BMETs may work with mechanical devices such as drills, grinders, and soldering irons. They should be familiar with the hazards associated the devices they handle, and use proper protective equipment as necessary. Eye goggles or shields (Figure 9.3), gloves, masks, or ear protection may be required.

D. Infection Control

Workers in any location can sometimes be exposed to infectious agents, but staff members in hospitals are especially at risk.

Infection control manuals should be located in each department, and everyone should have infection control training and be familiar with the material in the infection control manual.

Infection control is important to prevent illness in staff members, but also to avoid transmission of illnesses to and between patients.

Various means are used to help control infections.

Face masks prevent many infectious agents from moving in or out of the respiratory system (Figure 9.4). The mask should fit snugly around the mouth and nose and be secured so that it will not fall off or slip down inadvertently.

Frequent hand washing and the use of alcohol-based hand cleaners is important, especially before entering and when leaving a patient care area (Figure 9.5).

Gloves should be used when there is a possibility of hand contact with infectious agents, patients, or sterile fields (Figure 9.6). Some equipment may have infectious material on outer or inner surfaces, in which case proper precautions must be followed. If at all possible, contaminated equipment should be sent to the hospital's central processing area for cleaning and disinfection.

Certain areas of the hospital will require special infection control techniques to be implemented by staff members before they enter the area. Such areas include and isolation rooms where patients are known to have a contagious disease; special

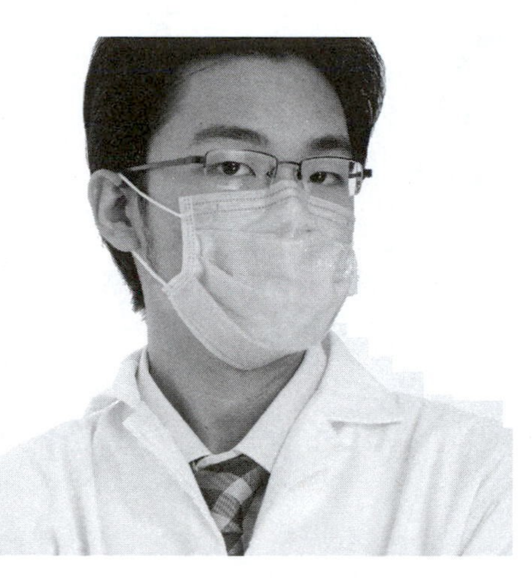

FIGURE 9.4 Surgical masks stop infectious agents going both ways. (Modified from Inmagine Corp, www.123rf.com, with permission.)

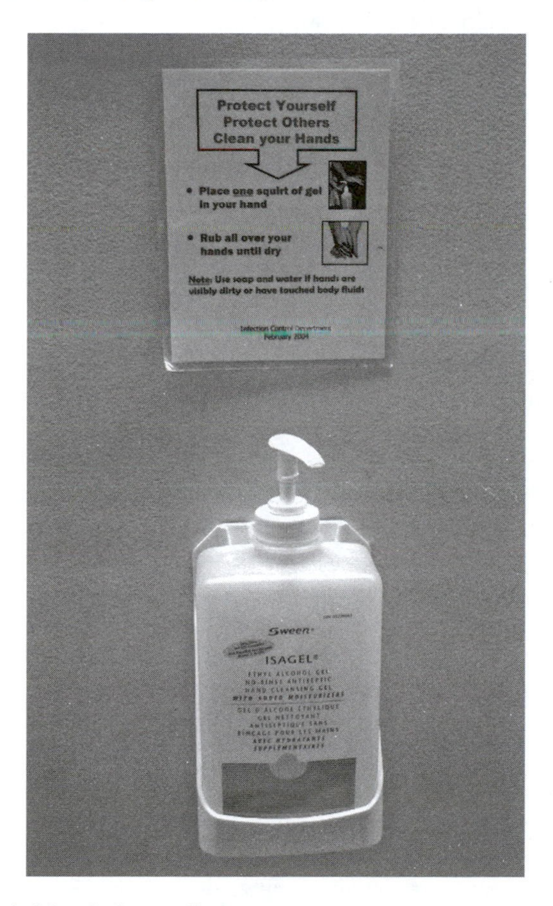

FIGURE 9.5 Alcohol hand cleaner dispenser.

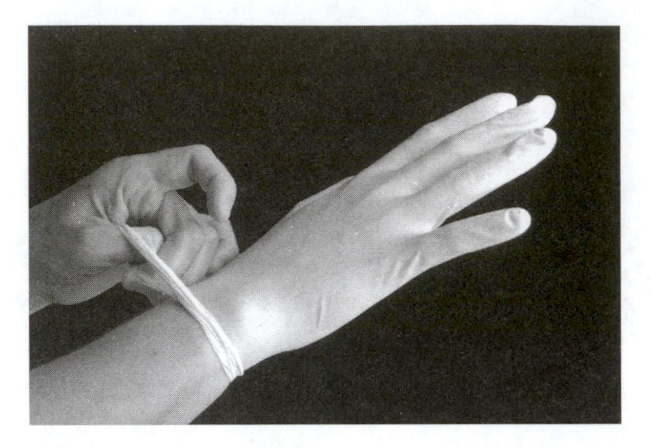

FIGURE 9.6 Surgical gloves on. (Modified from Inmagine Corp, www.123rf.com, with permission.)

procedure areas, such as endoscopy rooms; maternity delivery rooms; operating rooms; and sterile material handling areas.

Precautions may include the use of special foot coverings, head covers and gowns, or staff may need to change in to "OR greens," perform surgical hand washing, and wear head coverings, face masks, and surgical gloves (Figures 9.7 and 9.8).

Some special areas may require even more stringent infection control methods.

Staff should be familiar with the infection control requirements for the various areas of the hospital in which they may be working. If uncertain of the requirements for a particular area, nursing or other staff members will usually be willing to explain the procedures.

Cleanup of biohazardous material spills should be performed by staff members trained in proper procedures and using appropriate materials and instruments. Generally, biomed techs should avoid such spills and call cleaning staff.

E. Sharps Safety

The hospital environment contains many items that can cut or puncture skin, including hypodermic needles, scalpels, scissors, broken glass, and slivers of metal, wood, or plastic. These hazards should be handled in a safe manner, usually described in a policy and procedure or safety manual.

All areas of the hospital should have "sharps" containers that are specially designed to safely contain sharp hazardous objects until they can be disposed of properly. Such containers should be clearly marked with warning and instruction labels (Figure 9.9).

IV. PERFORMANCE ASSURANCE

For any device, the user wants it to function properly whenever it is used. When a device is used in the care of a patient, proper function is even more important and may be life-critical.

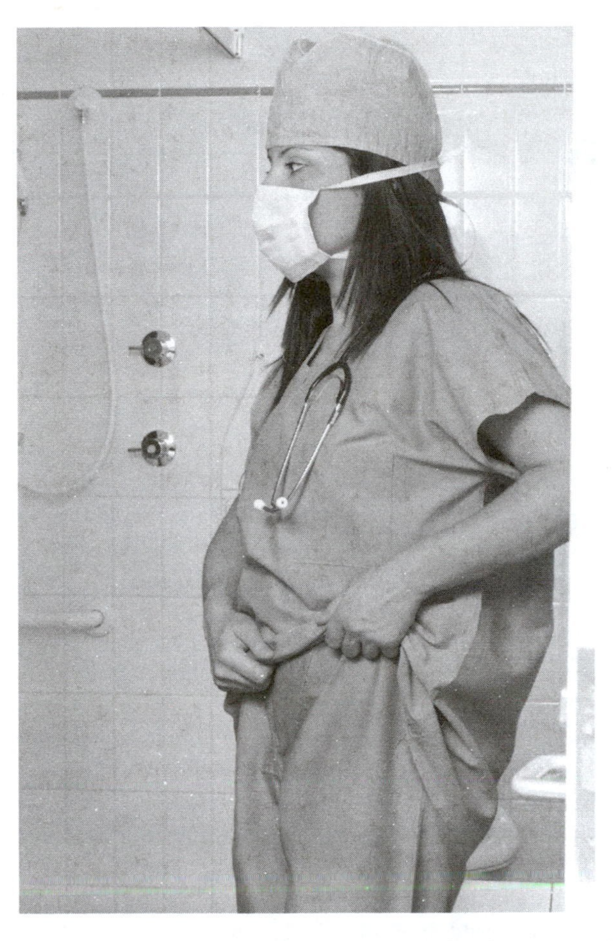

FIGURE 9.7 Ready to enter the OR. (Modified from Inmagine Corp, www.123rf.com, with permission.)

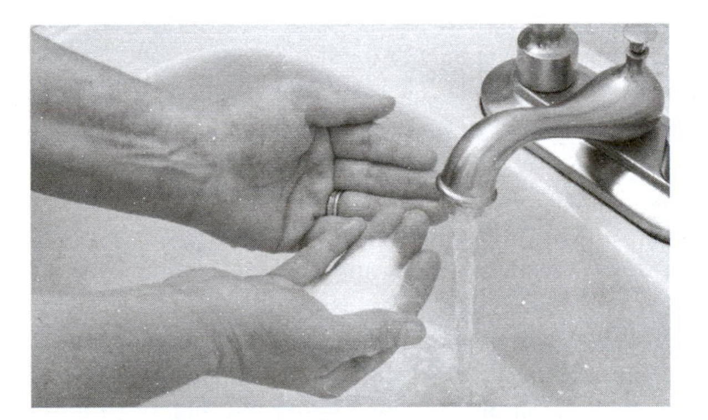

FIGURE 9.8 Hand washing is effective for disease prevention. (Modified from Inmagine Corp, www.123rf.com, with permission.)

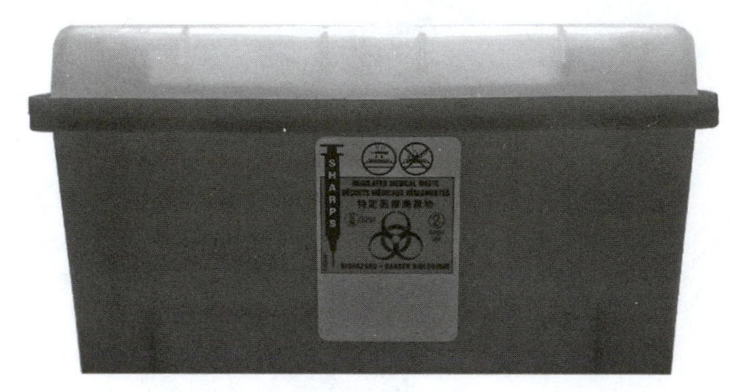

FIGURE 9.9 Sharps container. (Modified from Inmagine Corp, www.123rf.com, with permission.)

Effective performance assurance testing is the best means of ensuring that a given device will function as intended when it is called into use.

Note: the term "performance assurance" (PA) may be used interchangeably with or instead of "preventive maintenance" (PM), though PA is usually more comprehensive.

Most manufacturers provide a recommended PA procedure, and while such procedures are very thorough, they often include steps that are not critical to end-user performance. To complete full manufacturer-recommended performance assurance tests on a regular basis for all patient-care equipment would probably require that most biomed departments be quadrupled in size.

However, the manufacturer's guidelines can be used as a basis for a streamlined PA test procedure that still ensures proper performance. Some such procedures may be generic — for example, they may apply to all battery-powered defibrillator-monitors — while others may be model specific. Less critical equipment might only need a visual inspection and an electrical safety test.

PA test procedures can be developed in-house if done carefully. If a biomedical engineer is on staff, he or she should be involved in the process, if not arranging it entirely.

PA procedures may be available through third-party sources as well. The developers of equipment control software such as Fluke Biomedical's "Sentinel — Infinity" package or ECRI's "Health Devices IPM System" may have PA procedures included, as well as the facility for developing user-specific procedures (See Appendix F).

It is important for both equipment management and legal purposes to keep clear, accurate, and accessible records of PA test results. If, for example, a patient is injured during a course of treatment, a lawsuit may result, in which case it may need to be shown that proper procedures were followed to ensure safe and adequate equipment operation for any devices that were used with that patient.

When performing PA tests, the technologist must have a good understanding of both the theory of operation of the device under test and also the way in which the device is used with patients and any relevant physiological or anatomical effects. This gives more meaning to the tests and also enables the technologist to better evaluate test results.

There may be more than one PA test for a particular device: a shorter version to be repeated on a shorter schedule, and a longer version that is used for less frequent major tests or after significant repairs, or when the device is first received in the hospital. A separate "incoming inspection" procedure may be used, as well.

Joe Biomed sat at his workbench looking at two old Baxter 6201 infusion pumps (Figure 9.10).

One had come down to the lab with a note saying "Won't hold a charge," while the other had been giving an error message that indicated the interface board needed to be replaced. Joe had performed both repairs the day before, a quick battery change for the first unit and a longer, more involved job of replacing one of the major circuit boards in the second pump.

Because the battery change was a minor repair and the pump appeared to be in good condition, Joe ran it through a quick electrical safety test and then connected it to an IV pump tester. He purged the tester by allowing free flow of IV fluid through the test device, and then he threaded the IV tubing into the pump mechanism. Finally, he turned the pump on and programmed rate and volume-to-be-delivered settings into the pump.

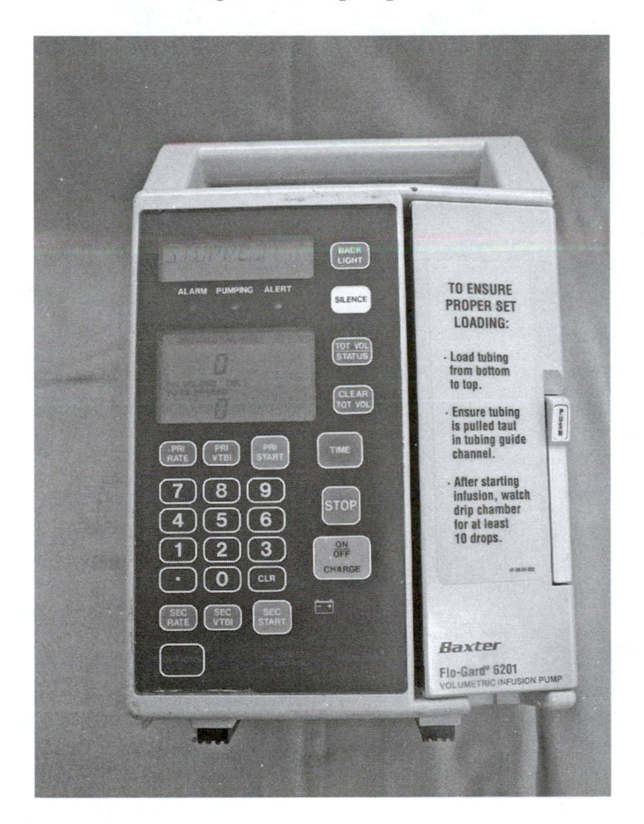

FIGURE 9.10 IV pump.

He first checked the flow rate of the pump at a few different flow rate settings and then used the tester's "occlusion test" function to check that the pump alarmed properly when the IV tubing was blocked. Finally, he started the pump at a medium flow rate and injected a measured bubble into the IV tubing above the pump and checked to see that an alarm sounded when the bubble entered the pump. Following this, Joe removed the tubing, put a sticker on the unit indicating when it was tested, and put it out for return to its home.

With the second pump, a major repair had been completed, so a more thorough test was called for (Figure 9.11). Joe repeated the basic tests that he had performed on the first pump, and then pressed a combination of keys on the pump's keypad to enter a test mode. In this mode, internal circuitry measured the upstream and downstream occlusion sensors and the air-in-line sensor and displayed unitless values on the LCD displays of the pump. Consulting the service manual for the pump, Joe noted the readings were within specifications. He then placed a Baxter calibrated metal disk in the upstream occlusion

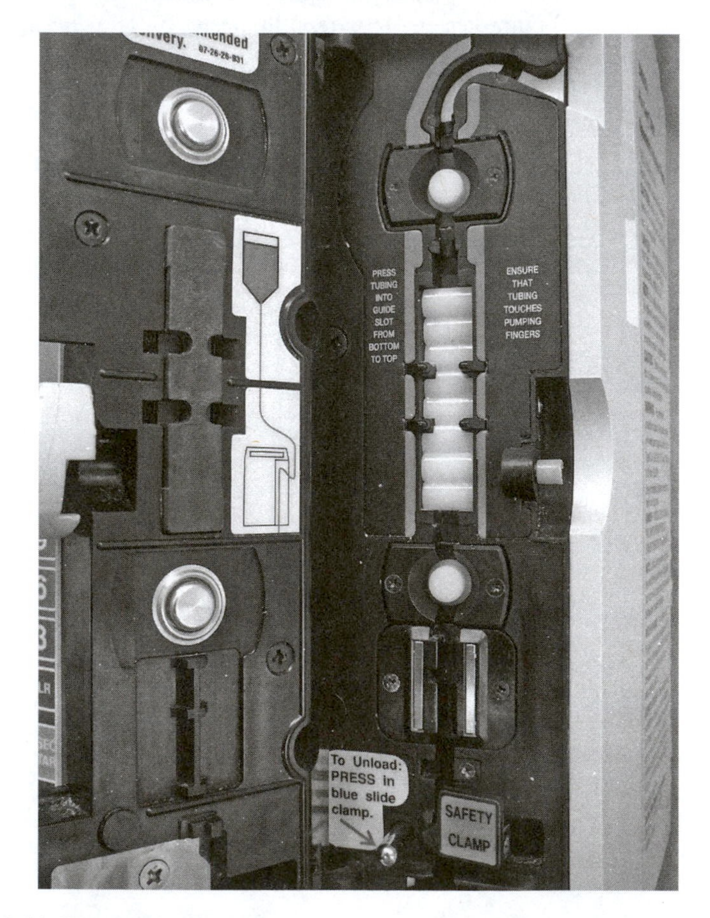

FIGURE 9.11 IV pump head open.

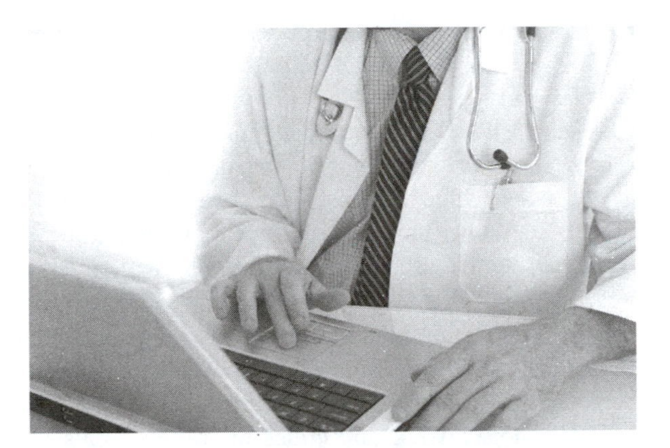

FIGURE 9.12 Performing data entry. (Modified from Inmagine Corp, www.123rf.com, with permission.)

sensor and noted the change in readings, again within spec. A repeat of this process with the downstream occlusion sensor was followed by a test in which an air-filled section of calibration was placed in the air-in-line sensor, then a water-filled section. Readings were noted for each step and compared to specified values.

With all tests in order, Joe labeled the second pump and took both to the central pump storage area, where they were catalogued and plugged in, ready for use.

Returning to the lab, Joe entered the work he had just done in the department's equipment control database (Figure 9.12) and went on to his next task.

V. TROUBLESHOOTING TECHNIQUES

Successful troubleshooting is the key to being able to diagnose problems and perform the right repair, returning the device in question to service as quickly as possible.

Good troubleshooting requires an organized approach, knowledge of specific troubleshooting techniques, and thorough familiarity with both the theory of operation and the construction and proper use of the device in question.

A calm and relaxed approach is always much more successful than a stressed-out panic method. Keep in mind that most problems are not as serious as they might first appear.

Troubleshooting in general has moved away from component-level diagnosis to more board or assembly diagnosis. It may be more expedient and in the long run more economical to replace a board or assembly than to try to isolate and replace a single faulty component. Fewer and fewer discrete components are being used in circuit design, and replacement of individual integrated circuits (ICs) is often difficult or impossible. Multilayer circuit boards and surface-mount technology require special tools for repair, if that is even deemed worthwhile at a factory depot.

Manufacturer service information often does not include component-level diagrams, descriptions, or parts lists, further adding to the difficulty of trying to go to the component level.

Some circuitry may still lend itself to component-level troubleshooting and repair, however, so such skills should not be abandoned.

Step Zero may be to determine if the device is covered under any kind of warranty or service contract. If so, and if the problem appears to be a real one, the problem is solved from your perspective. Ship it out, and let the manufacturer fix it!

Otherwise …

The first step in troubleshooting is to gather as much information about the failure as possible. This includes asking whoever was using the device about the conditions that were present when the failure occurred. Did the unit make any noises? Was there a smell or smoke? Were any codes or trouble lights displayed? What accessories were being used with the equipment? If possible, get the accessories! Was there anything else unusual just before the failure occurred? What other equipment was being used at the time?

This information is often impossible to obtain, as users either do not recall or did not notice details. "Someone else was using the equipment, and they are on night shift/away on vacation/died." Or nobody knows what happened or when.

Equipment will often arrive for repair with a scrap of paper taped to it saying, "Broken."

Step two involves reviewing information about the device. It may be something you work with often and know the common problems almost automatically, or it may be a device you have never seen before. If a service manual is available, it can be consulted. Are there troubleshooting tables or flow charts? Error code tables? Detailed and useful descriptions of the theory of operation? Sometimes the problem you are seeing is described in plain language in the manual, along with an outline of the steps needed to solve the problem.

On the other hand, service manuals may provide very little useful information for troubleshooting. They may have tables that describe a hundred other problems but not yours, or they may recommend solutions that do not work.

Service manuals may not be available, too. They may have been lost, or the equipment vendor may not have supplied them. In this case, your own troubleshooting skills come in to play.

Step three is to try to duplicate the problem. Some problems are intermittent, and just as your car never makes that funny noise when you take it to the garage, intermittent failures never seem to occur when you are testing a device in the lab.

Try to recreate the conditions under which the failure occurred, insofar as these are known. Patience and a methodical approach help to reach this goal, and some techniques only come with experience. If and when the problem crops up again, note in as much detail as possible the conditions preceding the failure and any symptoms of the failure itself. You may find that the original user's description was accurate, or it may be totally off base. In any case, repeating the failure in controlled conditions can provide vital clues as to the cause of the failure.

It may not be possible to duplicate a problem. The device may be totally inoperative, or it may continue to run without apparent problems. In the latter case

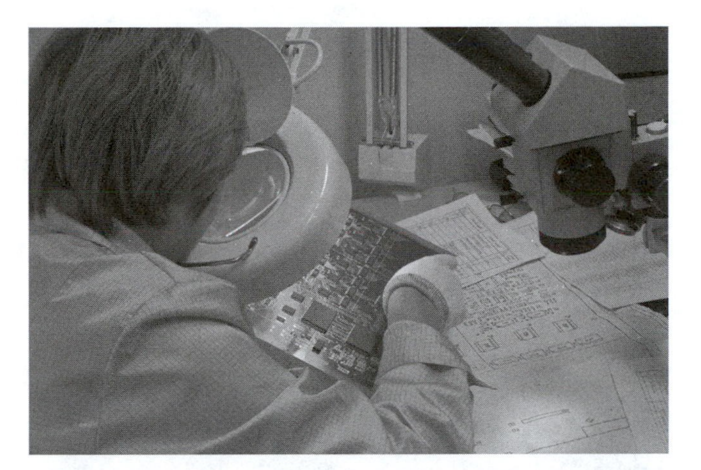

FIGURE 9.13 BMET examining circuit board. (Modified from Inmagine Corp, www.123rf.com, with permission.)

you may have to decide whether or not to return the unit to service without doing anything further. Your judgment is called into play, but if you are unsure, you might want to ask someone else or talk to factory service personnel. If the device is high risk, it may be prudent to arrange to have it returned to the manufacturer for testing and possible repair. If they cannot find a problem, it is then their responsibility if the device is returned to service and then causes problems.

With an inoperative device or if its operation is very erratic, you may need to go on to the next step ... after checking to be sure a good power cord is plugged in and any accessible fuses are intact. Oh, and that the power switch is turned on.

Step four: Observe! If the case of the unit is smashed, that can be a good clue that it was involved in an accident (even if the end users deny this possibility), and you may need to look for internal damage. Check the external of the device carefully for signs of damage, fluid entry, overheating, or tampering.

Opening the case and looking for obvious signs is next, and an experienced nose can often diagnose a problem simply by smelling the inside of the box (Figure 9.13). A fried resistor has a distinctive odor. Components may be obviously burned or discolored from overheating, or circuit board traces may be vaporized. Physical shocks can cause heavy components like transformers to pull loose from their normal locations, and liquids entering the device can leave obvious signs of corrosion or shorting. Some devices may have internal fuses that can be checked for continuity.

Replacing a burned-out component may solve the problem, but often this is only a symptom of the underlying problem. Sometimes replacing the component and powering up the unit can give further clues, if the bad part was not the actual problem.

Service manuals may provide good troubleshooting guides that take you methodically through the system, checking various things such as voltages or waveforms at test points or looking for specific responses from the device (Figure 9.14). In this case, the problem will usually become apparent eventually.

If no useful troubleshooting information is available, you may have to work through the circuit on your own. If possible, identify the power input section and

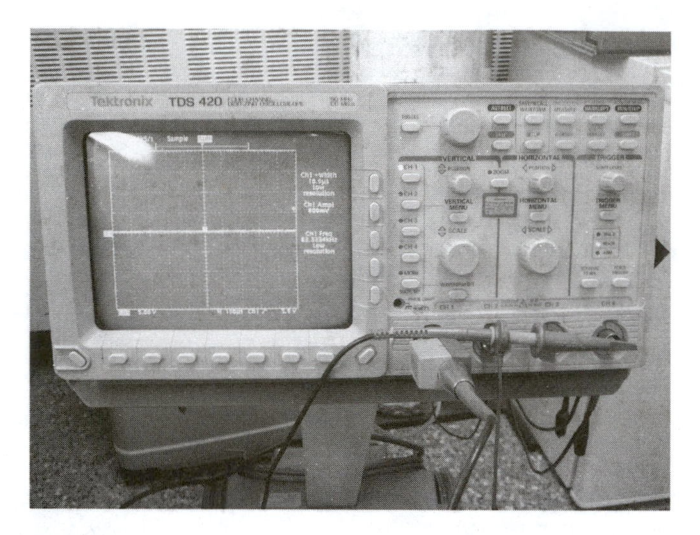

FIGURE 9.14 Oscilloscope.

power supply. Check for voltages — they may be marked on circuit boards, or you may be able to make an educated guess as to what voltages should be at various points in the circuit. Check switches for continuity, and also power supply transformer windings. If there appears to be no power coming from the power supply, it may need to be replaced.

Simple component faults can sometimes be diagnosed using a multimeter or component analyzer (Chapter 11). A faulty component can be replaced if parts are available, but again this may only be as symptom of another problem. On the other hand, replacing a bad diode may be a miracle cure.

If no individual component faults can be found, the next step may be called for.

Step five: If spare circuit boards or other assemblies are available for the device, and all other troubleshooting has failed to find the problem, you might try to replace boards/assemblies one at a time, beginning with the one you feel is most likely to be the source of the problem. A power supply board is a good place to start.

If no spare boards are available, you may want to order them, but this is a judgment call. Unless you are sure that a particular board is causing the problem, you may just be extending the down time of the equipment by such slow experimentation. Also, if circuit boards or assemblies are very expensive and the device itself is not, or if it is old and/or in poor condition otherwise, it may be more prudent to simply retire the device and tell the originating department that a new machine must be purchased (Step last!). The advice of a senior staff member or the head of the originating department may be in order; whoever holds the purse strings (Figure 9.15).

Step six: If, after following all courses of action available to you, the device is still not working, you may opt to send it to the manufacturer or approved repair facility. For large devices that are impractical to ship, an on-site service call would be required.

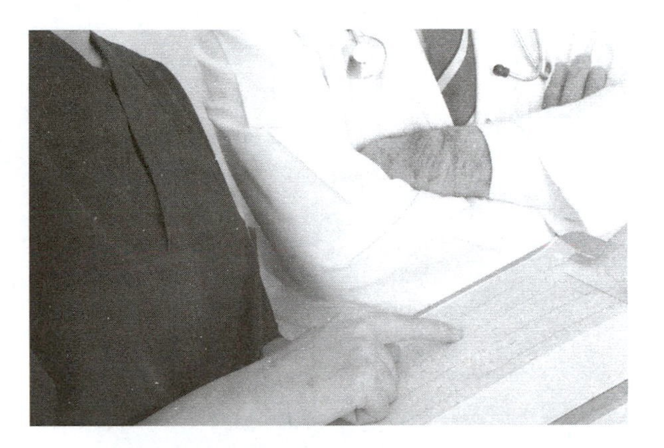

FIGURE 9.15 Consultation. (Modified from Inmagine Corp, www.123rf.com, with permission.)

Step six also means that you must hang your head in shame for the rest of the day, and place a large red "F" (for Failure) on the back of your lab coat. (Just kidding, of course — some problems are just not practically solvable in the lab.)

VI. ELECTROSTATIC DISCHARGE

Semiconductor devices are vulnerable to damage by electrostatic discharge (ESD). This damage may or may not cause immediate failure; if not, it may be cumulative, resulting in failure at some point in the future.

Failures caused by electrostatic shocks can be very expensive to repair and/or may result in extensive equipment downtime. Every precaution must be taken to prevent ESD damage.

Newer semiconductors and circuit designs have increased the resistance of equipment to ESD damage, but precautions must still be observed.

Components and circuit boards or assemblies that are vulnerable to ESD are shipped and stored in conductive plastic bags and/or with conductive foam sheets. These measures must be left in place until the part is about to be used.

When working on any device that may be damaged by ESD, one should wear an effective grounding wrist strap. These straps are connected to ground through a high-value resistor, which bleeds static electricity harmlessly to ground.

An antistatic desk mat is valuable as well; it will have a grounding connector like the wrist strap, with a resistor in line. Antistatic floor mats and grounded work chairs can further ensure protection.

VII. CHAPTER SUMMARY

Safety, electrical and otherwise, is one focus of Chapter 9. Other topics covered are performance assurance, troubleshooting techniques, and electrostatic discharge.

10 Testers and Tools

I. INTRODUCTION

A wide variety of test equipment is used in supporting medical equipment, and it is critical that the test devices provide accurate measurements. To ensure accuracy, test equipment should be calibrated on a regular basis, typically once a year. Calibration should be done by qualified personnel using equipment whose own calibration can be traced to a reliable standard that is recognized by the regulating authorities in your area.

Calibration records must be made and stored carefully.

II. GENERAL TEST EQUIPMENT

Much of the test equipment used in a biomed lab is the same as that used in any electronics repair shop, though it may tend to have somewhat higher specifications.

A. Digital Multimeters

An indispensable tool, a quality digital multimeter (DMM) performs a number of measurements (parameters will vary by model):

- AC and DC voltage and current
- Resistance
- Semiconductor junction state (working, open, or shorted) and polarity
- Continuity, indicated by a measured value and a tone
- Frequency
- Capacitance

Some models select the proper measurement range automatically, while others must be switched manually.

Measurements may be logged, high and low values recorded, and an interface to other devices may be included.

A wide variety of attachments and special probes are available (Figure 10.1 through Figure 10.3). These may allow the unit to measure temperature or humidity, high voltages, or current without direct contact. Some probes have very fine pincer tips that can connect to points on circuit boards without causing shorts.

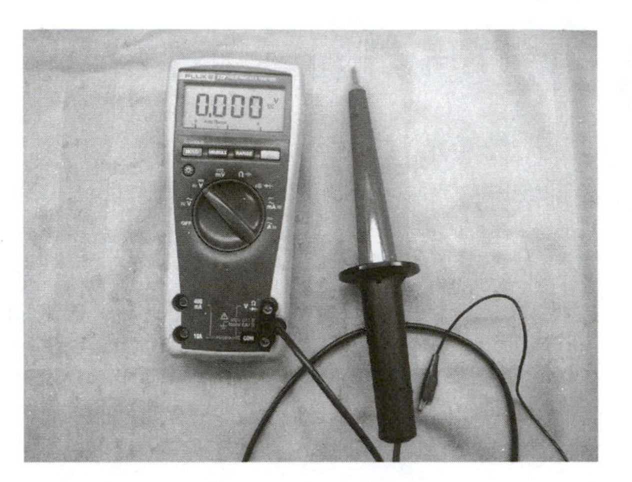

FIGURE 10.1 Digital multimeter with high-voltage probe

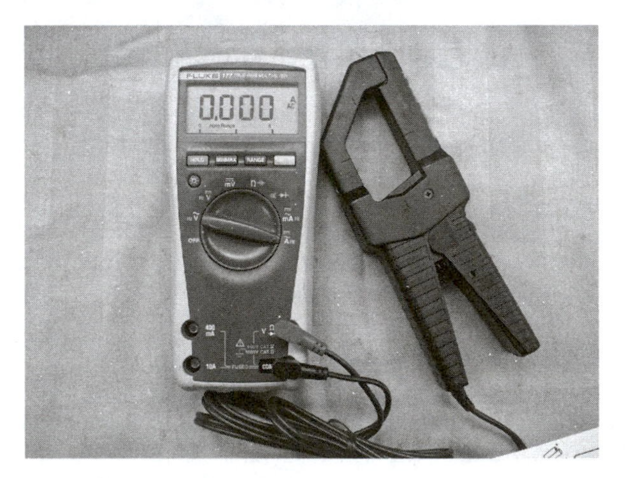

FIGURE 10.2 DMM with noncontact current probe.

B. Oscilloscopes

An oscilloscope (Figure 10.4) is a device that can display a graph of voltage vs. time. This is used to measure the signals found in electronic devices for troubleshooting or calibration. Oscilloscopes have a wide range of capabilities and may be specialized for particular applications such as television, radio, computer networking, or various industrial uses.

Scopes may use CRT or LCD displays and can be cart mounted, rack mounted, or even handheld. The latter may have some of the functions of a DMM included; these are referred to as "scopemeters."

A valuable feature of oscilloscopes is the ability to store waveforms. This can make waveform comparisons easier, and it also allows the capture of transient events.

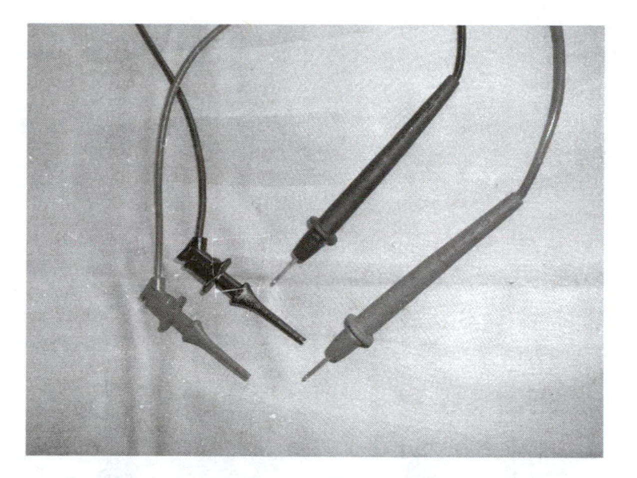

FIGURE 10.3 A few other types of probes.

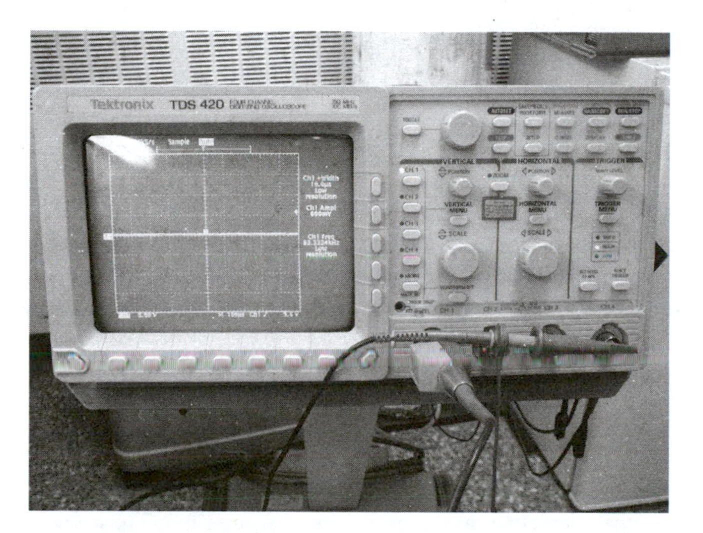

FIGURE 10.4 Oscilloscope.

Associated with storage functions is a delay feature that can help to visualize short-duration events that occur over a longer time period.

Color displays can help to differentiate between various signals being analyzed.

An automatic setup feature is useful when examining a wide range of signal types. The scope detects the signal to which it is connected and analyzes it to determine frequency and amplitude and uses this information to set time and voltage scales to provide the best possible waveform.

Some scopes can further analyze waveforms and perform various measurements, giving numeric values to such parameters as frequency, peak amplitude, rise and fall times, positive and negative pulse widths, and more.

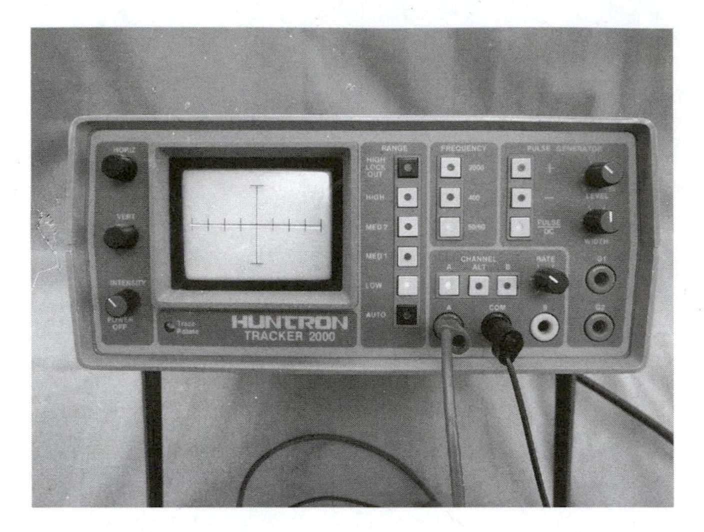

FIGURE 10.5 Component tester.

Learning to use an oscilloscope effectively is very much a hands-on endeavor, since features and special applications are so varied. Some manufacturers provide tutorials, which may even be built into the scope, to aid in learning how to use the unit.

A specialized type of oscilloscope can be very useful in troubleshooting electronic components (see Figure 10.5). This unit can apply specific signals to semiconductors and some other components and can display a graph of the response. Certain patterns are indicative of the state of the component being tested. A wide variety of semiconductors, capacitors, resistors, and inductors can be evaluated this way. Units may have a feature that allows the rapid alteration of views of two sets of probes, which means that a questionable component can be compared to a known good one.

C. Other Test Equipment

A number of other devices may be useful in a biomed lab. These include:

- Sound level meters (Figure 10.6), to provide a quantitative measure of sounds in various situations.
- Thermometers, used to check medical thermometers or to help locate overheating components. These may be stand-alone devices or a special attachment for a DMM.
- Tachometers, to measure the rotational speed of equipment such as centrifuges. Tachometers may operate by physical contact or by an optical sensor.
- Oxygen analyzers (Figure 10.7), to measure oxygen concentrations in devices such as infant incubators, oxygen concentrators, and ventilators.
- Manometers for pressure or vacuum measurement in ventilators, noninvasive blood pressure (NIBP) units, and suction machines.

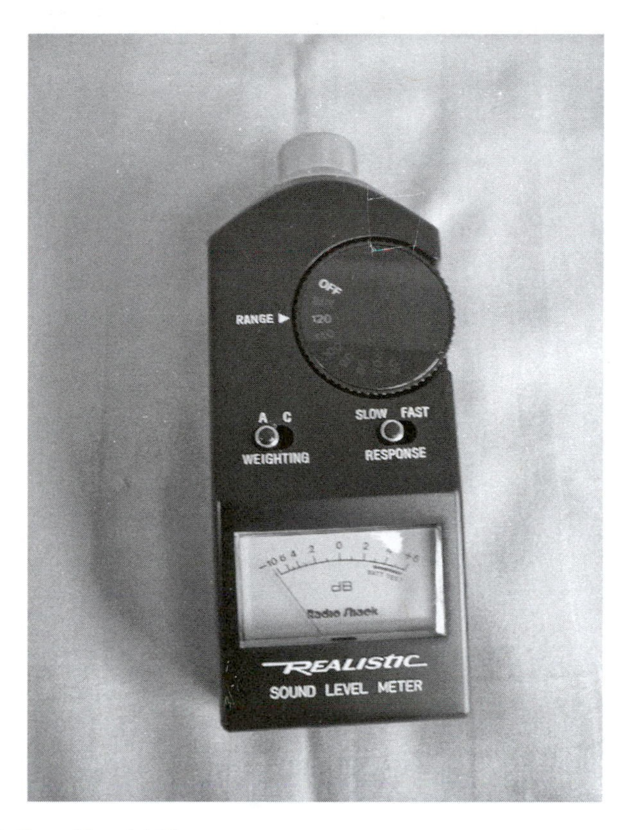

FIGURE 10.6 Sound level (dB) meter.

III. SPECIALIZED BIOMEDICAL TEST EQUIPMENT

Many types of medical equipment have specific parameters that need to be tested when doing PA tests. Test equipment manufacturers have designed units that integrate various functions so they can perform the necessary test quickly and accurately.

Most of these special testers have a printer port for making hard copies of test results, as well as a serial port for connecting to a computer. This may be used to interface the device with an equipment-control program.

As with all test equipment, these devices must be calibrated to a traceable standard on a regular schedule.

(Note: electrical safety analyzers were described in Chapter 9.)

A. ESU Analyzers

Electrosurgery machines put out high-powered electrical signals that must meet specific performance criteria for effective surgical function; ESU analyzers (Figure 10.8) measure these criteria. They include:

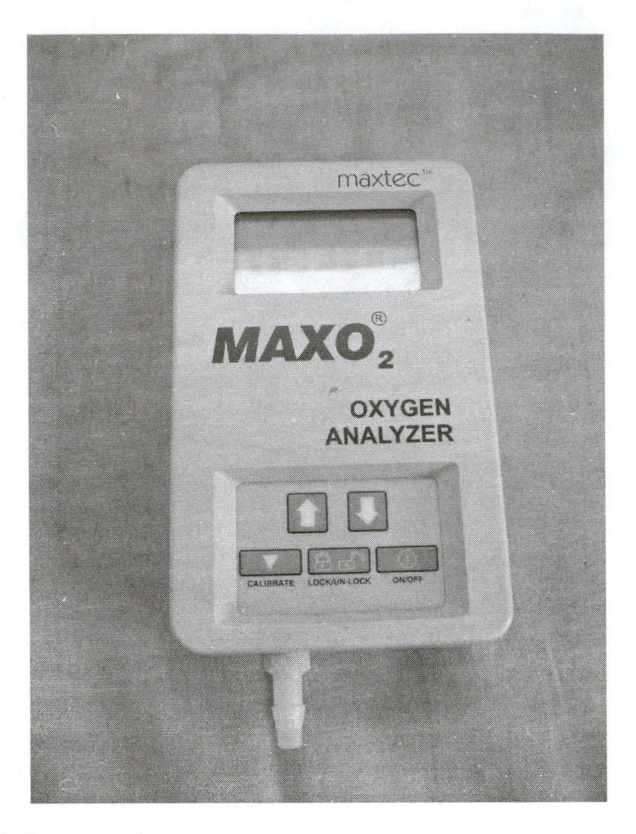

FIGURE 10.7 Oxygen analyzer.

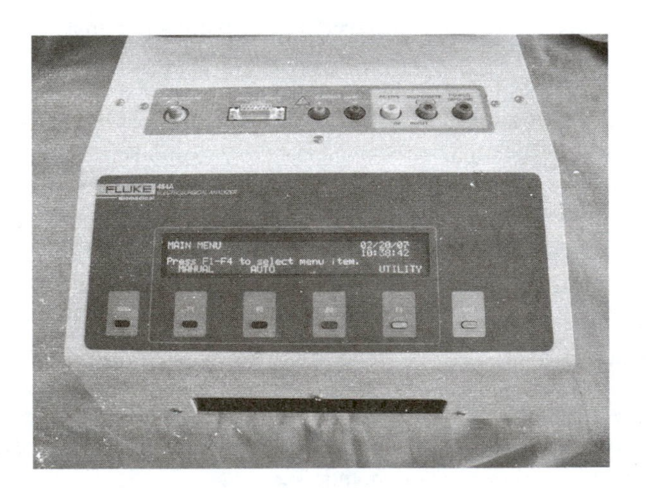

FIGURE 10.8 Electrosurgery unit analyzer.

- Power output — units selectable.
- Current.
- Peak-to-peak voltage.
- Crest factor, which is a unitless value equal to the peak amplitude divided by the RMS (root mean square or quadratic mean) value of a signal; it is a measure of the "purity" of the waveform.
- RF leakage, a measure of safety, since leakage can cause patient burns if it is high.
- Return electrode monitoring system upper and lower threshold values.

Since the impedance of tissue can vary greatly when undergoing ESU activity, ESU testers provide a number of different test load values to simulate changing loads. Power output and other parameters should stay within specified limits for the various loads.

Automated standard test procedures may also be built into the tester.

B. Infusion Device Analyzers

Infusion pumps must deliver fluids at a set rate and also meet safety requirements. Infusion device analyzers (Figure 10.9) measure flow rates and total volumes delivered so these values can be compared to pump settings.

Many pumps do not provide smooth fluid flow, especially at lower rates. The flow can be intermittent, with rates averaged over time. A pump analyzer must be able to measure such intermittent flows and accurately determine average flow rates.

Occlusion alarms are an important part of pump function, and testers have facilities for measuring pressures that are developed when an occlusion occurs.

C. Physiological Simulators

Testing and troubleshooting physiological monitors is much easier if realistic patient signals are available for connection to the monitor. Real patients can be hard to find, however, so simulators were developed to take their place (see Figure 10.10).

These units use microprocessor technology combined with digital-to-analog converters to generate accurate representations of many physiological signals.

ECG is the most basic of these signals, but a modern simulator will produce not only normal QRS complexes at various rates and amplitudes, but also a range of different arrhythmia patterns, plus sine, square, and triangle waves.

A set of color-coded posts allows various types of ECG electrode terminals to be connected to the simulator.

Respiration signals can be included with ECG signals for monitors with such capability; rate, amplitude, and impedance can all be modified.

Invasive pressure signals are another aspect of these simulators. Pressures include arterial blood pressure at various locations in the body, central venous pressure, and intracranial pressure. The rates for blood pressure waveforms are set by the ECG rate in use, and ECG arrhythmias will make for different pressure waveforms as well.

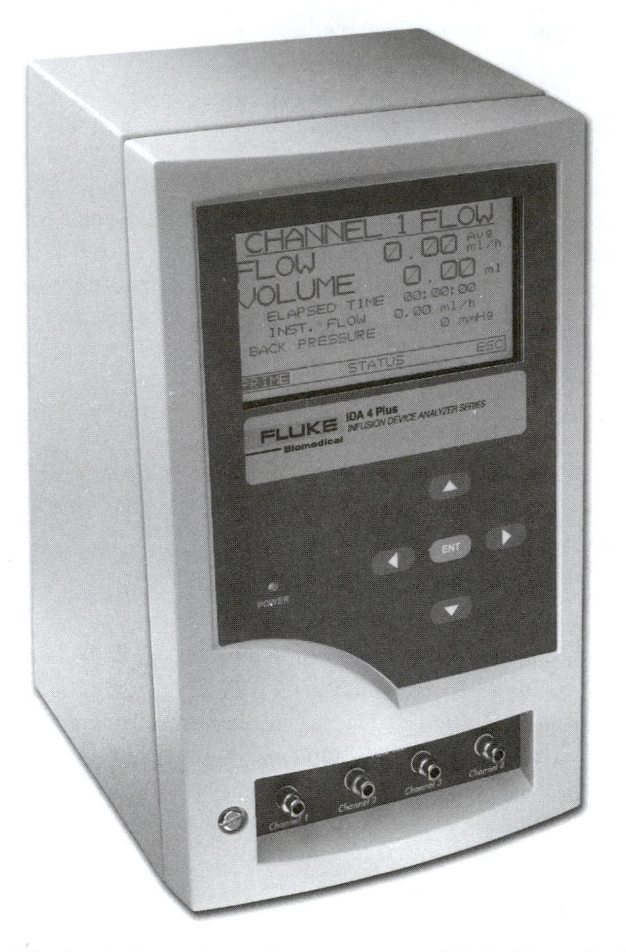

FIGURE 10.9 Infusion device analyzer. (Image courtesy of Fluke Biomedical.)

D. NIBP Analyzers

Noninvasive blood pressure monitors determine blood pressure by inflating a cuff until blood flow is completely occluded and then bleeding off pressure while noting when Korotkoff sounds start and end.

To test for proper function, NIBP testers (Figure 10.11) must be able to simulate the pulsatile pressure waveforms found in a real arm. An accurate manometer must be included, and the simulated pressure values displayed, so they can be compared to the values determined by the monitor being tested.

Since monitor accuracy may be different at different levels, the analyzer should be able to simulate a variety of blood pressure situations, including hypo- and hypertension and child or infant pressure patterns.

NIBP monitors must meet specific standards for leak rates, and analyzers have facilities for inflating the NIBP system to specific pressures and then holding, measuring the drop in pressure (leak rate) over a given time, usually one minute.

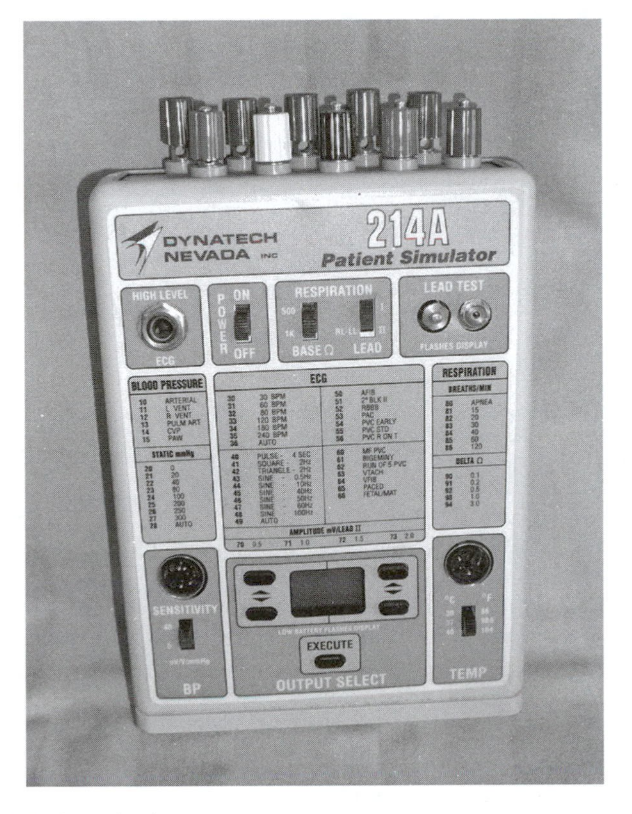

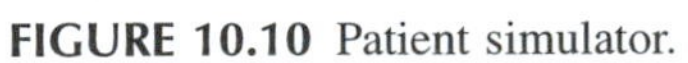
FIGURE 10.10 Patient simulator.

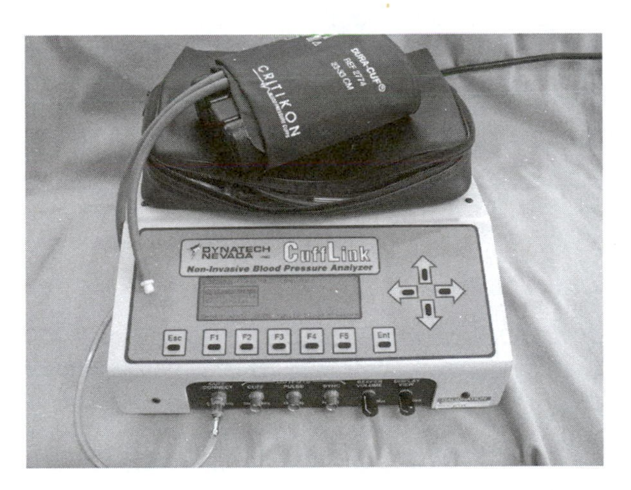

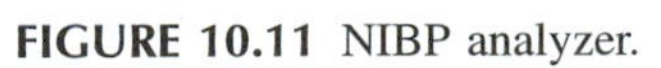
FIGURE 10.11 NIBP analyzer.

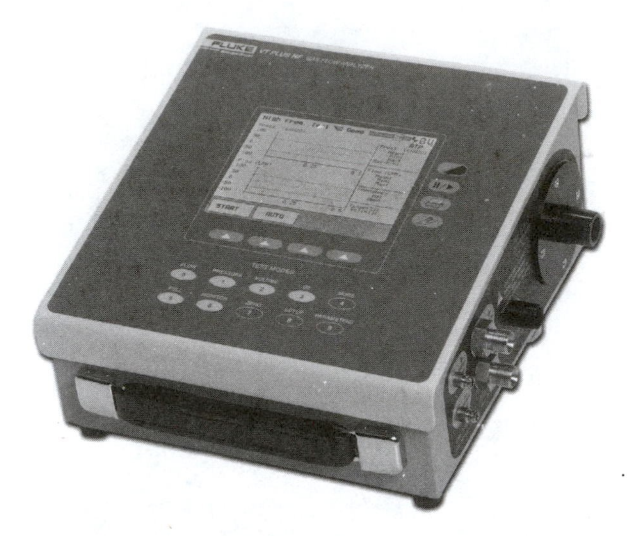

FIGURE 10.12 Gas flow analyzer. (Image courtesy of Fluke Biomedical.)

If the NIBP system has a self-test or calibration mode, the analyzer should be able to apply set pressures so they can be compared to monitor values. This may be used to perform calibrations of the monitor if such a feature is available.

E. Ventilator Analyzers

Gas control is the primary function of medical ventilators. Gas pressure, flow curves, and frequency in both directions are handled in order to provide optimal respiratory support to the patient. Ventilators can respond to certain patient conditions, possibly modifying their behavior depending on feedback from the patient.

In order to adequately test ventilator performance, an analyzer (see Figure 10.12) must be able to accurately measure gas flow and pressure and provide both numeric and graphic representations of these measurements so they can be compared to the expected performance of the ventilator. Range, accuracy, and response time of the analyzer must be sufficient to provide useful results.

The ability of the tester to simulate a patient may be useful; this involves the use of a model lung, such as a rubber bag having similar characteristics to a real lung.

F. Incubator Analyzers

Infant incubators provide an environment that causes minimal stress to babies, so that they can recover from medical or surgical conditions more easily. In conflict with this goal is the need to give access for caregivers so they can provide care and treatment to the infant.

Testing incubator performance focuses on the environmental factors, so an analyzer (Figure 10.13) must be able to measure various parameters to ensure environmental integrity.

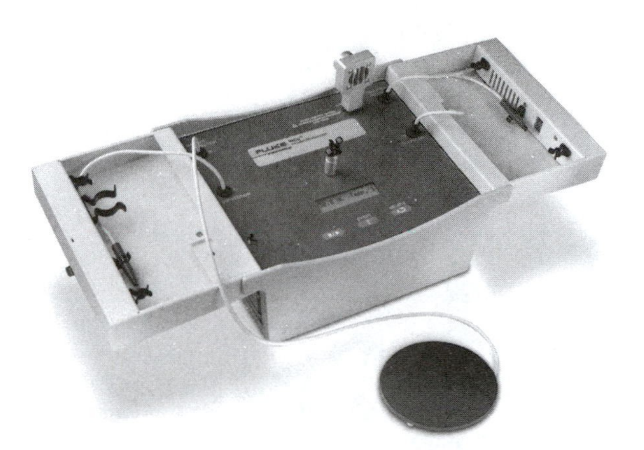

FIGURE 10.13 Incubator analyzer. (Image courtesy of Fluke Biomedical.)

Newborn infants often cannot adequately control their body temperature, so incubators must provide steady, even heat that can adjust rapidly to changing conditions such as opening and closing access doors. Temperature can vary throughout the interior or the incubator, so an analyzer should be able to monitor and verify temperature at multiple locations simultaneously.

Oxygen concentration, air flow rates, humidity, and sound levels are other important parameters that incubator testers should be able to analyze.

G. Ultrasound Analyzers

Both therapeutic and diagnostic ultrasound machines depend on having ultrasound power output within specifications. Ultrasound power meters convert sound energy into an electrical signal for measurement and display (Figure 10.14).

Meters contain a reservoir of degassed water into which the ultrasound head is immersed, a detection transducer, and associated electronics. Sound levels can be measured as pulsed or continuous, and a serial port allows communication with a computer.

H. Specialized Calibration and Testing Devices

Some manufacturers supply special test equipment to help field technologists to test and maintain their medical technologies.

As an example, IVAC Corp. produces the Core Calibrator for use with IVAC tympanic thermometers (Figure 10.15).

A cable connects the unit being tested to the calibrator, and the probe tip is inserted into a well containing a precisely controlled blackbody at 26°C. A measurement is triggered on the thermometer, and a value displayed on the thermometer screen. The process is repeated with a second well at 38°C. If both of these values are within specifications, the unit can be returned to service. If one or both is out of range, then "Calibration" is selected on the calibration unit. The probe is inserted into the 26°C well, and when the measure trigger is depressed, the unit is calibrated

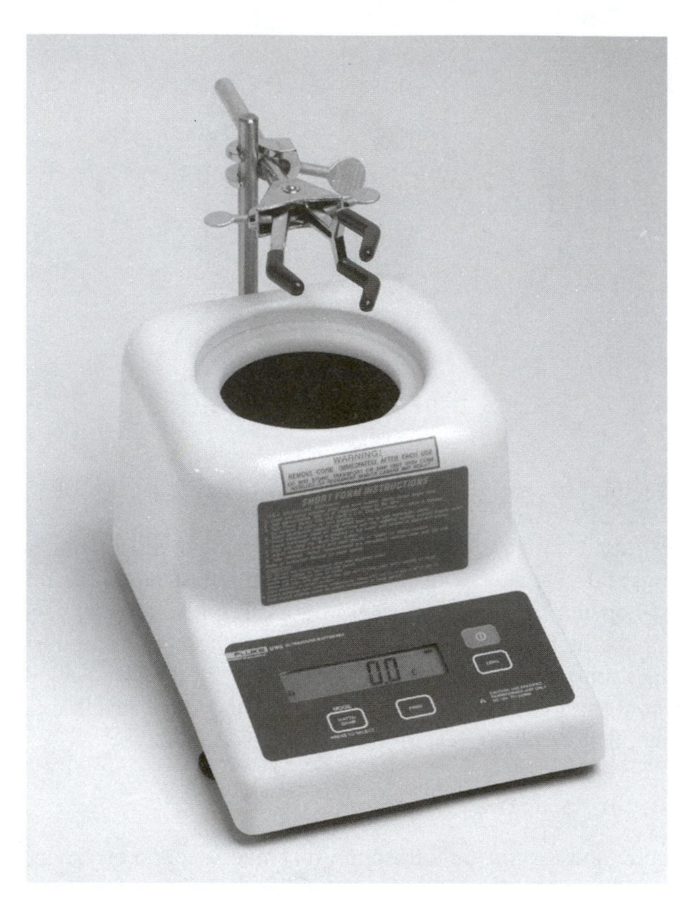

FIGURE 10.14 Ultrasound wattmeter. (Image courtesy of Fluke Biomedical.)

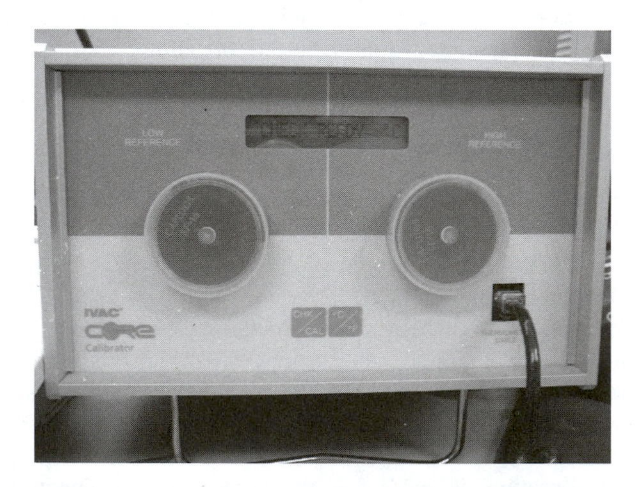

FIGURE 10.15 IVAC CoreChek thermometer test and calibration unit.

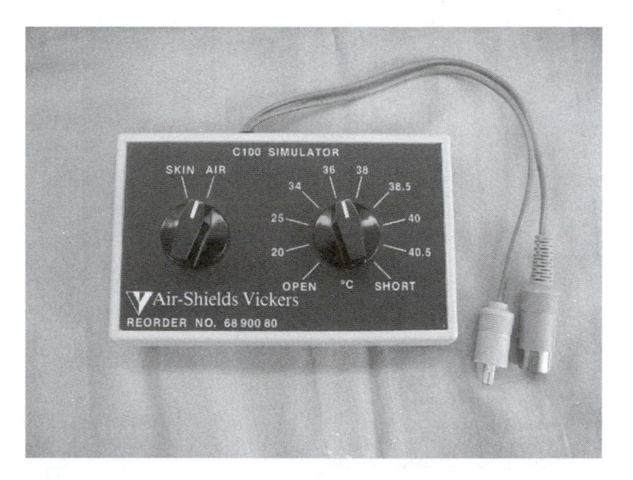

FIGURE 10.16 Incubator temperature probe simulator.

to exactly 26°C. Repeating at 38°C gives two reference points, so that accurate calibration can be performed.

Another example is the temperature probe simulator (Figure 10.16) used for testing some older Air-Shields infant incubators.

The device simply plugs into the incubator in place of the actual air and skin temperature probes. Internal resistors that simulate specific temperatures are selected by a rotary switch, which also has settings to simulate open or shorted probes. This allows a quick and accurate check of the temperature function of the incubator, as well as being used for calibration purposes.

IV. TOOLS

Working with a wide range of medical devices means that a wide range of tools is required. These may be ordinary hand and power tools, or they may be specialized devices intended for use with just one specific model of equipment.

Quality tools make a great difference in end use: they fit better, they last longer, they are harder and stronger, and they are less likely to damage hardware components. The extra initial price will be paid back many times over.

A. General

Hand tools include such things as screwdrivers, wrenches, hammers, pliers, cutters, and measuring devices.

Screwdrivers come in a tremendous variety of types and sizes (Figure 10.17), and eventually it seems you need just about every one in the course of your work. Different manufacturers favor particular types of fasteners — one may use mostly slotted screws, while another uses only Philips and a third prefers Torx or Bristol splines or Allan-type screws.

"Wrenches" includes everything from small open-end spanners, to adjustable "Crescent" wrenches, to metric and standard socket sets of every size (Figure 10.18).

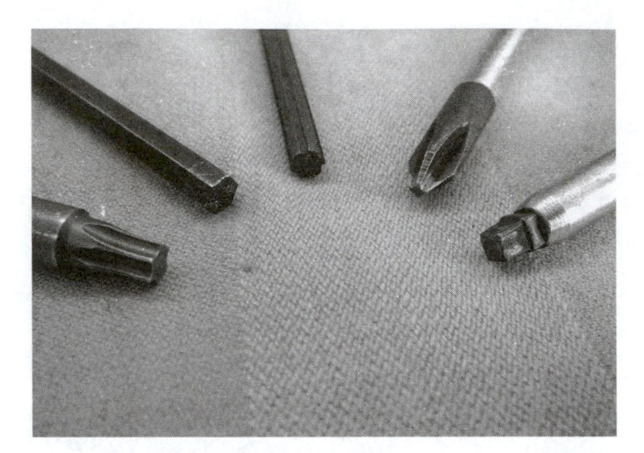

FIGURE 10.17 A variety of screwdriver tips.

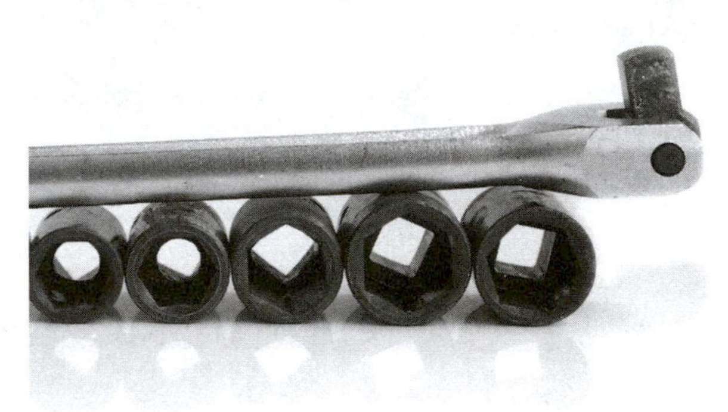

FIGURE 10.18 Socket wrench set. (Modified from Inmagine Corp, www.123rf.com, with permission.)

Some applications specify that fasteners be tightened to particular torque values, and this requires an accurate torque wrench handle.

Pliers and cutters again come in a wide variety, and many different types will be needed in the lab. Quality once more is key, as cheap pliers can bend and lose their grip, while poor-quality cutters simply mangle things instead of providing a clean, accurate cut.

A very specialized form of grabber is used to remove integrated circuits from sockets. These can be further specialized for removing microprocessor and other similar chips (Figure 10.19).

A good tape measure will be used often, for measuring cable runs or cabinet sizes, and a micrometer caliper can be invaluable for ordering parts that do not have part numbers.

B. Specialized Tools and Components

Certain pieces of equipment may utilize proprietary fittings that cannot be handled with off-the-shelf tools. In such cases, the manufacturer may supply or sell the special tools required, or a talented fabricator might be able to build them. This kind

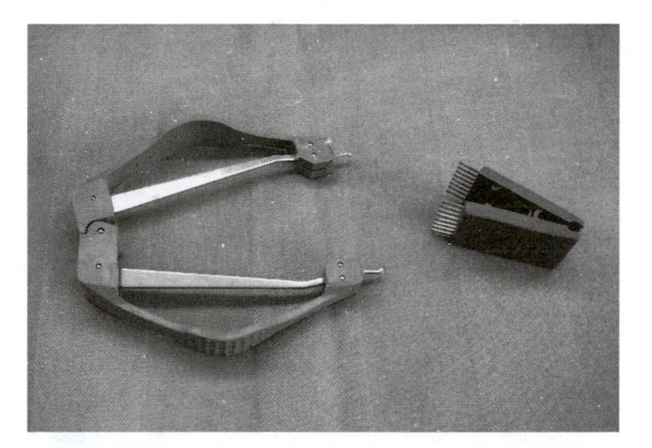

FIGURE 10.19 IC removal tool + chip contact extender.

of unique hardware tends to make manufacturing more expensive and can be frustrating for service personnel, and so it seems not to be found as much as it once was.

C. Power Tools

A few general power tools are essential in a biomed work area. These include power drills and high-speed rotary tools, drill presses, and grinding wheels.

V. SOLDERING

Though component repair is becoming less and less common with medical equipment, it still may be necessary to unsolder and replace a resistor or diode occasionally. Soldering wires and other connectors is also done often enough that a good soldering station is indispensable.

A simple but quality soldering station consists of a power supply, a handle with replaceable soldering tip, a holder, and a sponge/wiping reservoir (Figure 10.20). Tip temperature is not adjustable, but is set for the most common types of solder.

More sophisticated stations include adjustable temperature, a wider variety of tips, a solder suction/blower module, and perhaps a smoke removal system (Figure 10.21).

Solder comes in a variety of types and diameters. Most solder for electronic circuit repair has a rosin core that helps reduce oxidation on the parts to be soldered so that a better joint is produced.

Common solder is a lead–tin alloy, but some materials do not bond well with this type of solder. Specialty solders are available for particular applications, one of the more common being silver solder. Silver solder is still mostly lead and tin, but a portion of silver is added to modify its characteristics. Silver solder has a higher melting point than lead–tin solders.

Removing components from a circuit board involves melting the solder that was used to install it originally, and then getting rid of the excess. This can be done with a vacuum system that forms part of the soldering station, or it can be done using a mechanical "solder sucker" (Figure 10.22).

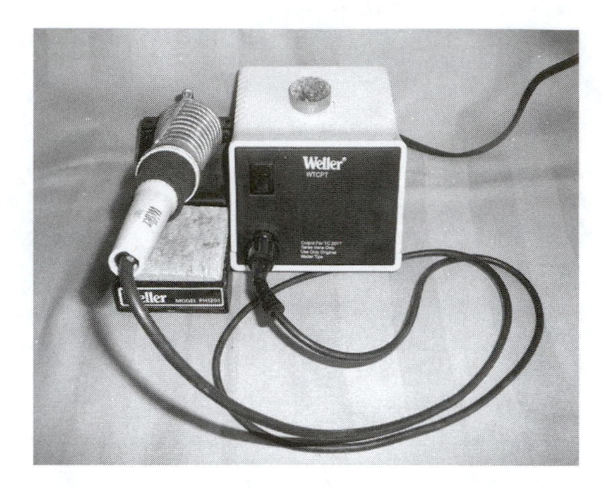

FIGURE 10.20 Basic soldering station.

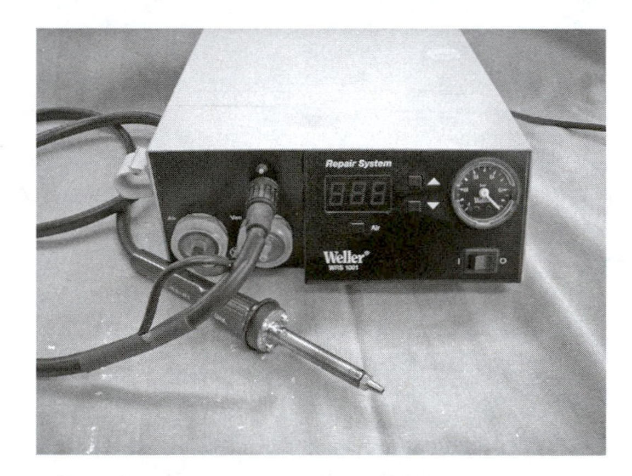

FIGURE 10.21 High-end soldering station.

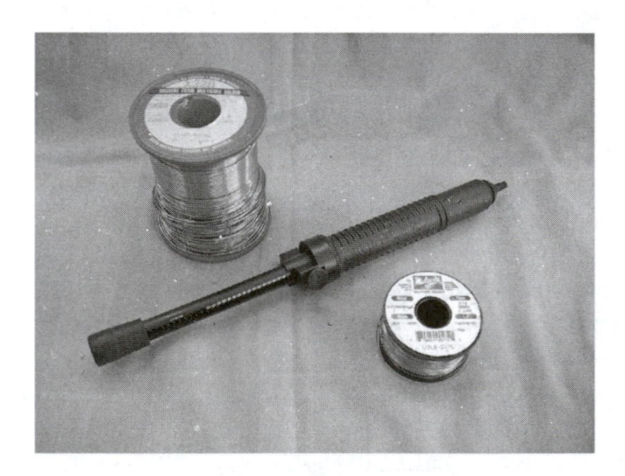

FIGURE 10.22 Different types of solder plus a solder sucker.

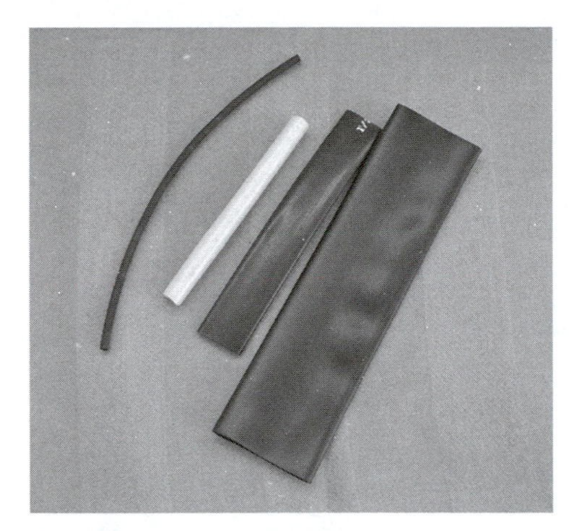

FIGURE 10.23 Heat-shrink tubing.

The process of soldering can produce considerable quantities of acrid smoke; prolonged exposure to such material is not recommended, so high-use soldering systems need to have s smoke removal mechanism. This is just a vacuum device that pulls air and smoke from around the soldering tip and filters out the smoke particles.

VI. OTHER

Many other materials are used in biomedical equipment support activities. Some of these include:

- Adhesives, such as silicone rubber glues and sealers, cyanoacrylate cements, epoxy cements, and thread-locking compounds. Plexiglas can be almost impossible to repair with other adhesives, but a few drops of methylene dichloride wicked into a joint will produce a strong bond.
- Lubricants include silicone greases, powdered graphite, specialty oils, and anti-seize compounds.
- Solvents for cleaning equipment include various alcohols, special adhesive tape and label removers, and special formulations to remove the glaze and dirt from rubber surfaces.
- Contact cleaners, which can remove dirt and oxidation from edge or pin connectors.
- Heat-shrink tubing (Figure 10.23), a special plastic tube material that reduces by one half or more in diameter but very little in length when heated; very useful for making tidy, long-lasting coverings for wires and other conductors.

VII. CHAPTER SUMMARY

This chapter is completely concerned with tools, from general and special testing units to hand and power tools.

11 Batteries, Radiation, and Computers

I. BATTERIES

Many medical devices incorporate batteries, either as their sole means of operation, as a power backup or bridge for times when line power is unavailable, or for data retention or clock functions.

Batteries can range from tiny button cells in clock circuits to banks of lead acid batteries weighing hundreds of kilograms used to power mobile C-arm x-ray machines.

Generally, batteries can be divided into rechargeable and nonrechargeable types, with a number of subtypes of each.

Batteries function by having two chemicals bathed in an electrolyte, with chemical reactions between the components producing an electrical potential. When a circuit is completed, current flows from one terminal of the battery, through the circuit components, and back into the other terminal. Chemical reactions within the cell replenish the electron supply, and current continues to flow. When the chemical reactions have used up all the available reactants, current flow stops. In rechargeable batteries, by applying a reverse voltage to the terminals, the chemical reaction can be forced to operate in reverse until the reactants are back to their original (charged) states.

This chapter will provide an overview of the chemistry and performance characteristics of some of the more common battery types, as well as some information about their applications in medical equipment.

Relevant performance characteristics include:

- Voltage per cell.
- Cell chemistry.
- Energy density, which is the amount of electrical energy contained in the battery per unit weight.
- Internal resistance, which determines how much current the battery can supply.
- Shelf life, how long a charge is maintained while the battery is disconnected.
- Voltage discharge curve, generally either flat or sloped, with a rapid or gradual drop-off at the end. This can be important since some devices require supply (battery) voltage to stay above a certain high level, while

others can continue to operate even when battery voltages drop to 75% of the fully charged level or even less.

A. Nonrechargeable Batteries

1. Alkaline

Volts/cell: 1.5 V
Chemistry
anode: zinc powder
cathode: manganese dioxide powder
electrolyte: potassium hydroxide
Energy density: high
Internal resistance: low
Shelf life: excellent
Discharge curve: sloped, rapid drop
Applications — photo flash, analog radios, flashlights, pulse oximeters, tympanic and probe thermometers

2. Mercury

Volts/cell: 1.35 V
Chemistry
anode: zinc
cathode: mercuric oxide
electrolyte: potassium hydroxide
Energy density: high
Internal resistance: high
Shelf life: excellent
Discharge curve: very flat, sharp drop
Applications — hearing aids, other small electronics; no longer commonly used because of the mercury content

3. Zinc/Air

Volts/cell: 1.65 V
Chemistry
anode: zinc powder
cathode: oxygen
electrolyte: potassium hydroxide
Energy density: high
Internal resistance: high
Shelf life: excellent if sealed, poor if opened
Discharge curve: very flat, sharp drop
Applications — hearing aids, telemetry transmitters

B. Rechargeable Batteries

1. Lithium or LiIon

Volts/cell: up to 4 V depending on design
Chemistry
anode: lithium
cathode: varies
electrolyte: organic liquids
Energy density: very high
Internal resistance: low
Shelf life: good
Discharge curve: sloped, gradual drop
# of charge cycles: very high
Applications — portable digital electronics such as cell phones, digital cameras, laptops, automatic external defibrillators, Mars Rovers

2. Nickel Metal Hydride or NiMH

Volts/cell: 1.35 V
Chemistry
anode: rare earth or nickel alloys
cathode: nickel oxyhydroxide
electrolyte: potassium hydroxide
Energy density: high
Internal resistance: low
Shelf life: good
Discharge curve: flat, gradual drop
# of charge cycles: high; very to extremely high if treated carefully
Applications — cell phones, digital cameras, camcorders, power tools, emergency backup lighting, laptops, Toyota Prius, satellites

3. Nickel Cadmium or NiCad, NiCd

Volts/cell: 1.3 V
Chemistry
anode: nickel
cathode: nickel oxyhydroxide
electrolyte: potassium hydroxide
Energy density: medium
Internal resistance: low
Shelf life: good
Discharge curve: flat, gradual drop
# of charge cycles: very high if treated carefully, otherwise medium to low
Applications — calculators, digital cameras, solar powered modules, laptops, defibrillators, electric vehicles (See Figure 11.1 for examples.)

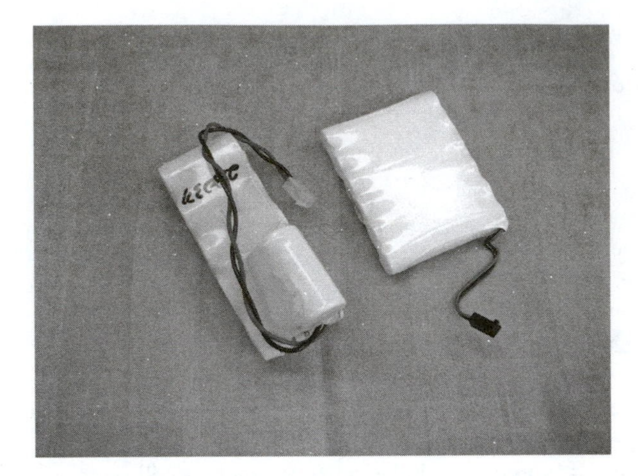

FIGURE 11.1 A few NiCd batteries.

4. Lead Acid

Volts/cell: 2.0 V
Chemistry
  anode: lead
  cathode: lead dioxide
  electrolyte: sulfuric acid
Energy density: medium
Internal resistance: low
Shelf life: poor
Discharge curve: gradual slope, slow drop
# of charge cycles: high
Applications — automotive batteries, solar and wind power storage, defibrillators, automatic external defibrillators (AEDs), IV pumps, portable monitors, transport incubators

Lead acid batteries (see Figure 11.2 for examples) may use a gelled electrolyte to allow operation in various orientations. This type is sometimes referred to as sealed lead acid, or SLA.

C. Battery Analyzers

The useful life of rechargeable batteries, especially nickel cadmium, nickel metal hydride, and lead acid types, can vary greatly depending on how they are handled. It is very difficult to get most end users to exercise battery packs regularly or to avoid deep discharges or overcharging.

Most medical charging circuits will not allow overcharging, and some manufacturers include battery conditioning circuits or charger systems with their equipment or even built into battery packs.

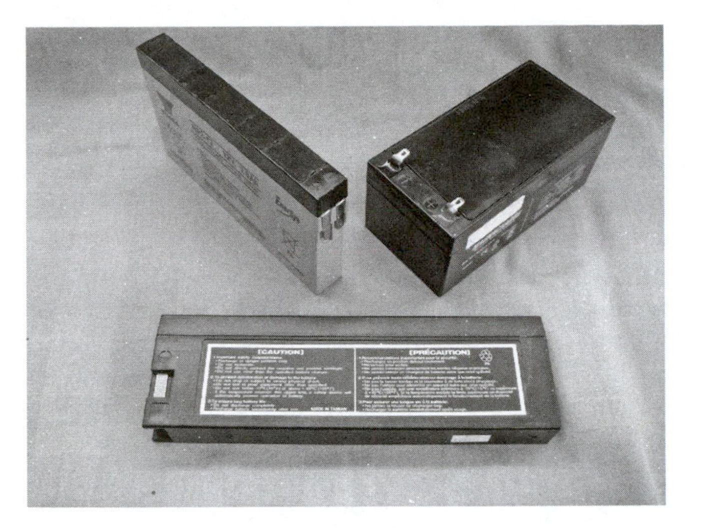

FIGURE 11.2 Some lead acid batteries.

Many other batteries, however, do not get treated in an ideal manner and often lose some of their original performance.

Battery analyzers (Figure 11.3) can help to overcome this problem by allowing biomed departments to take batteries from devices on a regular schedule and run them through a conditioning cycle. Analyzers can sense nonspec voltages, internal resistance, and nonstandard charge/discharge curves and apply a conditioning cycle tailored to their analysis. This can often restore much of the original capacity of the battery.

Analyzers can also perform a different conditioning and charging cycle on new batteries.

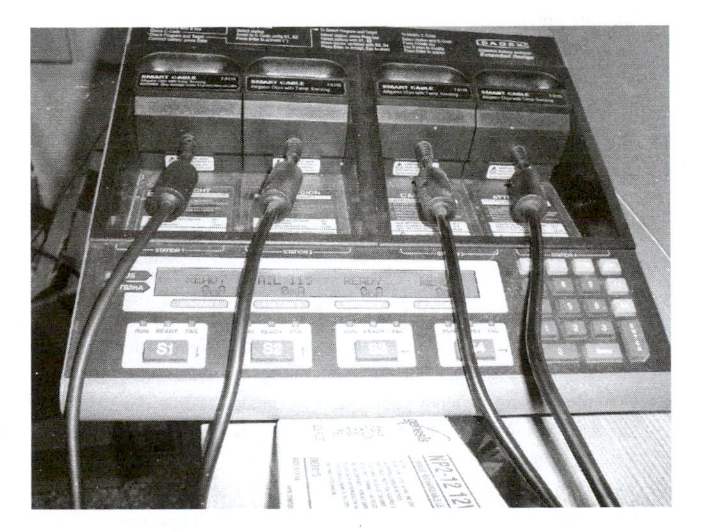

FIGURE 11.3 Battery analyzer.

Battery parameters (type, voltage, and specified amp-hour capacity) are entered into the analyzer, and a specific program or "auto" is selected. The analyzer performs its tests and routines; when finished, it reports on the battery condition and measured values. Data can be exported to a computer for collection and evaluation, and battery labels with the measured data printed out.

D. Battery Disposal

Mercury batteries are no longer used due to their use of toxic mercury, but most other batteries still contain chemicals that should not be released into the environment. Facilities are available to take used batteries and either recycle them or dispose of them safely. Some companies may even pay for used batteries.

Batteries — of all types — should never be placed in the regular garbage!

II. ELECTROMAGNETIC RADIATION

Certain physical actions, such as heating, can result in a photon being emitted from a substance. Photons are elementary particles that are the basis of all electromagnetic phenomena, including light, radio waves, x-rays, and gamma rays. Photons have no mass, and they travel at "the speed of light," 300,000 km/sec in a vacuum.

One of the major characteristics of photons is their wavelength (or inversely, their frequency), as seen in the following list:

Radiation Type	Wavelength
Gamma rays	1–10 pm
Hard X-rays	10–100 pm
Soft X-Rays	100 pm–1 nm
Extreme ultraviolet	1–10 nm
Near ultraviolet	10 nm–380 nm
Visible light:	
Violet	380–430 nm
Blue	430–500 nm
Cyan	500–520 nm
Green	520–565 nm
Yellow	565–590 nm
Orange	590–625 nm
Red	625–740 nm
Near infrared	740 nm–5 μm
Moderate infrared	5–12 μm
Far infrared	12–1 mm
Extremely high frequency radio (microwaves)	1 mm–1 cm
Super high frequency (microwaves)	1–10 cm
Ultrahigh frequency	10 cm–1 m
Very high frequency	1–10 m
High frequency	10–100 m
Medium frequency	100 m–1 km

Radiation Type	Wavelength
Low frequency	1–10 km
Very low frequency	10–100 km
Voice frequency	100–1000 km
Extremely low frequency	1000–10000 km

Note: pm = picometers, 10^{-12} m; nm = nanometers, 10^{-9} m; μm = micrometers, 10^{-6} m.

III. DIGITAL ELECTRONICS

Almost all current medical electronic devices involve digital circuitry, and so a brief discussion of digital is in order. This is a very complex field, and many resources are available to provide further information — see Appendix G.

A. Introduction

Natural signals are almost all analog; that is, if they are quantified, their measured values can be in any increment between the positive and negative extremes. A graph of signal vs. time would be a smooth curve at any magnification level.

Early electronic circuits dealt with signals in their analog forms, amplifying, filtering, or otherwise manipulating them but always with an infinite number of gradations between high and low.

As technology advanced, it became apparent that some manipulations of electrical signals would be very difficult if only analog signals were used. Counting or assigning whole-number values to a measurement required that discrete levels be considered, and values between those discrete levels had to be changed either up or down to fit the numbers.

If the number of steps is too few, important information about the signal can be lost. For any signal, however, there will be a point at which dividing a signal into many small, discrete levels will provide enough information about the signal for whatever purpose it is being analyzed.

Conversely, if the number of steps is too great, there is a "waste" of information: the gradations between steps are smaller than is significant in analysis.

B. Digital Signals

Dividing analog signals into a number of discrete values is the basis of digital electronics.

The term "digital" comes from "digit" or finger, meaning that values are represented as if you were using your fingers — in other words, whole numbers.

In practice, almost all "digital" electronics use as a base only two whole numbers, zero and one. This two-state model lends itself to electronics in that circuit components can be turned on (representing a one) or off (representing a zero. No intermediate values are needed, just on or off. In this way, perhaps devices should be called binary instead of digital, but the digital term is entrenched.

C. Binary Numbers

Individual binary values are referred to as bits (BInary digits), and larger decimal numbers can be represented by binary bits using the base two counting system. This places a value on the position of a bit in a larger number, just as in base ten.

A number in base ten may be made up of several digits, each of which carries more or less weight depending on its position in the number. For example, in the base ten number 3692, the digit 3 carries a weight of 1000, the 6 has a weight of 100, the 9 a weight of 10, and the 2 a weight of 1. This is shown in the way we would say such numbers: three thousand six hundred and ninety two. In this example, the three is the most significant digit, since it carries the most weight, while the two is the least significant digit.

Base two numbers work the same way, except that only two digits (or bits) are involved, 0 and 1, and the position weight of each bit is a multiple of two. For example, in the binary number 11010011, the right-most 1 carries a weight of one, while the next 1 carries a weight of two, and so on until the left-most 1 carries a weight of 128 (two to the power of 7; the right-most bit is two to the power of zero). The decimal equivalent of 11010011 would be:

$$1 \times 128 + 1 \times 64 + 0 \times 32 + 1 \times 16 + 0 \times 8 + 0 \times 4 + 1 \times 2 + 1 \times 1 = 211$$

By representing analog values as binary numbers, a great deal of manipulation becomes possible, as well as perfect data transmission, storage, and reproduction.

D. Analog to Digital Conversion

Converting analog signals to digital (binary) numbers requires that the end user decide how accurate the digital representation needs to be. This involves two factors: frequency and amplitude.

With any analog signal, there are frequency and amplitude components. Frequency is a measure of how rapidly the signal changes with time, and amplitude measures the size of changes.

To accurately represent frequency, an analog signal must be sampled often enough that important features of the signal are not missed. This feature is called sample rate.

At a certain point, small changes in amplitude become insignificant in a given application. As long as a single binary bit value can represent the smallest significant change in amplitude, the signal can be represented with sufficient accuracy. Once this determination is made, it can be calculated how many bits are required to represent the largest analog value. For example, if the smallest significant component of a signal was 1 millivolt and the largest signal amplitude was 75 millivolts, 75 separate binary values must be available. A seven-bit number can have 128 possible values, from 0, represented by 0000000, to 127, represented by 1111111. So seven bits would be more than adequate to accurately represent the analog signal. This feature is referred to as the resolution of the system.

In practice, binary numbers are almost always grouped in powers of two — 4, 8, 16, 32, 64, 128, etc., with groups of eight being a practical group — 8 bits equaling one byte.

Once the necessary sample rate and resolution are determined, the samples can be converted into digital values that are an adequate representation of the original signal.

In practice, sample rates and resolution values are usually chosen to be larger than the minimum that has been determined.

Analog signals are converted into digital data streams by devices called analog to digital converters (A/D). There are a number of different techniques for performing the conversion, and details of circuits are not particularly relevant. Most A/D converters used in medical equipment are off-the-shelf packages.

E. Microprocessors

Integrated circuits were developed to manipulate digital information, and while some system designs use only relatively simple digital integrated circuits (ICs), more and more use a special, complex type of IC called a microprocessor. These devices can take sets of digital information (data) and manipulate it in flexible ways controlled by a program, a series of commands that perform operations on the data.

Microprocessor systems consist of four basic parts: input, storage, processor, and output. Of course, this encompasses a huge range, from tiny, cheap calculators in which almost everything is condensed into a single IC chip, to room-filling super-priced supercomputers. In a way, the whole of the Internet could be considered a planetary microprocessor system.

F. Computers and Networks

General-purpose computers based on microprocessors are used for a variety of purposes in the biomedical engineering technology field (Figure 11.4). Equipment management, work order processing, calibration and troubleshooting, parts ordering,

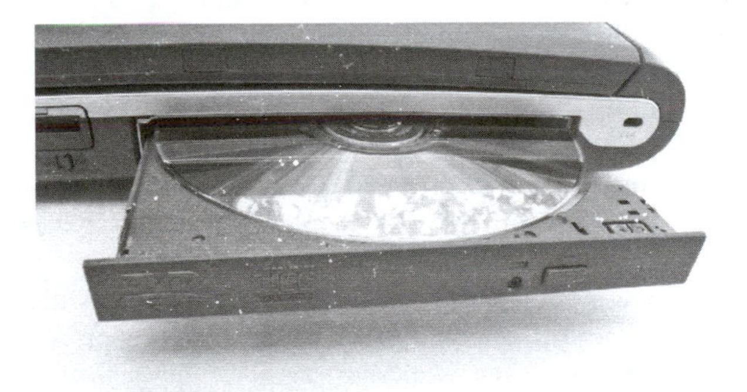

FIGURE 11.4 Laptop computer with CD. (Modified from Inmagine Corp, www.123rf.com, with permission.)

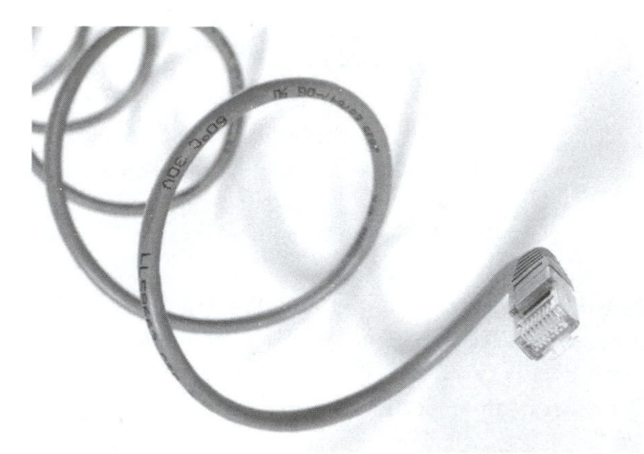

FIGURE 11.5 CAT-5 LAN cable. (Modified from Inmagine Corp, www.123rf.com, with permission.)

research, report writing, and communication using e-mail are routine functions that computers can be used for to help staff members be more effective in their roles.

Whether desktop, laptop, or palmtop, computers in hospitals are usually connected to an internal data network, which may be referred to as a local area network (LAN) or intranet (see Figure 11.5). This can allow communications with other hospital personnel, connection to various databases, including patient care systems, and connection to the Internet.

More and more medical devices are using microprocessor systems much like general-purpose computers as the basis of their design. Packaging is modified to suit the application, and input and output devices are often special-purpose designs, but the "guts" of the system are often standard components. Some manufacturers go a step further by using a quality off-the-shelf computer tower running a commercial operating system and adding their own software and proprietary input and output components to interface with their applications. This makes system design much easier and less expensive than designing everything from the ground up (often reinventing the wheel) and cuts development time and costs. Many systems use standard keyboards and mice, as well as commonly available (though usually high-end) display monitors and printers.

Instead of designing and building a unique data communication system, again equipment manufacturers use standard serial ports and networking systems for data communications. This makes it relatively simple for medical devices to connect to both in-hospital intranets and to the Internet (Figure 11.6).

Data sharing, whether in-house or open to the world, allows distant specialists to examine patient records, including ECG patterns, lab reports, x-ray and MRI images, medication regimes, and vital sign records. They can then contact local medical personnel to consult regarding diagnoses and courses of treatment; this contact is more and more likely to be via computers and networks.

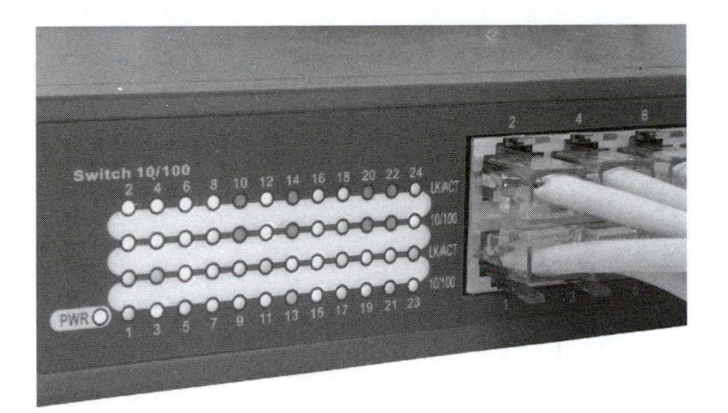

FIGURE 11.6 Network switch. (Modified from Inmagine Corp, www.123rf.com, with permission.)

Students can see real patient information and case histories, and different institutions can share epidemiological data, while researchers may have access to vast amounts of data for their studies.

Such connections must be used carefully, as medical systems often contain private patient medical and identity data. Robust security, regularly maintained, is vital. The responsibility for this security as well as other aspects of computer support may fall to biomed, or it may be taken over by the information management group, or there may be a division of labor.

IV. CHAPTER SUMMARY

Chapter 11 covers batteries, electromagnetic radiation, digital systems, and computers.

12 Technology Management

I. GENERAL CONSIDERATIONS

Even a small hospital will have a considerable number and variety of patient care technology devices, and for them to be supported fully and effectively, a management system must be in place.

Technology management includes everything about medical equipment: planning, evaluation, acquisition, incoming testing, installation and commissioning, staff education, performance assurance testing, repairs, ongoing evaluation, life-cycle cost analysis, utilization, vendor management, and decommissioning and retirement.

Effective management can provide benefits including obtaining the best value for money spent on equipment, maximizing uptime and minimizing risk, and optimal utilization of resources.

II. PLANNING

Equipment planning involves having a clear understanding of the needs of the patients who are being served by the hospital as well as the needs of medical staff. Budget considerations are critical, as is a broad knowledge of both the theory of medical equipment function and its application. Awareness of the range of equipment available plus the strengths and weaknesses of various manufacturers, vendors, and suppliers can help in making the best decisions regarding technology.

Education, awareness, and communication are vital.

III. SOFTWARE

Some aspects of equipment management can be made much easier with specialized software packages. Systems can be used to catalog equipment, track repair and maintenance costs, schedule PA testing, manage hazard and recall information, and track employee performance.

Some systems will interface with test equipment to generate work orders, identify equipment, control test procedures, and document and organize test results.

Appendix A: Normal Values

In the course of working with various devices in medicine, you will come across measurements of different values and parameters. This table is included to give perspective on some of the more common medical measurements. "Normal values" is the range of values found in healthy, normal individuals.

Hematology — Red Blood Cells (erythrocytes)	
RBC (Male)	4.2–5.6 M/µl (million cells/µl)
RBC (Female)	3.8–5.1 M/µl
RBC (Child)	3.5–5.0 M/µl
Hematology — White Blood Cells (leukocytes)	
WBC (Male)	3.8–11.0 K/mm^3 (thousand cells/mm^3)
WBC (Female)	3.8–11.0 K/mm^3
WBC (Child)	5.0–10.0 K/mm^3
Hemoglobin	
Hgb (Male)	14–18 g/dl
Hgb (Female)	11–16 g/dl
Hgb (Child)	10–14 g/dl
Hgb (Newborn)	15–25 g/dl
Hematocrit	
Hct (Male)	39–54%
Hct (Female)	34–47%
Hct (Child)	30–42%
General Chemistry	
Bilirubin, total	0.2–1.4 mg/dl
BUN	6–23 mg/dl
Calcium (total)	8–11 mg/dl
Carbon dioxide	21–34 meq/l (milliequivalents/l)
Carbon monoxide	symptoms at ≥ 10% saturation
Chloride	96–112 meq/l
Ethanol	0 mg%; Coma at ≥ 400–500 mg%
Glucose	65–99 mg/dl
HDL (Male)	25–65 mg/dl
HDL (Female)	38–94 mg/dl
Potassium	3.5–5.5 meq/l
Sodium	135–148 meq/l
Urea nitrogen	8–25 mg/dl
Lipid Panel (Adult)	
Cholesterol (total)	< 200 mg/dl desirable

Cholesterol (HDL)	30–75 mg/dl
Cholesterol (LDL)	< 130 mg/dl desirable
Triglycerides (M)	> 40–170 mg/dl
Triglycerides (F)	> 35–135 mg/dl

Urine

Specific gravity	1.003–1.040
pH	4.6–8.0
Na	10–40 meq/l
K	< 8 meq/l
Cl	< 8 meq/l
Osmolality	80–1300 mOsm/l
Glucose	≥ 180 mg/dl)

Cerebrospinal Fluid

Osmolality	290–298 mOsm/l
Pressure	70–180 mm H_2O

Hemodynamic Parameters

Cardiac index	2.5–4.2 l/min/m^2
Cardiac output	4–8 l/min
Stroke volume	60–100 ml/beat
Systolic arterial pressure	90–140 mm Hg
Diastolic arterial pressure	60–90 mm Hg
Central venous pressure	2–6 mm Hg
Ejection fraction	60–75%
Left atrial pressure	4–12 mm Hg
Right atrial pressure	4–6 mm Hg
Pulmonary artery (PA) systolic pressure	15–30 mm Hg
PA diastolic pressure	5–15 mm Hg
PA mean pressure	10–20 mm Hg
PA wedge pressure	4–12 mm Hg
PA end diastolic pressure	8–10 mm Hg
Right ventricular end diastolic pressure	0–8 mm Hg

Neurological Values

Intracranial pressure	5–15 mm Hg

Arterial Values

pH	7.35–7.45
$PaCO_2$	35–45 mm Hg
HCO_3	22–26 meq/l
O_2 saturation	96–100%
PaO_2	85–100 mm Hg

Venous Values

pH	7.31–7.41
$PaCO_2$	41–51 mm Hg
HCO_3	22–29 meq/l
O_2 saturation	60–85%
PaO_2	30–40 mm Hg

GLOSSARY FOR NORMAL VALUES

Bilirubin A by-product of the breakdown of red blood cells, it is normally destroyed by the liver. High levels can indicate liver problems. High concentrations of bilirubin in the body can cause the skin to turn yellow (jaundice).

BUN Blood urea nitrogen.

Cardiac index The amount of blood pumped by the heart per unit of time divided by body surface area, usually expressed in $l/min/m^2$.

Cardiac output A measurement of blood flow through the heart, expressed in l/min.

Central venous pressure The blood pressure in the right atrium or veins near the heart, mainly the vena cava.

Cerebrospinal fluid A clear, colourless fluid containing small amounts of glucose and protein. Cerebrospinal fluid fills the ventricles of the brain, spaces between the brain and the cerebral membranes, and the central canal of the spinal cord. It acts as a shock absorber as well as carrying some nutrients and materials involved in immune response.

Cholesterol A fatlike steroid alcohol found in animal fats and oils, in bile, blood, brain tissue, milk, yolk of egg, myelin sheaths of nerve fibers, the liver, kidneys, and adrenal glands. It is the main component of most gallstones and is involved in atherosclerosis (hardening of the arteries).

Diastolic arterial pressure The peak pressure reached in arteries close to the heart (such as the ascending and descending aorta), corresponding to the maximal contraction of the ventricles.

Ejection fraction A measure of the ability of the ventricles to contract.

HCO_3 Bicarbonate. A chemical produced in red blood cells, liberated through exchange with chloride. It may then be excreted by the kidneys.

HDL High density lipoprotein ("good cholesterol").

Hemoglobin (Hgb) A molecule involved in carrying oxygen in the blood; an iron atom forms part of the molecule.

Hematocrit (Hct) The relative volume of blood occupied by red blood cells.

Intracranial pressure The pressure exerted by cerebrospinal fluid within the skull.

O_2 saturation A measure of the amount of oxygen carried by the blood compared to the maximum theoretically possible, expressed as a percentage.

Osmolality The concentration of osmotically active particles in solution expressed in terms of osmoles of solute per kilogram of solvent.

$PaCO_2$ Partial pressure of carbon dioxide in the blood.

PaO_2 Partial pressure of oxygen in the blood.

pH A logarithmic measure of the activity of hydrogen ions in a solution, which also indicated relative acidity/alkalinity. pH 7 is neutral; pH 0 is extremely acidic; pH 14 is extremely alkaline.

Pulmonary artery wedge pressure The pressure measured in the pulmonary artery when blood flow in the artery is occluded, usually by a small balloon on the tip of a catheter. This catheter also contains a pressure transducer.

Specific gravity The density of a liquid compared to water, pure water having a specific gravity of 1.

Stroke volume The amount of blood pumped out of one ventricle of the heart as the result of a single contraction.

Triglycerides Glycerides in which the glycerol has three fatty acid molecules attached. They are the main constituent of vegetable oil and animal fats.

Appendix B: Regulations and Standards

A clear knowledge of regulations and standards regarding medical technology is vital to be able to provide full support to the equipment. Most regulations and standards pertain to patient and staff safety or to performance or manufacturing requirements.

These guidelines may be local (municipal, state, or provincial), or they may be national or international.

Local standards are too variable to cover here, but generally, local governments look to national and international bodies for guidance concerning such topics as medical technology.

National regulatory bodies include the Food and Drug Administration in the United States and Health Canada in Canada. Testing and standards agencies such as Underwriters Laboratories or the Canadian Standards Association carry no legal weight themselves, though their guidelines often form the basis of legal requirements.

Internationally, the Association for the Advancement of Medical Instrumentation (AAMI), the American National Standards Institute (ANSI), the Institute of Electrical and Electronics Engineers (IEEE), and the International Organization for Standardization (ISO) provide information and guidance on many technical matters.

CONTACT INFORMATION

AAMI

Association for the Advancement of Medical Instrumentation
http://www.aami.org/index.htm
Association for the Advancement of Medical Instrumentation
1110 North Glebe Road, Suite 220
Arlington, VA 22201-4795
From their Web site:

> The Association for the Advancement of Medical Instrumentation (AAMI), founded in 1967, is a unique alliance of over 6,000 members united by the common goal of increasing the understanding and beneficial use of medical instrumentation.
>
> AAMI is the primary source of consensus and timely information on medical instrumentation and technology.

AAMI is the primary resource for the industry, the professions, and government for national and international standards.

ANSI

American National Standards Institute
http://web.ansi.org/
American National Standards Institute
1819 L Street, NW
(between 18th and 19th Streets), 6th floor
Washington, DC 20036
Telephone: 202-293-8020
Fax: 202-293-9287
From their Web site:

ANSI facilitates the development of American National Standards (ANS) by accrediting the procedures of standards developing organizations (SDOs). These groups work cooperatively to develop voluntary national consensus standards. Accreditation by ANSI signifies that the procedures used by the standards body in connection with the development of American National Standards meet the Institute's essential requirements for openness, balance, consensus, and due process.

FDA — US

U.S. Food and Drug Administration
5600 Fishers Lane
Rockville MD 20857-0001
888-INFO-FDA (888-463-6332)
http://www.fda.gov/default.htm
From their Web site:

We are a team of 9,000 dedicated public health employees that includes physicians, nurses, consumer safety officers, lawyers, and scientists, with specialties ranging from biomaterials engineering to pharmacology. Decisions made by the FDA affect every American every day. In 2000, consumers spent $1 trillion—more than 20 percent of their income—on hundreds of thousands of products whose safety and effectiveness is our responsibility. Yet, the per capita cost of all FDA services is less than 2 cents a day!

The public trusts the FDA to ensure that:

1. Foods are safe, wholesome, and truthfully labeled.
2. Drugs for both humans and animals, and vaccines for humans are safe and effective.
3. Blood used for transfusions is safe and in adequate supply.
4. Medical devices, from scalpels to CT scanners, are safe and effective.
5. Transplanted tissues are safe and effective.

6. Equipment that uses radiant energy, such as X-ray machines and microwave ovens, is safe.
7. Cosmetics are safe and properly labeled.

Health Canada

Health Canada — Drugs and Health Products
http://www.hc-sc.gc.ca/dhp-mps/legislation/index_e.html
Health Canada
Address Locator 0900C2
Ottawa, Ontario
Canada
K1A 0K9
Telephone: 613-957-2991
Toll free: 866-225-0709
From their Web site:

> Health Canada develops and enforces regulations under Government of Canada legislation. The Department consults with the Canadian public, industry, and other interested parties in the development of laws that protect health and safety. We also prepare guidelines and policies in order to help interpret and clarify the legislation surrounding drugs and health products.

and

> The term Medical Devices, as defined in the Food and Drugs Act, covers a wide range of health or medical instruments used in the treatment, mitigation, diagnosis, or prevention of a disease or abnormal physical condition.
>
> Health Canada's Role: Health Canada reviews medical devices to assess their safety, effectiveness, and quality before being authorized for sale in Canada.

IEEE

Institute of Electrical and Electronics Engineers
http://www.ieee.org/portal/site
IEEE Operations Center
445 Hoes Lane
Piscataway, NJ
08854-4141
Phone: 732-981-0060
Fax: 732-981-1721
From their Web site:

The IEEE is a leading developer of standards that underpin many of today's technologies. Our standards are developed in a unique environment that builds consensus in an open process based on input from all interested parties. With nearly 1,300 standards either completed or under development, we are a central source of standardization in both traditional and emerging fields, particularly telecommunications, information technology, and power generation.

ISO

International Organization for Standardization — ISO
http://www.iso.org/iso/en/ISOOnline.frontpage
ISO Central Secretariat:
International Organization for Standardization (ISO)
1, ch. de la Voie-Creuse, Case postale 56
CH-1211 Geneva 20, Switzerland
Telephone: +41 22 749 01 11; Fax: +41 22 733 34 30
From their Web site:

> When the large majority of products or services in a particular business or industry sector conform to International Standards, a state of industry-wide standardization can be said to exist. This is achieved through consensus agreements between national delegations representing all the economic stakeholders concerned — suppliers, users, government regulators and other interest groups, such as consumers. They agree on specifications and criteria to be applied consistently in the classification of materials, in the manufacture and supply of products, in testing and analysis, in terminology and in the provision of services. In this way, International Standards provide a reference framework, or a common technological language, between suppliers and their customers — which facilitates trade and the transfer of technology.

Some Other Organizations

Underwriters Laboratories Inc.
http://www.ul.com/
Global Harmonization Task Force
http://www.ghtf.org/
International Electrotechnical Commission
http://www.iec.ch/
Nationally Recognized Testing Laboratory (NRTL) Program
http://www.osha-slc.gov/dts/otpca/nrtl/index.html
Newsletter Devoted to Electrical Product Safety Compliance
http://www.safetylink.com/
Therapeutic Goods Administration (TGA) is a unit of the Australian Government Department of Health and Ageing
http://www.tga.gov.au/manuf/index.htm
BSI British Standards is the National Standards Body of the UK
http://www.bsi-global.com/en/

Appendix C: Biomedical Engineering Technology Programs in the US and Canada

These institutions offer training programs for student wishing to become Biomedical Engineering Technologists. Thanks to AAMI for permission to reprint.

PROGRAM LISTINGS BY AREA

TWO-YEAR BIOMEDICAL EDUCATION PROGRAMS

United States

Alabama

Community College of the Air Force
Maxwell Air Force Base
Montgomery, AL 36112-6613
www.au.af.mil/au/ccaf/

Jefferson State Community College
Manufacturing Technology Center
2601 Carson Road
Birmingham, AL 36235
205-856-8517
www.jscc.cc.al.us

Northwest–Shoals Community College
P.O. Box 2545
800 George Wallace Boulevard
Muscle Shoals, AL 35662
256-331-5200
www.nwscc.cc.al.us

Arkansas

North Arkansas College
1515 Pioneer Drive
Harrison, AR 72601
870-743-3000
http://pioneer.northark.cc.ar.us

California

Los Angeles Valley College
5800 Fulton Avenue
Valley Glen, CA 91401
818-947-2600
www.lavc.cc.ca.us

Colorado

Aims Community College
Greeley Campus
5401 West 20th Street
P.O. Box 69
Greeley, CO 80632
970-330-8008
www.aims.edu

Arapahoe Community College
5900 South Santa Fe Drive
Littleton, CO 80120
303-797-4ACC (4222)
www.arapahoe.edu

Connecticut

Gateway Community College
North Haven Campus
88 Bassett Road
North Haven, CT 06473
203-285-2000
www.gwctc.commnet.edu

Delaware

Delaware Tech–Terry Campus
1832 North Dupont Parkway
Dover, DE 19901
302-741-2700
www.dtcc.edu

Florida

Broward Community College
North Campus
1000 Coconut Creek Boulevard
Coconut Creek, FL 33066
954-973-2292/2324
www.broward.edu

Florida Community College
Downtown Campus
101 West State Street
Jacksonville, FL 32202
904-633-8100
www.fccj.org

Santa Fe Community College
W-002
3000 Northwest 83rd Street
Gainesville, FL 32606
352-395-5650
www.santafe.cc.fl.us

Georgia

Central Georgia Technical College
3300 Macon Tech Drive
Macon, GA 31206
478-757-3400
www.cgtcollege.org

Chattahoochee Technical College
980 South Cobb Drive
Marietta, GA 30060
770-528-4545
www.chattcollege.com

Idaho

Boise State University
1910 University Drive
Boise, ID 83725-2070
www.boisestate.edu

Illinois

Parkland College
2400 West Bradley
Champaign, IL 61821-1899
www.parkland.cc.il.us

Richland Community College
One College Park
Decatur IL, 62521
217-875-7200
www.richland.cc.il.us

South Suburban College
15800 South State Street
South Holland, IL 60473
708-596-2000
www.ssc.cc.il.us

Indiana

Indiana State University
Department of Electronics and Computer Technology
School of Technology
Indiana State University
Terre Haute, IN 47809
812-237-3452; Fax: 812-237-3397
http://web.indstate.edu

IUPUI
425 University Boulevard
Indianapolis, IN 46202-5143
317-274-4591
www.iupui.edu/

Iowa

Des Moines Area Community College
2006 South Ankeny Boulevard
Ankeny, IA 50021-3993
515-964-6200 or 800-362-2127
www.dmacc.cc.ia.us

Western Iowa Tech Community College
4647 Stone Avenue
Sioux City, IA 51106
712-274-6400
800-352-4649
www.witcc.cc.ia.us

Kentucky

Madisonville Community College
2000 College Drive
Madisonville, KY 42431-9241
270-821-2250
www.madcc.kctcs.net

Louisiana

Delgado Community College
615 City Park Avenue
New Orleans, LA
www.dcc.edu

Louisiana Technical College
Sullivan Campus
1710 Sullivan Drive
Bogalusa, LA 70427
Telephone: 985-732-6640, 6641, 6642, 6643
Fax: 985-732-6603
www.ltc.edu/sullivan/

Maine

Southern Maine Technical College
Fort Road
South Portland, ME 04106
207-767-9500
www.smccme.edu

Maryland

Anne Arundel Community College
101 College Parkway
Arenold, MD 21012-1895
410-647-7100
www.aacc.cc.md.us

Howard Community College
10901 Little Patuxent Parkway
Columbia, MD 21044
410-772-4800
www.howardcc.edu

Michigan

Lansing Community College
P.O. Box 40010
Lansing, MI 48901-7210
517-483-1957
www.lcc.edu

Schoolcraft College
18600 Haggerty Road
Livonia, MI 48152
734-462-4400
www.schoolcraft.cc.mi.us

Minnesota

Anoka-Ramsey Community College
Coon Rapids Campus
11200 Mississippi Boulevard
Coon Rapids, MN 55433
763-422-3333
www.anokaramsey.mnscu.edu/

Dakota County Technical College
1300 145th Street East (County Road 42)
Rosemount, MN 55068-2999
651-423-8301
Toll-Free: 877-YES-DCTC (877-937-3282)

Missouri

St. Louis Community College
Florissant Valley
Engineering and Technology
3400 Pershall Road
St. Louis, MO 63135
314-595-4308; Fax: 314-595-2218
www.stlcc.cc.mo.us/fv/

Montana

Montana State University–Great Falls
College of Technology
2100 16th Avenue South
P.O. Box 6010
Great Falls, MT 59406-6010
406-771-4300 or 800-446-2698
Fax: 406-771-4317
www.msugf.edu

New Hampshire

New Hampshire Community Technical College
NH Biotechnology Center
c/o NHCTC
320 Corporate Avenue
Portsmouth, NH 03801
Telephone: 603-334-6306
Fax: 603-334-6308
www.nh.gov/nhctc

New Jersey

County College of Morris
214 Center Grove Road
Randolph, NJ 07869
Toll Free: 888-226-8001
973-328-5000
www.ccm.edu/

Thomas Edison State College
101 West State Street
Trenton, NJ 08608-1176
www.tesc.edu

New Mexico

Dona Ana Branch Community College of New Mexico State University
3400 South Espina
Las Cruces, NM 88003
http://dabcc-www.nmsu.edu/dabcc.asp

New York

Farmingdale State University of New York
Route 110
Farmingdale, NY 11735-1021
631-420-2000
www.farmingdale.edu

North Carolina

Caldwell Community College and Technical Institute
2855 Hickory Boulevard
Hudson, NC 28638
828-726-2200; Fax: 828-726-2216
www.caldwell.cc.nc.us

Stanly Community College
141 College Drive
Albemarle, NC 28001
704-982-0121
www.stanly.cc.nc.us

Ohio

Diagnostic Imaging Technical Education Center, Inc. (DITEC)
6864 Cochran Road
Solon, OH 44139
440-519-1555
info@ditecnet.com
www.ditecnet.com

Cincinnati State Technical and Community College
3520 Central Parkway
Cincinnati, OH 45223
513-569-1500
www.cinstate.cc.oh.us

Owens Community College
Toledo Campus
P.O. Box 10,000
Toledo, OH 43699
www.owens.edu

Oklahoma

Tulsa Community College
909 South Boston Avenue
Tulsa, OK 74119

Pennsylvania

Community College of Philadelphia
1700 Spring Garden Street
Philadelphia, PA 19130
215-751-8010
www.ccp.edu/site

Johnson College
3427 North Main Avenue
Scranton, PA 18508-1495
570-342-6404; Fax: 570-348-2181
www.johnson.edu

Penn State New Kensington
3550 Seventh Street Road – Route 780
Upper Burrell, PA 15068-1798
724-334-6712
www.nk.psu.edu/

Rhode Island

Community College of Rhode Island
400 East Avenue
Warwick, RI 02886-1807
401-825-1000
www.cc.ri.us

South Carolina

Florence–Darlington Technical College
2715 West Lucas Street
Florence, SC 29501-0548
800-228-5745
www.fdtc.edu/

South Dakota

Southeast Technical Institute
2320 North Career Avenue
Sioux Falls, SD 57107
Local: 605-367-7624
Toll-Free: 800-247-0789
TTY: 605-367-6040
www.southeasttech.com

Texas

St. Philip's College
1801 Martin Luther King Drive
San Antonio, TX, 78203
210-531-3200
www.accd.edu/spc/spcmain/spc.htm

Texas State Technical College–Harlingen
1902 North Loop 499
Harlingen, TX 78550-3697
956-364-4111; Fax: 956-364-5105
www.harlingen.tstc.edu

Texas State Technical College–Waco
3801 Campus Drive
Waco, TX 76705
www.waco.tstc.edu

Virginia

ECPI College of Technology
Main Campus
5555 Greenwich Road
Virginia Beach, VA 23462
757-671-7171
www.ecpi.edu/

Northern Virginia Community College
Annandale Campus
8333 Little River Turnpike
Annandale, VA 22003-3796
703-323-3000

Washington

Bellingham Technical College
3028 Lindbergh Avenue
Bellingham, WA 98225
www.btc.ctc.edu

North Seattle Community College
9600 College Way North
Seattle, WA 98103
206-527-3639
www.northseattle.edu/

Spokane Community College
1810 North Greene Street
Spokane, WA 99217-5399
www.scc.spokane.edu/

Wisconsin

Milwaukee Area Technical College
700 West State Street
Milwaukee, WI 53233
414-297-6600
www.milwaukee.tec.wi.us

Western Wisconsin Technical College
304 6th Street North
La Crosse, WI 54601
608-785-9200
www.witechcolleges.org/western.htm

Wyoming

Western Wyoming Community College
2500 College Drive
Rock Springs, WY 82901
307-382-1600
www.wwcc.cc.wy.us

US Armed Forces

Army Program Director
DOD BMET Training Course
382 TRS/XYBB
925 Missile Road
Sheppard AFB, TX 76311
www.cs.amedd.army.mil/details.aspx?dt=152

DeVry University
www.devry.edu/

Seattle Metro
Federal Way Campus
3600 South 344th Way
Federal Way, WA 98001

San Francisco Metro
Fremont Campus
6600 Dumbarton Circle
Fremont, CA 94555

Los Angeles Metro
Pomona Campus
901 Corporate Center Drive
Pomona, CA 91768

Los Angeles Metro
West Hills Campus
22801 Roscoe Boulevard
West Hills, CA 91304

Phoenix Metro
Phoenix Campus
2149 West Dunlap Avenue
Phoenix, AZ 85021

Denver Metro
Westminster Campus
1870 West 122nd Avenue
Westminster, CO 80234

Houston Metro
Houston Campus
11125 Equity Drive
Houston, TX 77041

Dallas Metro
Irving Campus
4800 Regent Boulevard
Irving, TX 75063

Kansas City Metro
Kansas City Campus
11224 Holmes Road
Kansas City, MO 64131

Columbus Metro
Columbus Campus
1350 Alum Creek Drive
Columbus, OH 43209

New York Metro
Long Island City Campus
3020 Thomson Avenue
Long Island City, NY 11101

Philadelphia Metro
Fort Washington Campus
1140 Virginia Drive
Ft. Washington, PA 19034

North Brunswick
North Brunswick Campus
630 US Highway One
North Brunswick, NJ 08902

Atlanta Metro
Decatur Campus
250 North Arcadia Avenue
Decatur, GA 30030

Miami Metro
Miramar Campus
2300 Southwest 145th Avenue
Miramar, FL 33027

Orlando Metro
Orlando Campus
4000 Millenia Boulevard
Orlando, FL 32839

Canada

Alberta

The Northern Alberta Institute of Technology
11762 – 106 Street
Edmonton, Alberta
Canada T5G 2R1
780-471-7400
www.nait.ca/programs/bet/

British Columbia

British Columbia Institute of Technology
3700 Willingdon Avenue
Burnaby, British Columbia
Canada, V5G 3H2
604-434-5734
www.bcit.ca/health/biomed/

Ontario

Durham College
Biomedical Technology Program
Oshawa Campus
2000 Simcoe Street North
Oshawa, ON L1H 7K4
905-721-2000
Fax: 905-721-3113
www.durhamc.on.ca

Fanshawe College
Biomedical Electronics
Manufacturing Division
1460 Oxford Street East
P.O. Box 7005
London, ON N5Y 5R6
519-452-4430 x4105
Fax: 519-452-1292
www.fanshawec.on.ca

Appendix D: Biomed Associations

For these organizations, only the group name and Internet addresses are listed. A listing of officers has been omitted, as they may change often.

If no URL is available, an e-mail address or surface address is given.

UNITED STATES

US Armed Forces

http://www.bmets-usa.org/index.html

Arizona

Arizona Bioindustry Association
http://www.azbioindustry.org/

Arkansas

Arkansas Association for Healthcare Engineering
http://www.aaheark.net/

California

California Medical Instrumentation Association
http://cmia.org/

California – Orange County

Orange County BMET Society (California)
http://ocbmet.com/

Colorado

Colorado Association of Biomedical Technicians
http://www.cabmet.org/

Connecticut

New England Society of Clinical Engineering
http://www.nesce.org./nesce.htm

Florida

Florida Biomedical Society
http://www.florida-biomed-society.org/

Gulf Coast Biomedical Society
http://www.geocities.com/gcbssec/

Georgia

Georgia Biomedical Instrumentation Society
http://www.biomedgbis.com

Indiana

Indiana Biomedical Society
http://www.indianabiomedical.com/

Maryland

Baltimore Medical Engineers and Technicians Society
http://www.bmets.org/

Minnesota and Surrounding Areas

North Central Biomedical Association
http://www.ncbiomed.org/index.php

Missouri (St. Louis Area)

Gateway Biomedical Society
http://gatewaybiomedsociety.org/

Nebraska and Surrounding Areas

Heartland Biomedical Association
http://www.hba.4t.com/

North Carolina

North Carolina Biomedical Association
http://www.ncbiomedassoc.com/

Pennsylvania

Philadelphia Area Medical Instrumentation Association
http://www.pamia.org/

Tennessee

East Tennessee Biomedical Association
http://www.etbiomed.org/index.shtml

Middle Tennessee Biomedical Association
http://www.geocities.com/midtenbiomed/index.html

Texas

North Texas Biomedical Association
http://www.ntba.org/

Southeast Texas Clinical Engineering Society
http://www.setces.org/

Virginia

Virginia Biomedical Association
http://www.vabiomed.org/

Washington, DC

National Capital Healthcare Engineering Society
http://www.nches.org/

Washington State

Washington State Biomedical Association
http://www.bmet.org/index.html

Wisconsin

Biomedical Associations of Wisconsin
http://www.baw.org/

Biomedical Electronics Technicians Association of Wisconsin
http://betawi.homestead.com/home.html

CANADA

Alberta

The Alberta Clinical Engineering Society
http://www.aces.ab.ca/

British Columbia

The Institute of Biomedical Engineering Technology
http://ibet.asttbc.org/

Ontario

The Clinical Engineering Society of Ontario
http://www.ceso.on.ca/

Quebec

l'Association des physiciens et ingénieurs biomédicaux du Québec
http://www.apibq.org/

INTERNATIONAL

International Federation for Medical and Biological Engineering
http://www.ifmbe.org/

NATIONAL BIOMED ASSOCIATIONS

Argentina

Sociedad Argentina de Bioingeniera
http://www.ibi.herrera.unt.edu.ar/sabi

Australia

Australian Federation for Medical and Biological Engineering
http://www.smbe.asn.au/index.htm

Austria

Österreichische Gesellschaft fur Biomedizinische Technik
http://www.oegbmt.at

Belgium

Belgian Society for Medical and Biological Engineering and Computing
www.biomengineering.org/

Brazil

Sociedad Brasileira de Engenharia Biomédica
http://www.sbeb.org.br
http://www.peb.ufrj.br~sbeb

Bulgaria

Bulgarian National Society of Biomedical Physics and Engineering
http://www.usb-bg.org/Bg/BG_society_of_biomedical_.htm

Canada

Canadian Medical and Biological Engineering Society
http://www.cmbes.ca

China

Chinese Society for Biomedical Engineering
http://www.csbme.org/

China, Taipei

Biomedical Engineering Society, Taipei, China
http://www.bmes.org.tw

Colombia

Colombian Association of Bioengineering and Medical Electronics
ingelmed@bioingenieros.com

Croatia

Croatian Medical and Biological Engineering Society
www.crombes.hr

Cuba

Sociedad Cubane de Bioingenieria
www.socbio.sld.cu

Cyprus

Cyprus Association of Medical Physics and Biomedical Engineering
www.campbe.org

Czech Republic

Czech Society for Biomedical Engineering and Medical Informatics
www.sbmili.cz/

Denmark

Danish Society for Biomedical Engineering
http://www.dmts.dk

Estonia

Estonian Society for Biomedical Engineering and Medical Physics
http://www.physic.ut.ee/ebmy/

Finland

Finnish Society for Medical Physics and Biomedical Engineering
http://www.lfty.fi

France

Societe Francaise de Genie Biologique et Medical
http://sfgbm.enst-bretagne.fr

Societe des Electricien et des Electroniciens
http://www.univ-paris12.fr/

Germany

Deutsche Gesellschaft fur Biomedizinische Technik E.V.
http://www.dgbmt.de or
http://www.vde.com/VDE_EN/Technical+Societies/DGBMT.htm

Greece

Greek Society for Biomedical Engineering
nipa@bme.med.uptras.gr or nipa@inbit.gr

Hong Kong

Hong Kong Institution of Engineers
http://www.hkie.org.hk/

Hungary

Society of Measurement and Automation Section Biomedical Engineering
http://www.mate.mtesz.hu/

Iceland

Icelandic Society for Biomedical Engineering
http://www.nervus.is/htfi

Ireland

Biomedical Engineering Association of Ireland
http://www.beai.org

Israel

Israel Society for Medical and Biological Engineering
http://www.eng.tau.ac.il/research/ismbe

Italy

Associazione Italiana di Ingegnaria Medica e Biologica
http://www.aiimb.it

JAPAN

Japan Society of Medical and Biological Engineering
http://www.jsmbe.or.jp

KOREA

Korean Society of Medical and Biological Engineering
http://www.kosombe.or.kr

LATVIA

Latvian Medical Engineering and Physics Society
http://www.cc.tut.fi/nbd/latvia/latvia.htm

MEXICO

Sociedad Mexicana de Ingeniería Biomédica
http://www.somib.org.mx

THE NETHERLANDS

Vereniging Voor Biofysica en Biomedische Technologie
www.vvb-bmt.nl

NIGERIA

Nigerian Institute for Biomedical Engineering
http://www.nibe.kabissa.org

NORWAY

Norwegian Society for Biomedical Engineering
http://www.medisinsktekniskforening.no/

POLAND

Polish Society for Biomedical Engineering
http://ptib.ibib.waw.pl

Polish Scientific and Technical Committee for Biomedical Engineering of Sep
palkot@mech.pw.edu.pl

Portugal

Speb-Sociedade Portuguesa de Egenharia Biomedica
ana@det.ua.pt

Serbia and Montenegro (Yugoslavia)

The Society of Biomedical Engineering and Medical Physics
Serbia and Montenegro
http://www.bimef.org.yu

Singapore

Biomedical Engineering Society (Singapore)
http://www.bes.org.sg

Slovakia

Slovak Society of Biomedical Engineering Medical Informatics
umertysl@savba.sk

Slovenia

Slovene Society for Medical and Biological Engineering
http://lbk.fe.uni-lj.si

South Africa

Biomedical Engineering Society of South Africa
dbee@cormack.uct.ac.za

Spain

Spanish Society of Biomedical Engineering
http://www.gbt.tfo.upm.es

Sweden

Swedish Society for Medical Engineering and Medical Physics
http://www.mtf.nu

Switzerland

Swiss Society of Biomedical Engineering
http://www.memcenter.unibe.ch

Thailand

Association for Medical Instrumentation
Faculty of Medicine and Siriraj Hospital
Div. of Medical Electronics, Dept. of Physiology
No. 2 Prannok Road
Bangkok 10700
Thailand

Ukraine

Institute of Medical Engineering and Clinics
may@citynet.kharkov.ua or may@univer.kharkov.ua

United Kingdom

Institution of Physics and Engineering in Medicine
http://www.ipem.ac.uk

United States

American Institute for Medical and Biological Engineering
http://www.aimbe.org

IEEE Engineering in Medicine and Biology Society
http://www.embs.org

Europe

European Society for Engineering and Medicine
http://www.esem.org

International

International Council on Medical and Care Compunetics – ICMCC
http://www.icmcc.com

Appendix E: Devices and Manufacturers

Given the large numbers of manufacturers of medical devices, the wide range of devices and the ever-changing face of the industry due to mergers and acquisitions, divestments, bankruptcies and start-ups, it would be of questionable value to provide an extensive listing of devices and manufacturers, and a limited listing would be no more useful. Internet access and excellent search engines have made the task of locating companies almost trivial, and so a listing has not been included in this text.

Appendix F: Test Equipment Manufacturers

BC BIOMEDICAL

http://www.bcgroupintl.com/BC_Biomedical_main.htm

BC Group has established a full line of Biomedical Test Equipment under the name of "BC Biomedical."

FLUKE BIOMEDICAL

http://us.fluke.com/usen/apps/Biomedical/default.htm

We are the world's leading manufacturer of quality biomedical test and simulation products. From stand-alone electrical safety testers to fully integrated and automated performance testing and documentation systems, we have a biomedical solution for every type and level of customer.

METRON BIOMED

http://www.metron-biomed.com/
See Fluke Biomedical.

NETECH CORPORATION

http://www.gonetech.com/

Netech Corporation has been designing, manufacturing, and distributing Biomedical and Industrial test instruments for over 17 years. Our products have established a reputation for high quality, reliability, and value.

Innovative products, ISO 9001-2000 Registration, a 2-year warranty, and excellent customer service, and technical support demonstrate an unyielding commitment to the medical industry.

TSI INCORPORATED

http://www.tsi.com/Default.aspx

TSI Incorporated designs and manufactures precision instruments used to measure flow, particulate, and other key parameters in environments the world over. TSI serves the needs of industry, governments, research institutions, and universities, with applications ranging from pure research to primary manufacturing. Every TSI instrument is backed by unique technical expertise and outstanding quality.

CLINICAL DYNAMICS CORPORATION

http://www.clinicaldynamics.com/

Clinical Dynamics designs, manufactures, and markets NIBP & SpO2 Analyzers for Patient Monitoring Management. Our customers include patient monitoring manufacturers, hospital biomedical engineering departments, and independent service organizations.

DATREND SYSTEMS INC

http://www.datrend.com/

Datrend Systems Inc. is dedicated to providing quality Biomedical Test Instruments (BTI) for biomedical and clinical engineering professionals. Additionally, we provide Product Development Services (PDS) on a contract basis for both medical and non-medical devices.

DALE TECHNOLOGY

http://www.daletech.com/

Today, Dale Technology is located in Everett, WA. The Dale Technology product line has expanded considerably and includes test instruments designed to verify the performance and calibration of medical devices. These devices include defibrillators, external pacemakers, infusion pumps, electrosurgical generators, rigid endoscopes, and even radiology equipment.

Appendix G: Bibliography and Internet Resources

This section is basically a collection of Web links that proved to be useful in compiling the book, grouped by topic.

ANESTHESIOLOGY/RESPIRATORY

http://www.virtual-anaesthesia-textbook.com/vat/equipment.html
http://www.virtual-anaesthesia-textbook.com/index.shtml
http://www.general-anaesthesia.com/index.html
http://www.anesthesiology.org/
http://www.frca.co.uk/article.aspx?articleid=100389
http://www.vivometrics.com/site/pdfs/find.php?file=wpRIPImped

ANATOMY

http://www.adam.com/index.html

BIOMEDICAL ENGINEERING

http://www.mymeta.org/bmetorgs/orglist.html
http://www.florida-biomed-society.org/Link's/Link1.htm#S
http://www.biomedical-engineering-online.com/content/1/1/5
http://www.biomedical-engineering-online.com/home
http://q.webring.com/hub?ring=bmetring
http://www.cs.amedd.army.mil/bmet/
http://www.aami.org/resources/education/ed.text.html
http://www.aami.org/resources/links/biomed.html
http://www.ingbiomedica.unina.it/aiimb/bme.htm
http://www.ceasa-national.org.za/ce_links.htm

BLOOD

http://www.abbottpointofcare.com/istat/
http://www.bodybio.com/main/products/bloodchem.htm
http://www.nlm.nih.gov/medlineplus/ency/article/003468.htm

CARDIOLOGY

http://www.anaesthetist.com/icu/organs/heart/rhythm/Findex.htm#arhythm.htm
http://www.medtronic.com/physician/tachy/icd/virtuoso.html
http://www.madehow.com/Volume-3/Pacemaker.html
http://www.heartstream.com/main
http://www.orau.org/PTP/collection/Miscellaneous/pacemaker.htm
http://www.nlm.nih.gov/medlineplus/arrhythmia.html
http://www.escardio.org/
http://www.ecglibrary.com/ecghist.html
http://www.mikecowley.co.uk/leads.htm
http://www.americanheart.org/presenter.jhtml?identifier=3034352
http://heart.health.ivillage.com/arrhythmia/arrhythmia.cfm
http://www.americanheart.org/presenter.jhtml?identifier=82
http://www.americanheart.org/presenter.jhtml?identifier=1200000
http://www.analog.com/library/analogDialogue/archives/29-3/low_power.html
http://www.acc.org/
http://www.pubmedcentral.nih.gov/articlerender.fcgi?artid=1502062
http://www.hrsonline.org/ep-history/topics_in_depth/topics/modecode history2.asp
http://www.pneupac.co.uk/Profile/Profile.htm
http://www.elecdesign.com/Articles/Index.cfm?AD=1&ArticleID=5951
http://www.hrsonline.org/
http://www.huntingtonhospital.com/body.cfm?id=39592
http://www.general-devices.com/particle.htm
http://www.emedicine.com/med/topic2968.htm
http://www.hoise.com/vmw/99/articles/vmw/LV-VM-01-99-26.html
http://www.physionet.org/physiotools/edr/cic85/
http://www.ctc.nhs.uk/ccm01.html

CHEMISTRY AND PHYSICS

http://www.bnl.gov/medical/Isotope_Distribution/Isodistoff.htm
http://www.ipj.gov.pl/~p2/POS/euinfo.htm
http://lbah.com/lasertheory.htm#Symptoms

EEG/BRAIN

http://www.epilepsyfoundation.org/answerplace/Medical/treatment/eeg.cfm
http://brain.web-us.com/brainwavesfunction.htm
http://www.pubmedcentral.nih.gov/articlerender.fcgi?artid=1413969

ENDO/ARTHROSCOPY

http://www.arthroscopy.com/
http://www.corexcel.com/rw/html/body_endoscopes_page1.htm
http://www.vet.uga.edu/mis/equipment/insufflator.php

EYES

http://www.prk.com/cataracts/history_of_lens_implants.html
http://www.bausch.com/en_US/default.aspx

GENERAL

http://www.meditec.com/normal-lab-values.html
http://en.wikipedia.org/wiki/Main_Page
http://www.gehealthcare.com/usen/index.html
http://health.allrefer.com/
http://www.mercksource.com/pp/us/cns/cns_home.jsp
http://www.medicalnewstoday.com/
http://eecindia.tripod.com/
http://www.meditec.zeiss.com/
http://cancerweb.ncl.ac.uk/cgi-bin/omd?action=Home&query=
http://www.ecri.org/

HARDWARE

http://www.powerstream.com/BatteryFAQ.html
http://www.mpoweruk.com/performance.htm
http://www.pubmedcentral.nih.gov/articlerender.fcgi?artid=1502062
http://zone.ni.com/devzone/cda/main
http://www.nano.com/
http://www.melexis.com/ProdMain.aspx?nID=615

HISTORY/INVENTIONS

http://inventors.about.com/library/inventors/blmedical.htm
http://www.thebakken.org/artifacts/categories.htm
http://www.medicaldevices.org/public/faq/default.asp
http://www.ecglibrary.com/ecghist.html
http://www.hrsonline.org/ep-history/timeline/1920s/

IMAGING

http://www.resonancepub.com/wroentgen.htm
http://www.brandx-ray.com/brand_x_ray_tube_co_inc_x_ray_tube_faq_page.htm

RENAL

http://www.courseweb.uottawa.ca/medicine-histology/English/Renal/Default.htm
http://www.emedicine.com/med/topic3024.htm

SURGERY

http://www.valleylab.com/education/poes/poes_10.html
http://www.hifu.ca/patient/about_ablatherm.php

Index

A

B

C

D

E

F

G

H

I

K

L

M

N

O

P

R

S

T

U

V

X

Z